Haemorrhagic
and
Thrombotic Diseases

Haemorrhagic
and
Thrombotic Diseases

Inga Marie Nilsson

Koagulationslaboratoriet,
Allmänna Sjukhuset,
Malmö, Sweden

A KABI book

JOHN WILEY & SONS
London · New York · Sydney · Toronto

First published under Inga Marie Nilsson, *Blödnings-och trombossjukdomar* by AB KABI, Stockholm 1971.

© I.M. Nilsson, L. Andersson, S. Cronberg, U. Hedner, H. Kjellman, B.R. Robertson.

English translation L. James Brown. Copyright © 1974, by John Wiley & Sons, Ltd.

Library of Congress Cataloging in Publication Data:
Nilsson, Inga Marie.
Haemorrhagic and thrombotic diseases.

"A Wiley–Interscience publication."
Rev. translation of Blödnings-och trombossjukdomar published in 1971.
Includes bibliographical references.
1. Haemophilia. 2. Blood—Coagulation, Disorders of.
I. Title.

RC642.N5413   616.1′5   73–14383
ISBN 0 471 64070 0

Photosetting in India by Thomson Press (India) Limited.
Printed in Great Britain by J.W. Arrowsmith Ltd., Winterstoke Road, Bristol.

Preface

It has been known from the earliest times that obstinate bleeding is a serious and life-threatening condition requiring immediate treatment. But until fairly recently it was often not possible to explain *why* bleeding occurred, except in those cases where the source of bleeding was demonstrable and controllable by surgery. In other cases the only therapeutic measure available was substitution of the blood lost.

Thrombo-embolic diseases and their complications have long been known. It is one of the commonest diseases of today. Though the ultimate cause of thrombosis still challenges research, certain aetiological mechanisms are beginning to emerge.

Thanks to intense basic and clinical research in haemorrhagic diseases this has raised the scientific status of coagulation and made it a new discipline. Our knowledge of the physiology and biochemistry of haemostasis has notably expanded during the last fifteen years.

Problems bearing on bleeding and thrombosis are now encountered in practically every branch of medicine. Methods are available for clearly distinguishing between different haemorrhagic diseases as well as for specific treatment.

Though the haemorrhagic and thrombotic disorders embrace so many vital problems, instruction in the subject has often been neglected and not confided to experts.

This book is primarily concerned with a survey of our knowledge of haemorrhagic and thrombotic diseases and their treatment. The survey is given against the background of the biochemistry of normal haemostasis with due reference to the latest advances in the relevant fields of research.

The book was written on the initiative of AB KABI, to whom I am indebted for their care and attention to its preparation.

Inga Marie Nilsson, 1971

Preface to the English Edition

The Swedish edition of this book was written in 1970. In the preparation of the English edition the content has been thoroughly revised and brought up to date. The chapters on Factor VIII, fibrinogen, Factor XIII, haemophilia, von Willebrand's disease, fibrinolysis and fibrin/fibrinogen degradation products have been rewritten with respect to the latest advances in the research in these fields.

Inga Marie Nilsson, August 1973

Contents

Mechanism of normal haemostasis

I. Introduction

Haemostasis is the combined effect of various mechanisms involved in the prevention of spontaneous haemorrhage and in the arrest of the escape of blood from injured vessels. The mechanism of haemostasis comprises the functions of four components:

      1) vessels   3) coagulation system
      2) platelets   4) fibrinolytic system

All four components must be functioning correctly if haemostasis is to be normal. A defect in any one of these functions may be sufficient to interfere with normal haemostasis. The relative importance attached to each of the components has varied with increasing knowledge. Some years ago, for example, coagulation was equated with haemostasis and all discussions on haemostasis were dominated by problems concerned with coagulation. Today, however, it is the platelets and problems bearing on fibrinolysis that are receiving most attention in this field of research. In the study of the mechanism of haemostasis, however, the mechanism must be regarded as a whole, i.e. as a process brought about by a balanced interplay of all four components.

II. Vessels

The vessel walls must be impermeable to the blood in order to prevent *spontaneous haemorrhage*. Some haemorrhagic diatheses, such as Schönlein-Henoch's purpura, are due to diffuse, widespread, minute vessel lesions. Such patients have widespread petechiae despite normal platelet function and normal blood coagulation.

Normal vessel function requires an adequate supply of vitamin C, but otherwise little is known about the factors necessary for such function. It is, however, known that allergic and toxic phenomena can interfere with vessel function.

Opinions differ on the role played by platelets in maintaining the impermeability of the vessel walls to blood. But according to the general consensus of opinion, platelets have a normal and continuous sealing function of purely mechanical nature. Patients with severe thrombo-cytopenia have widespread punctate haemorrhages in the absence of known trauma, a phenomenon accepted as evidence that a certain concentration of platelets is necessary to maintain the impermeability of the vessel wall and prevent spontaneous bleeding (for references, see

Hjort, et al., 1959; Hjort and Hasselback, 1961). An important argument in support of this theory of the sealing effect of platelets is that infusion of platelets can always arrest bleeding in patients with thrombocytopenia, regardless of the cause of the condition. Disrupted platelets, which contain all of the biochemical components of platelets, have no such haemostatic effect (Hjort, et al., 1959). Survival curves for labelled platelets suggest that the latter disappear from the circulation not only because of aging changes, but also owing to the effect of an extrathrombocytic mechanism, 'random destruction'. Hjort attributed this 'random destruction' to the death of platelets in the performance of their normal vessel-sealing function.

Traumatic vascular injury causes bleeding with subsequent contraction of the vessels involved. This contraction is probably a reflex reaction and of great importance for immediate haemostasis. The contraction is only temporary, but normally lasts long enough for a plug to form and seal the defect in the vessel. Serotonin is believed to be important in effecting such contraction of the vessel. It is, however, remarkable that partial or complete inhibition of serotonin by reserpine or the like does not interfere with the contraction of the vessel, it having been shown that administration of reserpine has no effect on the bleeding time or on vascular contraction (Hutchinson, et al., 1959; Witte, et al., 1961). It must therefore be assumed that vascular contraction is essentially a reflex action. Such contraction is of paramount importance for haemostasis, especially if the injured arteries and veins are large. One would naturally suspect the existence of haemorrhagic diseases due to reduced ability of the injured walls to contract when injured. In Osler's disease (teleangiectasia hereditaria) there is local injury to the vessels, whose contractility is impaired. A diffuse or widespread example of such a bleeding tendency is not known. It might therefore be concluded that in clinical practice there is no reason to consider impaired vascular contraction as a possible cause of abnormal haemostasis following traumatic injury.

III. Haemostasis and platelets
STIG CRONBERG

A. *Primary haemostasis*

Vessel injury is immediately followed by reactions which tend to stop the bleeding. Vascular factors, platelets and plasma factors are necessary for these reactions. The initial stage, *primary haemostasis,* leads to the formation of a platelet plug (Fig. 1). The fundamental morphological changes were described by Hayem in 1882, soon after the discovery of platelets by Bizzozero (Fig. 2). It was soon realised that platelets were involved in the development of thrombosis (Eberth and Schimmelbusch, 1886).

In vessel injury the endothelial cells are damaged with consequent denudation of the basement membrane and collagen fibres.

Platelets have a strong affinity to collagen, to which they adhere (Hugues, 1960). This adhesion results in the release of various platelet factors, such as adenosine diphosphate (ADP), epinephrine, serotonin and platelet factors 3 and 4 (Hovig, 1963). The first platelets attached to the collagen are soon covered by other platelets with the development of large aggregates, which form a loose plug. How this is possible despite the rapid flow of the blood stream is still largely unknown. *In vitro* experiments have shown that fibrinogen and divalent cations, such as calcium and magnesium (Cronberg and Caen, 1971b), are important for such aggregation (Cronberg, 1971). Judging from clinical experience, the von Willebrand factor is also essential. As mentioned, platelets contain active substances, particularly ADP (Gaarder, et al., 1961), which can initiate aggregation and may be regarded as transmitter substances. On the other hand, the coagulation factors play a subordinate role in the primary stage, since the primary bleeding time in haemophilia is normal. Thrombin forms from the platelet aggregates with consequent precipitation of fibrin which makes the loose platelet plug firm and impermeable.

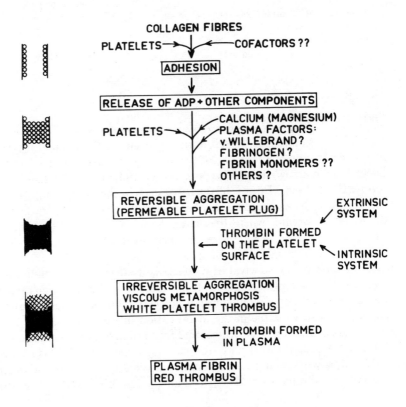

Fig 1. Schematic illustration of primary haemostasis.

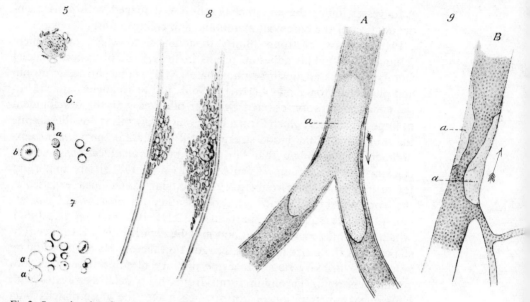

Fig 2. Some drawings from Bizzozero's publication in *Virchows Arch. Path. Anat.* 90 (1882) Taf. V.

5. White blood cell surrounded by platelets.
6. *a.* platelets seen from above and from the side.
   b. red blood cell.
   c. swollen platelets.
7. Fresh blood after addition of 1 per cent solution of acetic acid. The platelets are swollen and granular and a vitreous substance is seen.
   a. two haemolysed red blood cells.

8. Two thrombi attached to the wall of a small artery in the mesenterium of a guinea-pig. The larger thrombus contains a white blood cell among the platelets.
9. Guinea-pig mesenterium. *A.* a small artery with a thromboembolus consisting only of platelets. *B.* a small vein with two thrombi attached to wall and similarly made up of platelets.

B. *Platelets*

Formation and survival

Platelets are small discs, which normally occur in the circulating blood in a concentration of about 200000 per μl. They arise from megacaryocytes in the bone marrow. This process has been studied with electron microscopy (Ebbe, 1968). Fusion of micro-vesicles in the cytoplasm results in the formation of demarcation membranes for platelets, which are delivered to the blood stream, where they circulate for 9–11 days (Abrahamsen, 1968; Najean, et al., 1969). They are then taken care of by the reticuloendothelial system, mainly in the spleen.

Estimation of the survival of platelets is useful in the examination of patients with thrombocytopenia. It is particularly the turnover rate and the main site of destruction (spleen or liver) that are of interest. Turnover studies are also valuable in the investigation of other diseases in which increased destruction is suspected, and for finding out the best conditions for platelet preparations and storage (Aster and Jandl, 1964; Davey, 1966). Most workers have used platelets labelled *in vitro* with radioactive chromium (Abrahamsen, 1968; Kotilainen, 1969), but platelets labelled

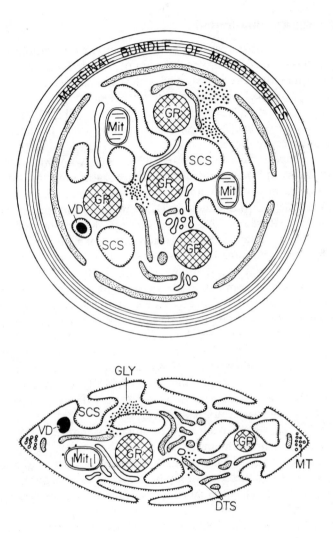

Fig 3. Diagram of a platelet. SCS = surface connecting system. MT = microtubules. Mit = mitochondria. GR = alpha granulae. VD = very dense granulae. GLY = glycogen granulae. DTS = dense tubular system.

After T. Hovig (*Ser. Haemat.* **I**, 2 (1968) p 7) modified from Behnke, O. *Anat. Rec.* **158** (1967) p 121.

with radioactive methionine and DFP (diisopropylfluorophosphate) have been tried also *in vivo*. It has, however, been objected that the labelling might injure the platelets (Kattlove and Spaet, 1970).

Morphology and ultrastructure

Platelets are incomplete cells with a cell membrane but without a nucleus. They are disc-shaped and have a diameter of 2–3 μm. In the living, unfixed, unstained state they are best studied with the phase contrast microscope. In recent years electron microscopic investigations have increased our knowledge of their ultrastructure (Hovig, 1968) (Figs. 3–7).

Some of the organelles of platelets are identical with those of other cells, and some are specific.

Platelets have a plasma membrane, which is 70–90 Å thick and consists of three layers. It is surrounded by a diffuse amorphous mass of varying thickness. Plasma proteins and coagulation factors such as factor V, factor VIII, factor XII and factor XIII, as well as fibrinogen are adsorbed to the surface (Roskam, 1922). The surface of the membrane is also rich in glycoproteins, which contain a large amount of sialic acid.

The plasma membrane forms pseudopodia, which can be clearly seen in the scanning electron microscope (Hovig, 1970) (Fig. 7).

The most typical granules of platelets are of two sorts, *viz.*, ordinary alpha granules and very dense granules. It is not certain whether this difference in density is due to differences in functional state or whether these granules differ in nature. A platelet usually contains 2–20 granules, 0·15–0·4 μm in diameter. They contain several important enzymes and active components (Day, et al., 1969). The alpha granules thus contain abundant acid phosphatases and other hydrolytic enzymes and are therefore often regarded as lysosomes. The very dense granules contain the major part of the serotonin and ADP.

Like other cells, the platelets also contain mitochondria (beta granules), which provide them with energy.

The platelets contain vacuoles and vesicles. They are connected with the surface of the platelet and may be regarded as invaginations of the plasma membrane. They are called the 'surface connecting system' (SCS) (Behnke, 1967).

Microtubules (Behnke, 1965) run in a bundle round the circumference of the platelet. They have a supporting function. They are thermolabile and disappear on exposure of the platelet to + 4°C, but reappear after warming the platelet.

Platelets also contain several other filaments, membranes and tubules ('dense tubular system') as well as a large amount of glycogen granules.

C. *Platelet factors*

The existence of platelet factors has long been accepted on the basis of physiological studies. Their chemistry is practically unknown. They are

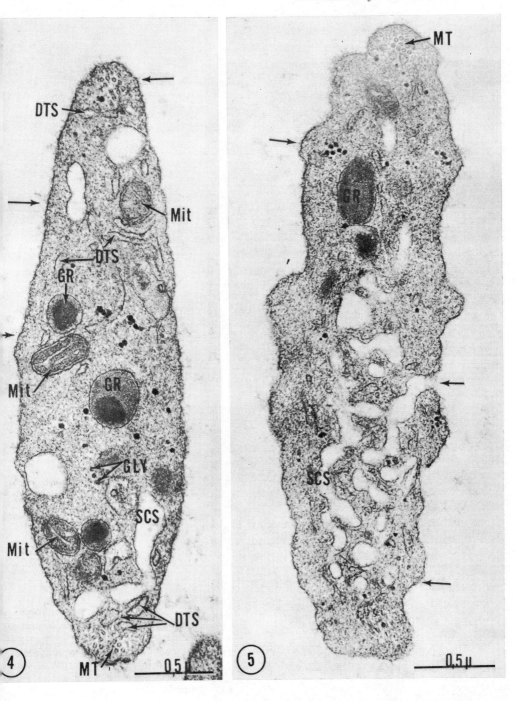

Figs 4 and 5. Human platelets. Symbols as in Fig 3. 15 000 ×. Photo T. Hovig (Hovig, T.: *Ser. Haemat.* **I**, 2 (1968) p 13).

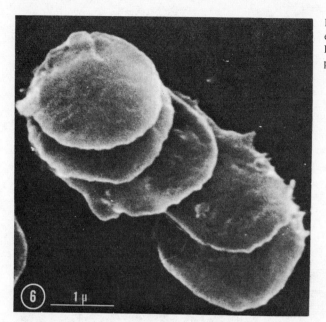

Fig 6. Normal platelets, as seen at scanning electron-microscopy. 21000 ×. Photo T Hovig (Hovig, T.: *Scand. J. Haemat.* **7** (1970) p 420).

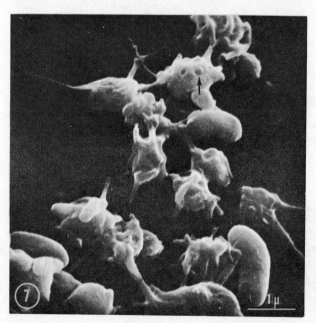

Fig 7. Scanning electron-microscopy of platelets from blood sample obtained two minutes after an infusion of latex particles. Platelets show changes in shape and formation of pseudopodia. A latex particle is seen in an invagination of the platelet surface (arrow). 15 000 ×. Photo T. Hovig (Hovig, T.: *Ser. Haemat.* **3** (1970) p 47).

designated by Arabic numerals to distinguish them from coagulation factors. The platelet factors, of which factors 3 and 4 are the most important, are given below.

Platelet factor 1 is identical with plasma factor V, which is adsorbed to the surface of the platelet.

Platelet factor 2 catalyses the coagulation of fibrinogen with thrombin.

Platelet factor 3 takes part in the formation of thromboplastin. It is probably an insoluble lipoprotein. It is believed to occur in the granules (White and Krivit, 1966) or in the membrane (Marcus, et al., 1967).

Platelet factor 4 is an antiheparin factor. It consists of a basic poly-peptide, which is readily soluble. Its release largely parallels that of ADP (Cronberg, Kubisz and Caen, 1970). Platelet factor 4 interferes with fibrinogen and early fibrinogen degradation products.

Platelet factor 5 is fibrinogen.

Platelet factor 6 is an antiplasmin.

Platelet factor 7 is identical with the coagulation factor VII.

ADP

Adenosine diphosphate (ADP) occurs in platelets and can activate them so that they aggregate (Gaarder, et al., 1961). It is not incorporated as such, but the platelets can take up labelled adenosine and adenine, which is afterwards converted to other adenine nucleotides, ATP and ADP. Holmsen (Holmsen, Day and Storm, 1969) has shown that adenine nucleotides incorporated in this way participate in the metabolism of platelets, but are not included in the storage pool of ADP that is liberated by the release reaction.

Serotonin

Platelets contain serotonin (5-hydroxytryptamine). It is not formed by platelets, but is taken up by them and labelled serotonin has been widely used in release studies (Jerushalmy and Zucker, 1966). Serotonin occurs in 'dense granules' (de Prada, et al., 1967).

Thrombosthenin

Platelets contain a contractile protein, thrombosthenin, made up of actine and myosine-like components (Bettex-Galland and Lüscher, 1961). Some authors believe that it occurs in the cytoplasm (Nachman, et al., 1967), while others contend that it is bound to the cell membrane (Rafel-son and Booyse, 1971).

D. *Physiology of platelets*

Adhesion

Platelets adhere to different surfaces. *In vivo* they adhere mainly to collagen fibres (Hugues, 1960) and the denuded basement membrane. Experimentally it has been shown that platelets adhere to glass and to plastic surfaces (Breddin and Bürck, 1963). They also adhere to siliconised surfaces. In some respects adhesion resembles phagocytosis. If small plastic particles are added to platelet-rich plasma, they may afterwards be detected inside the platelets (Mustard and Packham, 1968). On the other hand, on contact with a plastic surface that is too large to be incorporated, they spread out over the surface as far as they can. It has been suggested that glucosyltransferase in the platelets might mediate adhesion to collagen (Jamieson, et al., 1971).

Aggregation

The attachment of platelets to one another is called aggregation. After vessel injury, the platelet plug is rapidly built up by platelets. The aggregation differs when observed *in vitro* after addition of ADP, for example, in platelet-rich citrated plasma, where certain platelets are activated, and then unite to form an aggregate (Cronberg, 1970). The mechanism by which platelets are retained *in vivo* in the rapidly flowing blood stream is still largely obscure. ADP is probably involved in such a trigger mechanism, but can hardly serve as a transmitter until the platelets have first come into contact with one another.

Release reaction

Platelets release active products in response to certain stimuli (Grette, 1962). This liberation is not due to destruction of the cell, but to a specific reaction (Holmsen, Day and Stormorken, 1969). The substances released are mainly those bound to alpha granules and dense granules. They consist mainly of ADP, serotonin, platelet factor 4 and, to some extent, of the less soluble platelet factor 3 and hydrolytic enzymes. Some of them have the character of a transmitter substance and some influence the coagulation process. The release can be initiated by adhesion. Then the release does not require the presence of other cofactors, but under certain circumstances Ca^{2+} has a potentiating effect (Cronberg and Caen, 1971a). Also large aggregates can induce the release. Thus, ADP and adrenaline do not by themselves initiate any release, but if platelets are first aggregated by stirring and plasma factors are present, platelets will release their active products (Cronberg, Kubisz and Caen, 1970) (Figs. 8 and 9). Proteolytic enzymes, such as thrombin, can directly stimulate such liberation (Grette 1962, Holmsen, Day and Stormorken, 1969).

E. *Methods for studying platelets*

Bleeding time

The bleeding time according to Ivy is more sensitive than the bleeding time according to Duke (see Methods, page 211).

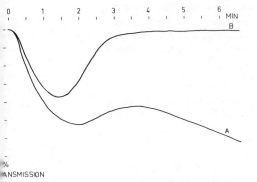

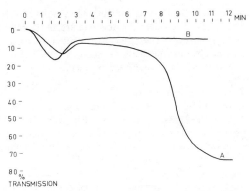

8. Aggregation in platelet-rich citrated plasma
er addition of ADP $(6 \times 10^{-7}\text{M})$ before (A) and
er (B) 1·6 g acetyl-salicylic acid is administered
ally. Observe first and second wave of aggregation
fore administration of acetyl-salicylic acid and
w this agent inhibits the second wave.

Fig 9. Aggregation in platelet-rich citrated plasma
with epinephrine $5·5 \times 10^{-6}\text{M}$ before (A) and after
(B) acetyl-salicylic acid by mouth. Observe how the
aggregation normally occurs in two waves, but how
the second wave is inhibited by the acetyl-salicylic
acid.

Platelet count

Determination of the platelet count requires the use of a reliable method. We recommend Björkman's method, in which blood is collected with EDTA and the blood cells are haemolysed with dilute potassium rhodanide solution (Björkman, 1959). Brecher and Cronkite's method with 1 per cent ammonium oxalate is also good and is widely used (Brecher and Cronkite, 1950). If a Coulter Counter or Ljungberg's celloscope is used for automatic counting, the red cells must first be sedimented off (Bull, et al., 1965). An automatic counter using an optical technique has also been described (Simmons, et al., 1971).

Direct microscopy

It is often possible to obtain a rough impression of the appearance of platelets and their ability to adhere and form aggregates by direct inspection of platelet-rich citrated plasma in the phase contrast microscope (Cronberg, 1968).

Wright's method

This was the first method to find clinical use (Wright, 1941). In this method a glass bottle is rotated slowly for twenty minutes, after which the number of residual platelets is compared with the original number. Owing to the long incubation time, complicating reactions may occur, such as adhesion, aggregation and release.

Breddin's aggregation method

This is a variant of Wright's method but uses platelet-rich citrated plasma instead of whole blood and a rotation time of ten minutes (Breddin and Bauke, 1965). The specimen is fixed and stained on a slide and the degree of aggregation is estimated.

Hellem's method

In the original method citrated blood is allowed to flow through a plastic tube containing small glass beads under strictly standardised conditions (Hellem, 1960). During this passage of the blood some of the platelets adhere to the beads, and the number of platelets before and after the passage are compared. The passage takes 30 seconds. A new variant using native or heparinised blood has since been elaborated (Hellem, 1970).

Salzman's method

In this method blood is rapidly sucked, directly from a blood vessel through a plastic tube (Vacutainer®) containing glass beads (Salzman, 1963). The platelets require about 3 seconds to pass through the tube, and the entire sampling takes about 45 seconds (Cronberg, 1968). The relative number of platelets retained in the filter is calculated in the same way as in Hellem's method. The results are in better agreement with the bleeding time than those obtained by other methods, but standardisation of the procedure offers difficulties. Bowie, et al. (1969) have standardised the method for heparinised blood.

Born's aggregation method

ADP is added to platelet-rich citrated plasma and is stirred, while the platelets aggregate. Light is then passed between the aggregates. The light intensity can be measured with a photometer and recorded graphically using a pen-recorder. The stirring and the temperature are standardised (Born, 1962; Cronberg, 1970). Information is obtained by recording the scattered light (Michal and Born, 1971).

ADP activates the platelets, which then begin to aggregate with the development of a primary wave of aggregation. If the dose is carefully chosen, the aggregates will disintegrate after little more than a minute. Under optimal conditions reactions occur inside the large aggregates with the result that ADP and other components are released. These activate the free platelets again and initiate a second wave of aggregation (MacMillan, 1966; Cronberg, Kubisz and Caen, 1970) (Figs. 8 and 9).

If collagen is used intead of ADP, aggregation does not begin until after a certain lag-period. This is because some platelets must first adhere and release their ADP before aggregation can begin.

In the choice of methods for studying platelet function it is obvious that the various methods only measure part of the total function and no single method can completely replace another. A striking example is the finding that a small dose of acetyl-salicylic acid seriously disturbs aggregation and several release tests, but produces at most negligible bleeding symptoms in normals, while in von Willebrand's disease it is only the Salzman test or modifications of it that can demonstrate an abnormality of platelet function *in vitro*.

IV. Mechanism of coagulation and the various coagulation factors

A. *Mechanism of coagulation*

The following 13 coagulation factors are now recognised.

    I Fibrinogen
    II Prothrombin
    III Thromboplastin (thrombokinase)
    IV Ca^{2+}
    V Factor V (proaccelerin, Ac-globulin)
    VI Accelerin (activated factor V)
    VII Proconvertin
    VIII AHF (AHG, 'antihaemophilic globulin')
    IX Haemophilia B factor (PTC, 'Christmas factor')
    X Stuart factor
    XI Haemophilia C factor (PTA)
    XII Hageman factor
    XIII Fibrin stabilising factor (FSF)

Fig 10. The classical coagulation theory.

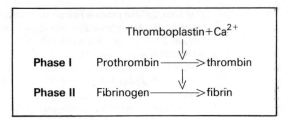

A genetic or acquired deficiency of any one of these factors leads to a coagulation defect or coagulopathy. Inherited coagulopathies are, as a rule, due to deficiency of only one factor; acquired coagulopathies, to two or more.

The foundation stone of our knowledge of the mechanism of coagulation was laid more than 100 years ago by Alexander Schmidt of the Virchow Institute in Berlin (for references, see Quick 1942). The names fibrinogen, prothrombin and thromboplastin were also coined at that time. In 1890 Arthus and Pages discovered that Ca^{2+} is necessary for coagulation. In 1905 Morawitz, Fuld and Spiro formulated a coagulation theory, which is now generally known as the classical theory (Fig. 10). According to this theory, thrombin is formed from prothrombin in the presence of thromboplastin and Ca^{2+}. The thrombin thus formed converts fibrinogen to insoluble fibrin.

The discovery of heparin by MacLean and Howell in America in 1916 and of vitamin K at the beginning of the 1930s by Henrik Dam in Copenhagen did not cause any revision of the classical theory of coagulation, though it did raise the status of prothrombin from simply that of a factor in the coagulation process to that of an important blood component. The methods devised by Smith and coworkers in the 1930s (Warner, Brinkhous and Smith, 1936) in Iowa, and by Quick (1935) in Milwaukee for the quantitative determination of prothrombin proved important in the expansion of our knowledge in the field.

Several other factors participating in the coagulation of blood were afterwards discovered. These discoveries complicated Morawitz's classical coagulation theory which, however, still constitutes the framework of most modern concepts of coagulation. Most of the new factors were discovered in the investigation of coagulation in patients with haemorrhagic diatheses. Since these factors were revealed at roughly the same time in different parts of the world, each haemorrhagic diathesis and the missing factor have been given different names. The following list of names that have been used for a single coagulation factor, AHF, is an illustrative example :

> Factor VIII (Koller)
> Antihaemophilic Globulin = AHG (Patek and Taylor)
> Antihaemophilic Globulin A (Cramer)
> AHF—Antihaemophilic Factor (Brinkhous)
> PTF—Plasma Thromboplastic Factor (Ratnoff)

Plasma Thromboplastic Factor A (Aggeler)
TPC—Thromboplastic Plasma Component (Shinowara)
Facteur Antihaemophilique A (Soulier)
Thromboplastinogen (Quick)
Prothrombokinase (Feissly)
Platelet Cofactor I (Johnson)
Plasmokinin (Laki)
Thrombocatalysin (Lenggenhager).

In 1954 an International Committee on Blood Clotting Factors was appointed to clear up this confusion. The committee recommended that the factors be designated by Roman numerals, followed by the name, in brackets, by which a given factor is generally known in a given country. For a factor to be recognised and given a Roman numeral several properties of it should, according to the committee, be known. Its thermostability or lability, its adsorption to $BaSO_4$, kaolin and Celite, its dialysability, its occurrence in various plasma fractions and electrophoretic properties must be defined. A well described haemorrhagic diathesis due to deficiency of the factor is necessary. A reproducible method isolating the factor must be available as well as reproducible methods for measuring its activity. Its survival *in vivo* must also be known. The role it plays in the coagulation process must be described. On the other hand, chemical identification of the substance is not necessary. So far, the committee has recognised 13 factors.

Various coagulation theories have been suggested, but no unanimity has been achieved concerning the actual coagulation process.

Before considering the most modern concepts of the coagulation mechanism it might be convenient to recall that there are two types of thromboplastin, the thromboplastin occurring in the tissues (tissue thromboplastin, tissue factor or 'extrinsic thromboplastin') and the thromboplastin ('intrinsic thromboplastin', 'blood thromboplastin' or 'plasma thromboplastin') that forms in plasma on coagulation of the blood. Tissue thromboplastin is preformed and occurs in all tissues,

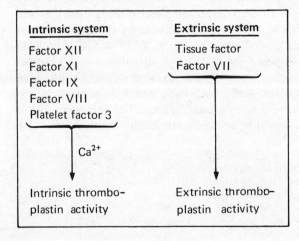

Fig 11. Intrinsic and extrinsic thromboplastin activity.

Fig 12. Coagulation scheme. Modified after Macfarlane, 1964 (*Nature* **202** (1964) p 495).

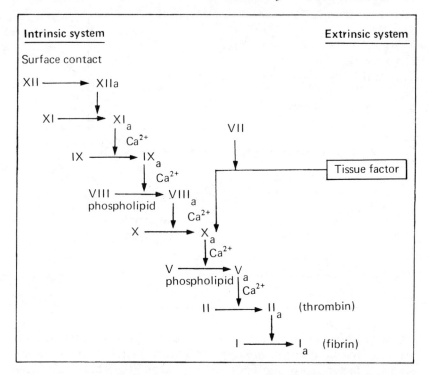

particularly in the lungs, brain and placenta. It is released by tissue injury. It has been shown that the active components of this tissue factor are lipoproteins (Deutsch, et al., 1964; Nemerson, 1969; Nemerson and Pitlick, 1970). Today all coagulation schemes distinguish between an intrinsic system, in which the tissue thromboplastin does not take part, and an extrinsic system, in which coagulation is initiated by tissue thromboplastin (Fig. 11).

Macfarlane and coworkers of Oxford (Macfarlane, 1964) proposed a coagulation theory, which they called the 'enzyme cascade', and Davie and Ratnoff (1964) a theory called the 'waterfall sequence' (Fig. 12). According to these theories, which have attracted wide attention, the coagulation process consists of a series of enzymatic reactions in which one coagulation factor successively activates the next. The names— cascade theory and water-fall theory—naturally strengthen the impression of acceleration in the system. According to Macfarlane, contact of the blood with glass activates Factor XII. One must assume that the activation by contact *in vivo* occurs in those parts of the vessel where the intima is damaged. The activating Factor XII, in turn, activates Factor XI. This results in the formation of a contact-activating product that activates Factor IX. Activated Factor IX, in turn, activates Factor VIII, which activates Factor X. In cooperation with Factor V and phospholipids, Factor X finally converts prothrombin (Factor II) to thrombin, which converts fibrinogen to fibrin. This, according to Macfarlane, explains the activation of prothrombin in an intrinsic system, i.e. without addition

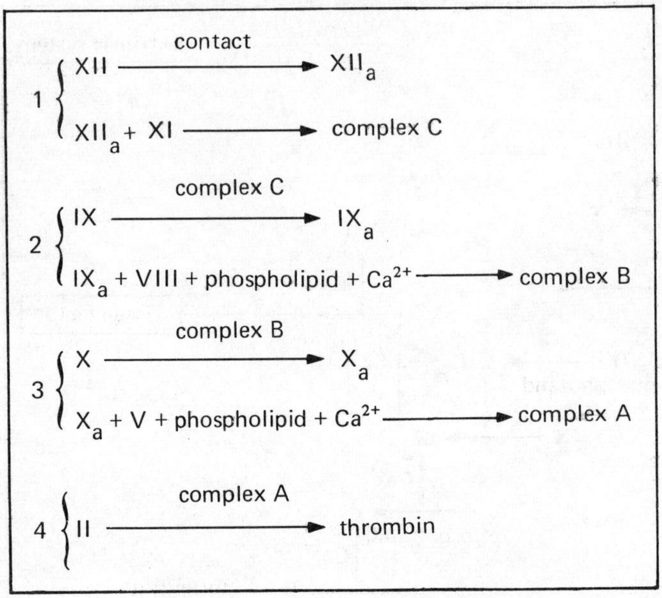

Fig 13. Coagulation, 4-stage cascade scheme, according to Hemker, et al. (1970).

of tissue thromboplastin. But prothrombin can also be activated in an extrinsic system. In the extrinsic system activated Factor VIII is replaced by tissue factor and by a plasma factor (Factor VII). This results in the formation of an active product, extrinsic thromboplastin, which activates Factor X to active Factor X. Calcium ions appear to be necessary for most of the above-mentioned reactions. Except for Ca^{2+}, phospholipids and fibrinogen, all coagulation factors are believed to act as specific proteolytic enzymes. Macfarlane also believes that the active enzymes produced at various stages are rapidly destroyed since they are not found in serum. This means that sufficient active product must be produced to activate the next stage in a relatively short time.

But evidence produced in recent years suggests that several reactions in coagulation are mediated by adsorption of coagulation factors to phospholipids. For example, there is much evidence that phospholipids adsorb activated Factor X and Factor V to their surface and that this complex together with Ca^{2+} is the thrombin-activating enzyme. The adsorption of factors to phospholipids is believed to be essential to the formation of the enzymatically active structure (Barton, et al., 1967; Hemker, et al., 1967; Deggeller and Vreeken, 1969; Hemker, et al., 1970). Hemker, et al. (1970) have recently reported experiments suggesting that Factor VIII and Factor IX react analogously with phospholipids. They thus believe that Factor VIII and Factor IX are adsorbed to a phospholipid micelle and that this complex is the active enzyme that activates Factor X. According to this conception, we have a 4-stage cascade scheme (Fig. 13) instead of Macfarlane's 7-stage scheme. Activated Factor X occupies a key position in blood coagulation and is the link between the extrinsic and intrinsic systems.

As mentioned, there are several hypotheses on the coagulation of the blood. The one deviating from most others is that proposed by Seegers of Detroit (Seegers, 1962; Seegers, 1967). He recognises only Factor VIII, prothrombin, thrombin, Factor V, fibrinogen and fibrin and claims that Factor VII, Factor IX and Factor X are only derivatives of prothrombin.

B. Blombäck (1966) proposed a coagulation scheme based on Macfarlane's cascade theory, according to which it is possible to divide the coagulation process into three phases (Fig. 14). In his scheme, on contact Factor XII is activated and in turn activates Factor IX. The active Factor IX together with Factor VIII, Ca^{2+} and phospholipids from platelets (platelet factor 3) form a third activating product, which may be called intrinsic thromboplastin or plasma thromboplastin. This product then activates Factor X to active Factor X. Active Factor X together with Factor V forms a prothrombin activator which apparently, according to the rules of an enzymatic reaction, converts prothrombin to thrombin. In the extrinsic system, intrinsic thromboplastin is replaced by tissue factor and Factor VII. An advantage of this scheme is the possibility to divide the coagulation process into three phases, which is most convenient in the investigation of coagulation defects.

Fig 14. Hypothetical coagulation scheme according to B. Blombäck 1966).

a. first phase = plasma thromboplastin formation phase.

b. second phase = conversion of prothrombin to thrombin.

c. third phase = conversion of fibrinogen to fibrin.

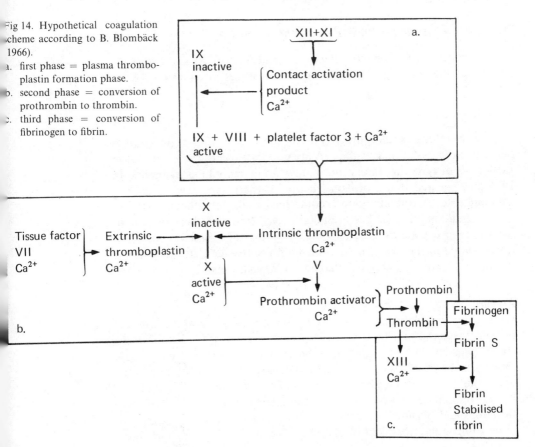

The first phase of the coagulation process is the formation of plasma thromboplastin in which Factor XII, haemophilia factors XI, IX and VIII and platelet factor 3 participate. This process, which normally takes 8–12 minutes, is the longest phase and the one which largely decides the duration of the coagulation time (Biggs, et al., 1953a, b). Defects in this first phase are characterised by retarded formation of plasma thromboplastin (prolonged coagulation time, prolonged recalcification time, prolonged cephalin time or partial thromboplastin time, prolonged activated partial thromboplastin time and defective 'prothrombin consumption'), but by normal coagulation time after addition of tissue thromboplastin (see Methods, page 214).

The second phase consists of the conversion of prothrombin to thrombin, which takes only 10–15 seconds. Factors X, V and VII take part in this phase. Defects of the coagulation process in this phase are characterised by a prolonged coagulation time on addition of tissue thromboplastin (one-stage prothrombin time or thromboplastin time).

The third phase consists of the conversion of fibrinogen to fibrin. In the presence of Factor XIII and Ca^{2+} the fibrin formed is converted to a more stable form.

B. *Phase I—plasma thromboplastin formation*

Some remarks on Factor VIII, Factor IX and Factors XI and XII participating in the first phase of the coagulation process are given below.

1. AHF (Factor VIII)

The antihaemophilic globulin (AHF) is the coagulation factor that is deficient in classical haemophilia A. It was Patek and Taylor (1936) in Boston who gave this factor the name 'antihaemophilic globulin'. In 1936 they claimed that a protein fraction in the plasma was missing in haemophiliacs. A globulin fraction containing a substance that normalised the coagulation time in haemophiliacs had, however, been produced from human plasma as early as 1911 by Addis. The discovery of AHF thus resulted in the abandonment of the former belief that the cause of haemophilia was pathological changes in the platelets.

Preparation and purification of AHF
During the second world war Cohn devised a method in which different plasma proteins could be separated by fractionation with alcohol in the cold. Together with his coworkers he found that the active principle missing in haemophiliacs was precipitated together with the fibrinogen in fraction I in Cohn's method 6. Fraction I consists mainly of fibrinogen. It is contaminated with other coagulation substances, including prothrombin and plasmin, which makes the fraction labile. It has proved of no value in the treatment of bleeders, it is readily coagulable when the

Fig 15. Preparation of fraction I–0, containing AHF, von Willebrand factor and
fibrinogen.

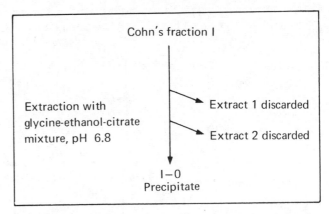

Fig 15. Preparation of fraction I–0, containing AHF, von Willebrand factor and fibrinogen.

prothrombin is converted to thrombin. The contaminating plasmin also breaks down Factor VIII.

Since then various attempts have been made to isolate and purify AHF.

Fraction I-O. In 1956, when Birger and Margareta Blombäck devised their glycine method for purifying fibrinogen we tested the AHF activity of various fractions (Nilsson, Blombäck, Blombäck and Svennerud, 1956; Blombäck, B. and Blombäck, M., 1956; Nilsson, 1957; Blombäck, M. and Nilsson, 1958). We found that the AHF of the original plasma could be almost quantitatively recovered in the fraction called I-O (Fig. 15). Fraction I-O was obtained by eluting Cohn's fraction I with 1 M glycine solution containing ethanol and citrate. Fibrinogen and AHF remained as precipitates, while prothrombin, plasmin and other proteins were washed off. This fraction was then stable. It consisted to 85–95 per cent of fibrinogen. The fraction also contained the factor lacking in von Willebrand's disease. Fraction I-O was afterwards prepared under sterile conditions, and has been used since 1956 in Sweden in the treatment of haemophilia A.

Only if a certain number of conditions are filled, can one expect to obtain a good yield of AHF in fraction I-O (Blombäck, M., 1958). When possible, the plasma should be prepared from fresh human citrated blood obtained with the silicone technique. For AHF is a labile plasma component and 40–50 per cent of the AHF in the blood can thus be inactivated within twelve hours' storage of citrated blood at room temperature (Rapaport, et al., 1959). The stability of AHF can also be increased considerably if the plasma is stored in the cold, though some of the activity is lost in association with freezing and thawing. It should also be added that the storage temperature is of great importance. Thus, a temperature of $-20°$C is not satisfactory for plasma to be used for the preparation of AHF; such plasma should be stored at $-30°$C or at a still lower temperature (Pool and Robinson, 1959; Blombäck, M., et al., 1960; Weaver and Langdell, 1966; Britten and Grove-Rasmussen, 1966). AHF is also inactivated by contact with glass surfaces and by mechanical handling of the blood. The stability of AHF depends also on the way

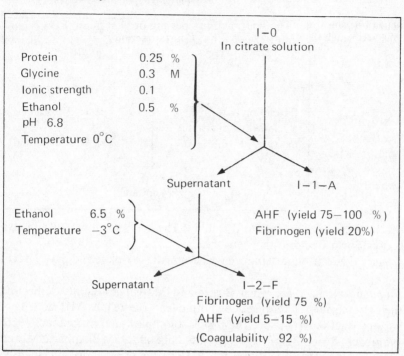

Protein   0.25 %
Glycine   0.3   M
Ionic strength   0.1
Ethanol   0.5   %
pH   6.8
Temperature 0°C

I−0
In citrate solution

Supernatant   I−1−A

Ethanol   6.5 %
Temperature −3°C

AHF (yield 75−100 %)
Fibrinogen (yield 20%)

Supernatant   I−2−F
Fibrinogen (yield 75 %)
AHF (yield 5−15 %)
(Coagulability   92 %)

Fig 16. Separation AHF from fracti I-0.

the blood is collected, for coagulation, if any, is accompanied by prompt reduction of the AHF activity from the blood (Penick and Brinkhous, 1956). Admixture of tissue factors during sampling must therefore be avoided. Preservation of a high AHF activity in the blood or plasma requires good venesection, rapid collection of the blood and immediate mixing of the blood with anticoagulants.

In the best batches of fraction I-O the AHF yield has been 90–100 per cent of the AHF content of the plasma used (Blombäck, M. and Nilsson, 1958; Blombäck, M., 1958; Blombäck, M., et al., 1960). The purification of AHF per mg protein in fraction I-O compared with fresh plasma is about 20–40 times and the AHF activity per unit of volume is 4–8 times that in the original plasma.

Attempts have been made to purify AHF further from fraction I-O. Fraction I-O has been separated into an AHF fraction (I-1-A) and a fibrinogen fraction (I-2-F) according to a method devised by M. Blombäck (1958) (Fig. 16). The AHF activity in fraction I-1-A per mg protein is about 200 times that in plasma. Fraction I-1-A has also been tried clinically, and *in vivo* the activity agrees with that *in vitro* (Blombäck, M. and Nilsson 1958; Nilsson, Blombäck and Blombäck, 1959). Fraction I-1-A still contains fibrinogen. From fraction I-1-A AHF has been purified further (Blombäck, B., Blombäck, M. and Nilsson, 1958). The AHF activity in fraction I-1-A has been adsorbed to tricalcium citrate, and then the fibrinogen remained in the supernatant fluid. The AHF activity could then be eluted with 0·1 M Na-EDTA at pH 6·8 from the tricalcium citrate precipitate. The AHF activity per mg protein in the EDTA eluate was ten times as high as that in fraction I-1-A. This means that the yield of AHF per mg protein was 2.000 times that in the original plasma.

AHF by ether fractionation. By ether fractionation of human plasma Kekwick and Wolf (1957) of England have isolated a fibrinogen fraction containing AHF. The AHF content of this fraction corresponds to that in fraction I-O. It has been successfully used in the treatment of haemophilia A (Maycock, et al., 1963). But side-effects in the form of fall in blood pressure and even shock have been observed, and it is therefore no longer used.

Animal AHF. Bidwell (1955) of Oxford has isolated an AHF preparation from animals' blood, particularly bovine and porcine blood. The blood AHF activity in these animals is much higher than that in human beings. Bidwell used precipitation with phosphate buffer and 20 per cent Na_3-citrate. She purified AHF from bovine plasma 100–400 times. The preparation still contained fibrinogen. The Oxford-group (see Biggs and Macfarlane, 1966) used these preparations in the treatment of haemophilia. The haemostatic effect was good. But a disadvantage of these preparations is their antigenicity. After some days the patients begin to develop antibodies to the foreign protein and then serious anaphylactic reactions may occur if treatment is continued. Animal AHF can thus be used only for short treatment of a patient. Treatment may, however, be prolonged to a certain extent by the use of AHF from different species.

Cryoprecipitate. Pool and Robinson (1959) discovered that cryoprecipitate from human plasma contains AHF. They thus found that the cryoprecipitate that formed when freshly frozen human plasma was gradually thawed ($+4°C$) contained considerable AHF activity (Fig. 17). Pool and coworkers studied this cryoprecipitate and its clinical value as a substitute for AHF (Pool, et al., 1964; Pool and Shannon, 1965; Hershgold, et al., 1966; Pool, 1969). The yield is said to be about 46 per cent of

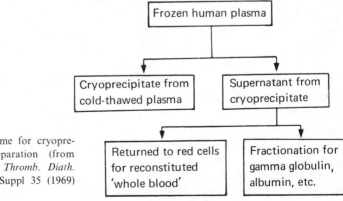

Fig 17. Scheme for cryoprecipitate preparation (from Pool, J.G.: *Thromb. Diath. Haemorrh.*, Suppl 35 (1969) p 35).

the AHF activity in the starting plasma and its purity per mg protein is 8–20 times that in the original plasma. Several workers have used cryoprecipitate as a starting material for further purification of AHF.

Glycine precipitation of AHF. Wagner, et al. (1964) and Webster, et al. (1965) found that at 0°C amino acids, such as glycine and β-alanine, could precipitate AHF in plasma that had first been adsorbed with Al(OH)₃ and Florigel. The yield per mg protein was 20–30 times that in the original plasma. Such AHF preparations have been used in the treatment of haemophilia A (Abildgaard, Ch., et al., 1966).

In recent years much more active AHF preparations have been obtained with the use of glycine precipitation (Brinkhous, et al., 1968; Wagner, et al., 1969). The starting material was cryoprecipitate. To this was added polyethylene glycol and the bulk of the fibrinogen was selectively precipitated (Johnson, et al., 1966). The AHF was afterwards precipitated by addition of glycine. In this way AHF was purified 100–400 times. About two-thirds of the preparation still consisted of fibrinogen. After administration of this AHF preparation the AHF values reached *in vivo* corresponded to those obtained *in vitro* (Brinkhous, et al., 1968).

Ethanol and polyethylene fractionation. Johnson and coworkers (Johnson, et al., 1969a, Newman, et al., 1971) obtained a highly purified AHF preparation. As a starting material they used freshly frozen plasma precipitated with 3 per cent ethanol during thawing. Contaminants were removed by Al(OH)₃ adsorption. An 'intermediate-purity AHF' was obtained. Part of the fibrinogen was afterwards removed by addition of polyethylene glycol. This resulted in a purification of more than 200 times. The preparation is called 'high-purity AHF'. Both preparations have been tried clinically and found to have a good clinical effect (Johnson, et al., 1971). By ultracentrifugation or by agarose gel chromatography they obtained a fibrinogen-free AHF purified 10.000 times (Johnson, et al., 1967).

Agarose gel filtration. Other workers have also used agarose gel filtration for purifying AHF. Using this method Paulssen, et al. (1969) separated AHF from fibrinogen in plasma. Ratnoff, Kass and Lang (1969) obtained an AHF preparation that contained 67 units of AHF per mg protein, which meant a purification of 3.360 times. van Mourik and Mochtar (1970) filtered cryoprecipitate through Sepharose 6 B in the presence of dextran and the preparations obtained were found to have a specific activity of 125–625 units per mg protein. Hershgold, et al. (1971a, b) used a cryoprecipitate which they adsorbed with Al(OH)₃, Fuller's earth, bentonite, ammonium sulphate fractionation and polyethylene glycol precipitation. Owen and Wagner (1972) used as a starting material a precipitate obtained by dialysis of plasma against polyethylene glycol. None of these preparations have been tried *in vivo*.

Arvin. Green (1971a) coagulated cryoprecipitate by addition of snake venom, Arvin, and then filtered the product through Sepharose. The filtrate had an AHF activity of 124 units per mg protein. The preparation has not been tried clinically.

Characteristics of AHF

Traces of AHF normally occur in the plasma. Its concentration is not higher than 10–20 mg/l. As mentioned above, AHF is a labile substance, and on storage at room temperature in citrated blood it rapidly decreases in activity. AHF is not adsorbable to $BaSO_4$ or other earth alkaline metal salts. AHF is consumed on coagulation. Serum therefore has no AHF activity (see Biggs and Macfarlane, 1962). AHF is broken down or inactivated by proteolytic enzymes, such as plasmin and thrombin.

Many attempts have been made to purify AHF. Particularly separation of AHF from fibrinogen has proved difficult. Denaturation of fibrinogen by heating, coagulation of fibrinogen with thrombin and Arvin, separation with Fuller's earth, kaolin, bentonite and polyethylene glycol, respectively, and precipitation with aliphatic amino acids have been used. Earlier chromatography on cellulose and ion exchanger was also used (van Creveld, et al., 1961; Michael and Tunnah, 1963; Veder, 1966). Michael and Tunnah (1963) who used chromatography of a concentrate of porcine plasma on an ion exchanger, obtained a preparation whose specific activity was 25.000 times that of plasma. But this highly active product still contained fibrinogen.

The introduction of gel filtration implied a further advance in the isolation and chemical characterisation of AHF. It is especially chromatography in agarose gel that has proved particularly valuable. This method was first described by Hershgold, et al. (1967) and Johnson, et al. (1967).

Ratnoff, et al. (1969) obtained a fibrinogen-free AHF which was, however, contaminated by other plasma factors. When the plasma was lipaemic, the fraction also contained lipids. β-lipoprotein was not detected. van Mourik and Mochtar's (1970) preparation was free from fibrinogen and other coagulation factors and did not contain lipids. Hershgold, et al. (1971a, b) prepared fibrinogen-free AHF, which had a specific activity 10.000 times higher than that of plasma. They claim that 90 per cent of the preparation consisted of AHF and that it contained 76 per cent amino acids, 10 per cent carbohydrates, and 11 per cent lipids (the AHF activity could be inhibited by addition of phospholipase).

The molecular weight of AHF had been given earlier as 180.000 to 200.000 (Shulman, et al., 1960; Aronson, et al., 1962; Bidwell, et al., 1966a; Hershgold and Sprawls, 1966). But in view of the behaviour of the substance on agarose gel filtration and ultracentrifugation, its molecular weight is now thought to be 2×10^6 or higher (Ratnoff, et al., 1969), The high molecular weight might perhaps be due to aggregation of subunits or a varying degree of complex formation. Barrow and Graham (1971) have given a molecular weight of 20.000 for an AHF-like substance prepared from renal tissue by filtration on Sephadex G-200. Weiss and

Kochwa (1970) ultracentrifuged plasma at increasing ionic strengths and found a shift of the AHF activity from fractions with a very high molecular weight to fractions with a low molecular weight, a shift suggesting dissociation. Holmberg and Nilsson (1973c) examined a purified AHF fraction prepared according to van Mourik and Mochtar, with SDS acrylamide electrophoresis. After reduction of the disulphide bonds a main component appeared with a molecular weight of 200.000. Marchesi, et al. (1972), who used a similar technique, found a molecular weight of 240.000. The heterogenous nature of AHF is demonstrable by electrophoresis in agarose. In cross-immuno-electrophoresis of plasma against an antiserum specific to the AHF protein, there appears a broad precipitation line extending from the anterior border of fibrinogen to the α_2 region (Holmberg and Nilsson, 1973c).

Using an immunological technique, Zimmerman, et al. (1971a) showed that in patients with haemophilia A the plasma invariably contains a cross-reacting protein, while patients with von Willebrand's disease have only a low content of this protein. Bouma, et al. (1972) found that the purified AHF fraction obtained by chromatography of cryoprecipitate on Sepharose 6 B in the presence of dextran also corrected the abnormal platelet adhesiveness in von Willebrand's disease *in vitro*. These findings suggest that the von Willebrand factor and the AHF activity in plasma are linked to one and the same molecular complex, which is in part structurally changed in haemophilia, but which occurs in low concentrations in von Willebrand's disease.

The site of synthesis of AHF has been widely discussed and is to some extent illuminated by what is said above about AHF and the von Willebrand factor. Formerly the liver was thought to be the site of synthesis. But cumulative data now suggest that AHF is produced not only in the liver, but also elsewhere. The AHF activity does not fall in liver disease (Hallén and Nilsson, 1964). Neither is the AHF activity reduced by the hepatocellular injury induced by chloroform in dogs or by carbon tetrachloride in rats (Pool and Spaet, 1954). The AHF activity may be markedly raised in acute liver necrosis (Meili and Straub, 1970), and such AHF has the same chromatographic characteristics on Sepharose as normal AHF (Holmberg and Nilsson, 1973c). Weaver, Price and Langdell (1964) and others, who used cross circulation experiments on normal and haemophilic dogs, produced evidence suggesting that the spleen is of importance for storage of AHF, and they feel that the reticulo-endothelial system is the site of synthesis of this coagulation factor. Niléhn (1962) studied symptomatic AHF deficiency. He, too, concluded that AHF is produced outside the liver and probably in the bone marrow. He based this conclusion on the finding that the AHF was decreased in osteomyelosclerosis as well as in other bone marrow diseases, but not in liver cirrhosis.

Gardikas, et al. (1965) found that the concentration of Factor VIII is higher in venous blood from the liver than in the general circulation. In perfusion experiments of the liver and spleen Norman, et al. (1967,

1968) found that the liver, and particularly the spleen, can store or release considerable AHF activity. They concluded that the spleen was the main site of synthesis or activation of AHF. But since the AHF is not abnormally low in splenectomised patients, they felt that AHF must presumably be formed also in the liver, bone marrow and lymph nodes. Dodds (1972) found perfusate from isolated rabbit liver to stimulate the formation of AHF and Factor IX activity in the spleen. The stimulating component was located in a fraction with a molecular weight of 115.000 to 300.000.

On the basis of these hypotheses splenic transplantation was tried in haemophilia in dogs and in one patient with haemophilia A (Norman, et al., 1968; Hathaway, et al., 1969; Penick, et al., 1970). Owing to severe bleeding complications the transplanted spleen had to be removed from the recipient and then under the protection of AHF concentrate. The findings in the animal experiments are difficult to interpret, but they may suggest a certain increase in the AHF. Several dogs died of haemorrhage after rejection of the spleen. Recently also liver transplantation has been tried in which the livers in haemophilic dogs were replaced by the livers from normal dogs and *vice versa* (Veltkamp, et al., 1971; Webster, et al., 1971). But owing to the shortness of the survival of the animals it is difficult to say anything about the effect on the AHF. According to the authors, however, the findings suggested that AHF can be produced both in and outside the liver. The spleen is believed to be the most important AHF depot.

Bouhasin, et al. (1971) described a patient with mild haemophilia A who developed acute lymphoblastic leukaemia with a rise of the AHF to normal level. They also found AHF activity in lysate from cultured white blood cells from normals, while such activity was missing or very low in white blood cells from patients with haemophilia A. Ponn, et al. (1971) feel that the splenic macrophages play a role in the synthesis of AHF.

The half-life of human AHF has been given as 6–9 hours (Biggs and Denson, 1963; Abildgaard, Ch., et al., 1964; Bowie, et al., 1967; Johnson, et al., 1971).

2. Haemophilia B factor (Factor IX)

Pavlovsky (1947) in Buenos Aires found that blood from a haemophilic patient could be normalised by blood from another haemophilic patient. Similar observations have been made by Koller, et al. (1950), Biggs, et al. (1952) and Aggeler, et al. (1952). It was therefore concluded that besides the classical haemophilia there is a coagulation defect caused by deficiency of a plasma protein that differs from the ordinary antihaemophilic globulin. The new haemophilic factor was called haemophilia B factor, 'Christmas factor' or plasma thromboplastin component (PTC) and it has been designated Factor IX by the nomenclature committee.

Properties of Factor IX

Factor IX is much more stable than AHF (F.VIII). It thus retains its activity unchanged in citrated blood stored for fourteen days at $+ 4°C$ (Geratz and Graham, 1960). Factor IX occurs in fraction IV-4 obtained by Cohn's fractionation. In plasma, Factor IX migrates with the α_1-globulins (Meyer, et al., 1969).

Factor IX in plasma is believed to occur in an inactive form and to be activated in association with coagulation (Ratnoff and Davie, 1962). Factor IX activity in the plasma increases also on contact with glass because the inactive form is activated to the more labile form. Factor IX activity is higher in fresh serum than in plasma, because the serum contains activated Factor IX, which is not stable and disappears much quicker from the circulation than does the inactivated form.

Factor IX is characterised by its adsorption to $BaSO_4$ and other alkaline earth metal salts. Also prothrombin, Factor VII and Factor X are adsorbed to these salts (see Biggs and Macfarlane, 1962).

Recently procedures for the preparation of highly purified human inactivated Factor IX have been devised (Aronson, 1973; Suomela, 1973; Østerud, 1973; Andersson, et al., 1973). These preparations do not contain any other coagulation activities. The purification of Factor IX is about 10.000-fold. The molecular weight is 72.000, and the amino acid composition has been determined. Activated Factor IX has a molecular weight of about 50.000 indicating that Factor IX is undergoing a significant molecular weight change with the activation. There is no evidence that activated Factor IX is a serine protease similar to the other members of the prothrombin complex.

Factor IX activity decreases during dicoumarol therapy and in liver diseases. It is agreed that Factor IX is formed in the liver (Ratnoff, 1960a).

The half-life of Factor IX is somewhat longer than that of Factor VIII. Loeliger and Hensen (1961b) and Ménaché (1964a) have determined the half-life as 20–40 hours and Biggs and Denson (1963) as 18–30 hours.

Preparation of Factor IX

The adsorbability of the factor to various metal salts has been utilised in the preparation of Factor IX.

Fraction PPSB. Soulier and coworkers (Soulier, Blatrix and Steinbuch, 1964; Soulier, Ménaché, Steinbuch, Blatrix and Josso, 1969; Josso, et al., 1970) have isolated a concentrate of Factors II, VII, X and IX (fraction PPSB) from human plasma by first adsorbing human EDTA-plasma with $Ca_3(PO_4)_2$. This precipitate is then eluted with 0·18 M Na_3-citrate solution. From the eluate, Factor IX activity is precipitated with 25 per cent ethanol at $−5°C$ and at pH 5·2. The Factor IX activity per mg of protein is about 100 times that in plasma. The activities of prothrombin, Factors VII and X and of Factor IX in the fraction are roughly equal. It has a good clinical effect. Shanbrom (1970) used Cohn's fraction III as a starting material and a modification of Soulier's method for further isolation. He obtained Factor IX in a concentration 200–400 times that in plasma.

Oxford method. Bidwell and coworkers (Bidwell, et al., 1967; Biggs, 1970) have devised a method for isolating Factor IX from globulin fractions obtained by alcohol fractionation of plasma. They used $Ca_3(PO_4)_2$ adsorption and citrate elution. Heparin is added to the eluate, which is afterwards dialysed and freeze-dried. They reported that they obtained a 200–300 purification of Factor IX. However, the final solution used for clinical use contains only 10 units of Factor IX per ml.

DEAE-cellulose fractionation. Tullis and coworkers (Tullis, et al., 1965, Tullis, 1970) have devised a method for isolating Factor IX from plasma with the use of DEAE-cellulose. They obtained Factor IX concentrated about 100 times. This fraction contains prothrombin, Factors VII and X in roughly equal concentrations.

Pert, et al. (1970) started from Cohn's fraction III and afterwards used DEAE-cellulose and $Ca_3(PO_4)_2$.

Dike, Bidwell and Rizza (1972) have prepared a concentrate of Factors IX, II and X and a separate concentrate of Factor VII by adsorption of the factors on DEAE-cellulose from plasma or from the supernatant after removal of Factor VIII. The yield of Factor IX *in vitro* is about 50–75 per cent and the purification about 300-fold.

3. Factor XI (haemophilia C Factor, PTA) and Factor XII (Hageman Factor)

Rosenthal and coworkers (1953) of New York described a new haemorrhagic diathesis which differed from classical haemophilia and occurred in both males and females. The bleeding symptoms of this disease are not so severe as in classical haemophilia. They felt that the bleeding defect is due to deficiency of a previously unknown plasma factor, which they called 'plasma thromboplastin antecedent' or PTA. This type of haemophilia is now called haemophilia C.

Ratnoff and coworkers (Ratnoff, 1954; Ratnoff and Colopy, 1955) described another new coagulation defect. They called this defect after the name of their first patient 'Hageman trait' and the missing factor, Hageman factor. Patients with Hageman factor deficiency have a genetically prolonged coagulation time in glass tubes as well as in siliconised tubes, but no increased bleeding tendency.

In 1961 the nomenclature committee gave PTA and Hageman factor the names Factor XI and Factor XII.

Factor XI and Factor XII form a complex that influences the reaction of the blood to contact with glass. It has long been known that blood coagulates much faster in glass tubes than in siliconised tubes. In recent years these effects of contact with foreign surfaces on coagulation have received relatively wide attention (Waaler, 1959; Soulier, Prou-Wartelle and Ménaché, 1959; Margolis, 1959a, 1961; Rapaport, et al., 1961:

Ratnoff, 1960b, 1965; Rosenthal, 1961; Biggs and Macfarlane, 1962; Ollendorff, 1962; Nossel, 1964; Niewiarowski, et al., 1965; Veltkamp, et al., 1965; Haanen, et al., 1965; Wilner, Nossel and Le Roy, 1968; Girolami, 1969). Our knowledge of Factor XII is greater than that of Factor XI. This is because the study of Factor XI is impaired to some extent by the fact that Factor XI deficient plasma is partly normalised by freezing.

Factor XI and Factor XII are characterised by the fact that they are adsorbed to glass, kaolin, Celite and barium carbonate. This results in activation of Factor XI and Factor XII and initiation of coagulation. Opinions differ on the mechanism of activation by contact with glass. According to one opinion, inactive Factor XII is bound to an inhibitor. On contact with glass Factor XII is believed to be separated from this inhibitor and become active (Ollendorff, 1962). According to most other authors, Factor XII is activated directly by contact with glass. The chemical changes in Factor XII induced by contact with glass are unknown (Ratnoff, 1965). It has been assumed that glass produces 'a molecular rearrangement' in the Factor XII molecule. A characteristic common to all agents capable of activating Factor XII is that they are negatively charged. It has also been shown that ellagic acid and cellulose sulphate solutions can activate Factor XII even in the absence of contact with glass (Ratnoff, 1965; Kellermeyer and Kellermeyer, 1969). Wilner and coworker (1968) have shown that purified human collagen can activate Factor XII. These authors produced evidence for the assumption that in collagen it is the free carboxyl group in glutamic acid and asparagine that are responsible for the activation. Recently Walsh (1972) studied the coagulation reactions in which collagen-stimulated platelets participate. Using an albumin density gradient separation method for washing platelets free of adsorbed coagulation factors he found that collagen can induce a coagulant activity in platelets, which initiates intrinsic coagulation. This capacity was independent of Factor XII, provided that Factor XI was available. He suggested that this alternative pathway might explain the absence of a haemostatic defect in the Hageman trait.

It is otherwise generally believed that when Factor XII is activated, Factor XI is converted from an inactive to an active form (see Waaler, 1959; Nossel, 1964; Ratnoff, 1965). How Factor XII changes Factor XI in this activation is unknown. Activated Factor XI afterwards converts Factor IX to an active form. This requires the presence of Ca^{2+} (Ratnoff and Davie, 1962).

Factor XII is believed not only to activate Factor XI, but also to have other functions. According to Margolis (1959b), Factor XII is associated with the kininogen-kinin system and 'the capillary permeability factor'. Activated Factor XII in plasma thus releases a factor that increases the vascular permeability of the skin in guinea-pigs. This is accompanied by a reduction of kininogen (Gautvik and Rugstad, 1967). In addition, some authors believe that Factor XII can activate the fibrinolytic system (Iatridis and Ferguson, 1962; McDonagh and Ferguson, 1970). Nilsson and Robertson (1968) have, however, shown that the content of Factor XII is not correlated with the local fibrinolytic activity that develops on venous occlusion of the arms.

Many attempts have been made to isolate Factor XII from normal plasma. Hageman factor or the activation product has been eluted from glass tubes with borate buffer of pH 9–11. The active substance has afterwards been purified further by acid precipitation and fractionation with $(NH_4)_2SO_4$. The activation product has also been eluted from Celite with 7 per cent NaCl solution and afterwards precipitated by addition of $(NH_4)_2SO_4$ to 33–50 per cent saturation (Haanen, et al., 1960). Ratnoff and Davie (1962) have purified Factor XII from human plasma by chromatography on various cellulose columns. Schoenmakers, et al. (1963, 1965) have prepared bovine Factor XII by elution from glass and chromatography on CM-Sephadex and DEAE-Sephadex. Homogeneity was observed on polyacrylamide gel electrophoresis, on disc electrophoresis and on ultracentrifugation. Its specific activity was increased 6.000-fold. They regarded Hageman factor as a sialoglycoprotein with a molecular weight of about 80.000. Speer, et al. (1965) purified Hageman factor by adsorption and elution from Celite, iso-electric precipitation, precipitation with $(NH_4)_2SO_4$, chromatography on CM-Sephadex and on phosphocellulose. A 10^6-fold purification was obtained on ultracentrifugal analysis. The product obtained was found to be homogeneous. It is, however, not clear how Hageman factor was separated from Factor XI. Speer, et al., gave the molecular weight of their preparation as 160.000, but their preparation, in contrast with that of Schoenmakers, was activated. Grammens, et al. (1971) have recently purified bovine Factor XII by adsorption to glass, various precipitation methods and DEAE-cellulose chromatography and obtained a homogeneous preparation. They have studied the physico-chemical and immunological properties of this bovine Factor XII. The molecular weight was determined as 140.000. Factor XII has both estero-lytic and proteolytic activity (Schoenmakers, et al., 1965). It is inactivated by chymotrypsin (Ratnoff and Davie, 1962). On electrophoresis it migrates between β- and γ-globulins (Ratnoff, 1965).

So far no method is available for purifying Factor XI. Partial purification is, however, believed to be possible by repeated chromatography on cellulose (Kingdon, et al., 1964). Barth, et al., (1969) purified activated Factor XI from porcine plasma by adsorption and elution from Celite, followed by chromatography on DEAE-cellulose and DEAE-Sephadex. On disc electrophoresis the purified material produced two bands, but its identity is not certain. In electrophoresis, Factor XI is recovered as well as Factor XII between β- and γ-globulins (Rosenthal, 1955). According to Kingdon, et al. (1964) Factor XI is a hydrolytic enzyme and splits TAMe. Otherwise its nature is unknown.

As for other properties of Factor XI and Factor XII, it might be mentioned that both factors are said to be stable during storage. Both factors can also be detected in serum. Factor XI is not adsorbed to $BaSO_4$ but Factor XII is to some extent, and this property is of importance when measuring the activity of these factors. Factors XI and XII are, as mentioned, characterised by the fact that they are adsorbed to glass, kaolin and Celite. According to Soulier and Prou-Wartelle (1959), adsorption of Factor XII requiries larger amounts of Celite than does Factor XI (15 mg Celite/ml plasma adsorbs Factor XI; 30 mg Celite/ml plasma adsorbs Factors XI and XII). Both factors are more thermostable than other coagulation factors. They are not inactivated by exposure to temperatures up to 56°C (see Wright, 1962).

As mentioned, much or our knowledge of Factor XI is still vague. Biggs, et al. (1968) have discussed 'the coagulant activity of platelets'. After separation of platelets from platelet-rich plasma which had been incubated for 16–20 hours at 37°C, a coagulation accelerating factor developed which shortened the coagulation time of plasma deficient in Factors XII, XI and VIII. According to Biggs and coworkers, development of this platelet activity requires only access to Factor XII. Is this 'coagulant activity of platelets' possibly identical with Factor XI activity?

Factors XI and XII are not influenced by dicoumarol therapy. According to Rapaport (1961) Factor XI activity may be reduced in liver cirrhosis. This is the only condition known with acquired deficiency of Hageman factor and PTA.

The half-life of Hageman factor (Factor XII) has been given as 52 hours (Veltkamp, et al., 1965). Nossel (1964) has stated that the half-life of Factor XI in the circulation is about 60 hours.

C.   *Phase II—conversion of prothrombin to thrombin*

Some remarks on Factor V, Factor VII, Factor X and prothrombin in the second phase of the coagulation process are given below (see Fig. 14).

1. Factor V

In 1943 Owren of Oslo described a patient with a congenital haemorrhagic diathesis and with prolonged one-stage prothrombin time (thromboplastin time), as in prothrombin deficiency. He found that the one-stage prothrombin time could be normalised by prothrombin-free plasma. He also showed that the condition was due to deficiency of a factor normally occurring in the blood and necessary for normal conversion of prothrombin to thrombin. He called it Factor V or proaccelerin and designated the coagulation disorder Factor V deficiency or parahaemophilia (Owren, 1947). The same observation was made at roughly the same time by Quick (1943), Fantl and Nance (1946) and Ware and Seegers (1948), who respectively called the new factor 'labile factor', prothrombin accelerator and accelerator globulin.

Factor V has been conceived as a proenzyme that is activated by activated Factor X with the formation of a prothrombin activator, which enzymatically converts prothrombin to thrombin (Breckenridge and Ratnoff, 1966; Denson, 1967). But recent research has produced much evidence that phospholipids adsorb Factor V as well as Factor X and that this complex, together with Ca^{2+} constitutes the enzyme (prothrombinase) that converts prothrombin to thrombin (Papahadjopoulos and Hanahan, 1964; Barton, et al., 1967; Deggeller and Vreeken, 1969; Esnouf, 1969). Thrombin increases the reactivity of Factor V about three-fold (Barton, et al., 1967). It has been shown that a fraction in Russell viper venom reacts stoichiometrically with Factor V and accelerates its effect in the conversion of prothrombin (Schiffman, et al., 1969; Prentice and Ratnoff, 1969; Kahn and Hemker, 1972).

Factor V is a labile substance, which is rapidly inactivated during storage. Factor V activity disappears within a few hours from oxalated plasma, but less rapidly from citrated plasma. Factor V is not adsorbed to $BaSO_4$ or other alkaline earth metal salts. Factor V is consumed on coagulation and is thus not found in serum. The denaturation of Factor V in human plasma is, however, a process that is essentially different from the activation of Factor V in the course of the coagulation process. The disappearance of Factor V activity from human plasma may be regarded as denaturation of a protein. In the course of coagulation, Factor V activity is believed to be inactivated because a second molecule of Factor V combines with the prothrombinase molecule (Hemker and Kahn, 1972). Factor V is not affected by dicoumarol (Owren, 1947). Factor V is inactivated by plasmin and trypsin (Colman, 1969). Thrombin destroys human Factor V activity after the initial phase of potentiation. Factor V can be recovered in Cohn's fraction III (Biggs and Macfarlane, 1962).

Ware and Seegers (1948) devised a method for isolating Ac-globulin or Factor V. Their purest preparation contained 50 per cent of Factor V. Partially purified Factor V preparation has also been prepared by Owren (1948) and Surgenor, et al. (1961). In these methods the prothrombin, Factor VII and Factor X were removed by absorption to $BaSO_4$ or some other alkaline earth metal salt. The plasma fractions were afterwards fractionated with $(NH_4)_2SO_4$ and other precipitating methods. The value of these methods was limited by the lability of Factor V. Purification of human Factor V has proved to offer still greater difficulties than that of bovine Factor V. Blombäck, B. and Blombäck, M. (1963) have worked out a method for purifying and stabilising Factor V. With human Cohn's fraction VI-1 M as a starting material they found that it was possible to stabilise Factor V in this fraction by addition of Mg^{2+}, Ca^{2+} or Si^{2+} ions. This was followed by gel filtration on Sephadex G-200. Esnouf and Jobin (1967) have isolated and purified Factor V from bovine plasma. They used DEAE-cellulose eluate from $BaSO_4$-adsorbed bovine plasma as starting material. Chromatography of DEAE eluate on cellulose was afterwards performed. Contaminants of S_{20} components were removed by ultracentrifugation. They obtained an immunologically homogeneous preparation with a molecular weight of 290.000 and a sedimentation constant of 5·8. The amino acid content of Factor V was also determined. The purification concentrated the protein 6.000 times. Their preparation showed no increase in activity on incubation with thrombin. Colman, et al. (1970), who used $(NH_4)_2SO_4$ precipitation and cellulose, reported native bovine Factor V to occur in three forms differing in molecular size, the oligomeric inconvertible forms A and C, and a phospholipid-containing complex designated form L. But Day and Barton (1972) have recently produced evidence suggesting that the L and C forms were artifacts of the preparative procedure. They also pointed out that concentrations of Ca^{2+} higher than 0·001 M suppress the activity. Kahn and Hemker (1972) found the molecular weights of inactivated and activated bovine Factor V to be 400.000 and 195.000, respectively, suggesting the dissociation into a dimer in the process of activation. Kahn and Hemker (1970) used a method similar to that of Esnouf and Jobin for preparing human Factor V with chromatography on cellulose and addition of Ca^{2+} and Mg^{2+} and glycerol for stabilisation. They reported a purification of only 30 times. They found inactivated human Factor V to have a molecular weight of 410.000 and when activated (by Russell viper venom) to have a molecular weight of 110.000 suggesting dissociation of a tetramer (Kahn and Hemker, 1972).

Factor V is synthesized in the liver and is therefore reduced in liver diseases. *The half-life of Factor V* has been given as about 36 hours (Webster, et al., 1964).

2. Factor VII (proconvertin)

As early as 1947 Owren reported that conversion of prothrombin required not only Factor V, but probably also a further accelerator. Later he encountered a coagulation picture of the type he had predicted in a patient lacking such an accelerator (see Owren, 1951). Owren called this factor proconvertin. At roughly the same time both Alexander and coworkers (1949) and Koller and coworkers (1951) in Zürich reported that serum normally contained an accelerator, which Alexander called 'serum prothrombin conversion accelerator (SPCA)', while Koller called it Factor VII. It has been designated Factor VII by the nomenclature committee.

Factor VII is a plasma factor, which does not take part in the conversion of prothrombin in the intrinsic system, but only in the extrinsic system. In the presence of tissue factor and Factor VII, then, an active product, extrinsic thromboplastin, is formed and this product activates Factor X to active Factor X. This can then participate in the ordinary way in the activation of prothrombin (Fig. 14). Østerud, et al. (1972) recently investigated the mechanism of activation of Factor VII by bovine thromboplastin and Ca^{2+}. Factor VII was isolated in an activated state after incubation with tissue thromboplastin and Ca^{2+} and subsequent destruction of all thromboplastin activity by phospholipase C. The activated state was dependent upon the presence of phospholipid bound to Factor VII, since the activation was reversible by prolonged treatment with phospholipase C. Binding of Factor VII to tissue thromboplastin membranes was thus not necessary in the activation of Factor X by Factor VII, provided the latter had previously been exposed to tissue thromboplastin.

In factor VII deficiency the one-stage prothrombin time is prolonged. In the investigation of coagulation defects in phase II it is the rule to determine not only the one-stage prothrombin time, i.e., the coagulation time found on addition of tissue thromboplastin to plasma, but also the coagulation time on addition of Russell viper venom to plasma. The preparation of Russell viper venom commonly used is called Stypven. The coagulation time on its addition to plasma is known as the Stypven time. Macfarlane (1961) has shown that Russell viper venom reacts with a serum factor, Factor X, and Ca^{2+} and forms a product that afterwards reacts with phospholipids and Factor V with the formation of a potent prothrombin activator. Williams and Esnouf (1962) have succeeded in isolating the active component of Russell viper venom, which enzymatically activates Factor X. It has later been shown that Russell viper venom contains not only this component, but also a separate component which can activate Factor V (Prentice and Ratnoff, 1969; Schiffman, et al., 1969). Russell viper venom or Stypven plus phospholipids thus has an effect corresponding to that of tissue thromboplastin plus Factor VII. *The Stypven time is thus normal in Factor VII deficiency.*

Factor VII is a stable factor. It is not consumed during coagulation and can thus be recovered in the serum. It is adsorbed to $BaSO_4$ and other alkaline earth metal salts. Factor VII is decreased in patients receiving dicoumarol, in vitamin K deficiency and in liver diseases. Factor VII is said to be β-globulin (Owren 1954). Factor VII is purified with largely the same methods as prothrombin. It has not been possible to recover one of them without simultaneous loss of the other. Prydz and coworkers (Prydz, 1965c; Gladhaug and Prydz, 1970; Prydz and Gladhaug, 1971) have devised a method for purifying Factor VII from human plasma and serum. The adsorbable factors were purified by elution from a column of $BaSO_4$ and Sephadex G-25. The eluate was then purified further by chromatography on DEAE-Sephadex. They claimed to have purified Factor VII about 1.300 times and to have a preparation free from prothrombin and homogeneous when examined with immunoelectrophoresis and disc electrophoresis. Estimates of the molecular weight of the human plasma material are of the order of 60.000, while the protein obtained from serum has a molecular weight of about 45.000. Prydz also stated that he had prepared an antiserum against Factor VII (Prydz, 1965a). Further, in tissue culture experiments he has shown that Factor VII is synthetised in rat liver cell suspensions (Prydz, 1965b).

Marder and Shulman (1964) and Loeliger, et al. (1960) reported a *half-life* of 5 hours for Factor VII; Owen, et al. (1964) reported an initial half-life of 4 hours and a subsequent half-life of 23 hours.

3. Factor X (Stuart Factor)

In 1957 Graham and coworkers (Hougie, Barrow and Graham, 1957; Graham, Barrow and Hougie, 1957) of Chapel Hill noticed that the coagulation of blood samples from some of their patients with Factor VII deficiency could be normalised *in vitro* by addition of blood from other patients with Factor VII deficiency and *vice versa*. Since then several patients with prolonged one-stage prothrombin time have been examined, and it has been found that they fall into two groups, namely those lacking Factor VII and those lacking Stuart factor. Stuart was the name of Graham's first patient. Graham and coworkers also showed that patients with Stuart factor deficiency have a prolonged Stypven time and defective thromboplastin generation, in contrast with patients with Factor VII deficiency. Telfer, Denson and Wright (1956) had as early as 1956 described a patient who was regarded as being deficient in a new plasma factor, which they called Prower factor after the patient's name. Duckert and coworkers (1955) also arrived at the conclusion that serum contained a factor necessary for thromboplastin formation and that this factor was not identical with Factor VII or Factor IX. They called it Factor X. Later comparative studies have shown that Stuart factor, Prower factor and Factor X are obviously identical. In 1959 Stuart factor was designated Factor X by the nomenclature committee. It is important to remember that *both the one-stage prothrombin time and the Stypven time are prolonged in Factor X deficiency*.

Factor X is a stable factor, which is adsorbed to $BaSO_4$ and alkaline earth metal salts. It persists in the serum. Factor X is decreased in patients treated with dicoumarol, in vitamin K deficiency and liver diseases (Hougie, et al., 1957).

As mentioned above, most authors now believe that activated Factor X together with Factor V, phospholipid and Ca^{2+} forms a dissociable complex, which acts as a prothrombin activator (prothrombinase). Factor X can be activated both by the components of the intrinsic system and of the extrinsic system. Factor X can also be activated by trypsin and, as mentioned previously, by a component of Russell viper venom and Ca^{2+}. It has been shown that Factor X also has esterase activity (see Esnouf, 1969). Its coagulative activity as well as its esterase activity can be inhibited by di-isopropyl fluorophosphate and soybean inhibitor (Leveson and Esnouf, 1969).

Factor X has been electrophoretically identified as an α-globulin (Denson, 1958). Esnouf and Williams (1962) have focused most interest on the purification of Factor X. They used citrate eluate from $BaSO_4$ adsorbate from bovine plasma as a starting material and DEAE-cellulose for fractionation. The authors claim that they purified the substance 4.000 times and that the preparation is homogeneous in the ultracentrifuge and has a sedimentation constant of 4·23. The molecular weight has been given as about 54.000 (Esnouf, 1969). But this preparation contains also Factor IX and Factor VII activity. Aronson, et al. (1969) have purified Factor X further by chromatography on hydroxiapatite and subsequent preparative disc electrophoresis and DEAE-cellulose chromatography. They gave the molecular weight as 86.000. They also showed that the major part of the peptides in Factor X differ from those in prothrombin. They interpreted this as direct evidence against Factor X being a derivative of prothrombin.

The half-life of Factor X has been given as 48 hours (Biggs and Denson, 1963).

4. Prothrombin (Factor II)

Prothrombin is the substrate in the second phase of coagulation. In the beginning of the 1930s Henrik Dam of Copenhagen discovered that vitamin K is necessary for the synthesis of prothrombin. This raised the status of prothrombin to that of a clinically important blood component. Another mile-stone in the history of our knowledge of prothrombin is Link's (see Jorpes, 1955) isolation of 3:3'-methylene bis-(4-hydroxi-coumarin), dicoumarol, and his discovery that this substance inhibits prothrombin formation.

With the exception of fibrinogen, prothrombin is the coagulation plasma protein that has been best purified, thanks especially to the work of Seegers in Detroit. Since 1940 Seegers has published by himself or in cooperation with other investigators more than 200 papers on prothrombin. He has also published several monographs of his investigations (see Seegers, 1940; Seegers, 1952; Seegers, 1962; Seegers, 1964; Seegers, 1967; Seegers, et al., 1967; Seegers, Murano and McCoy, 1970). He purified prothrombin with a method in which diluted plasma was adsorbed with $Mg(OH)_2$ and in which the eluate was afterwards fractionated. These preparations had an activity of 15.000 to 33.000 thrombin units (Iowa-units) per mg tyrosine. Seegers and Smith (1942) defined one Iowa-unit of thrombin as the amount of thrombin that coagulates one ml of one per cent fibrinogen solution in 15 seconds at $28°C$. Thrombin is now measured in NIH units. One NIH unit of thrombin corresponds to 1·25 Iowa-units.

Seegers has purified prothrombin further by chromatography on DEAE-cellulose, but further purification did not increase its specific activity. According to Seegers, prothrombin is a stable glycoprotein with a molecular weight of about 63.000. Prothrombin migrates in the electro-phoretic field as a α_2-globulin. The amino acid composition of prothrombin has been determined. It has been found that prothrombin has only one N-terminal amino acid group, namely alanine. Prothrombin can be adsorbed to insoluble salts of alkaline earth metals, from which it can afterwards be eluted with citrate. Seegers succeeded in activating prothrombin to thrombin by addition of concentrated citrated solution alone. He regarded the conversion of prothrombin to thrombin as a degradation process, and he has shown that activation by citrate splits off a component which contains carbohydrate and which is not thrombin. The thrombin obtained by citrate activation was isolated by Seegers who found it to be an electrophoretically homogenous preparation with a molecular weight of 30.000.

Landaburu, et al. (1968) used Seegers' original method, but later purified the bovine prothrombin further by chromatography on Amberlite AG_3-X_4. This preparation had an activity of more than 40.000 Iowa-units per mg tyrosine. On iso-electric fractionation of purified prothrombin,

Landaburu and Albado (1969) obtained a fraction with Factor X activity. They therefore thought that a physical interaction had probably occurred between prothrombin and Factor X.

A series of publications on prothrombin and thrombin has been published by Magnusson since 1965 (see Magnusson, 1971). He has shown that Seegers' bovine prothrombin contains impurities, and he estimated its purity at 90–95 per cent. Using ionic strength gradient elution after adsorption on DEAE-cellulose he succeeded in separating Seegers' material into four components, one of which was prothrombin, which proved homogeneous on starch electrophoresis in three different buffer systems. With another method in which human fraction II + III was used as a starting material, Magnusson isolated an apparently homogeneous human prothrombin. In addition, he succeeded in obtaining homogeneous bovine and human thrombin. These prothrombin preparations could not be activated to thrombin on incubation with citrate solution. Non-activated prothrombin preparations, both human and bovine, were found to have one mole N-terminal alanine per mole. After activation he was able to demonstrate 2 (or 3) moles isoleucine, one mole treonine and minor amounts of other N-terminal amino acids per mole. The molecular weight of thrombin was estimated at 40.000 and that of prothrombin at 74.000. Magnusson also tried to determine the primary structure of bovine and human prothrombin and thrombin. Prothrombin is a single polypeptide chain and it is cleaved, by the prothrombin-converting complex, to thrombin, which consists of two polypeptide chains, A and B. A single disulphide bridge connects the A-chain with the B-chain. Magnusson determined the sequence of the A-chain (bovine thrombin) and found 49 amino acids and no carbohydrate. So far 265 amino acids have been identified in the B-chain. This chain includes carbohydrate. Thrombin is in many respects similar to trypsin and chymotrypsin in structure and in effect, but it also has some peculiarities which are of interest from a chemical point of view. While trypsin generally splits all arginyl bonds and lysyl bonds in a protein or a peptide, thrombin attacks only certain bonds.

Opinions differ on the kinetics of the conversion phase of prothrombin during normal coagulation, as witnessed by several publications (see Seegers, 1962; Seegers, et al., 1967; Seegers, et al., 1970; Cole, et al., 1965; Biggs and Macfarlane, 1962; Ratnoff and Davie, 1962; Kline, 1965; Prentice, et al., 1967; Barton, et al., 1967; Esnouf, 1969; Hemker, et al., 1967; 1970). Most authors believe that the processes involved in the first stage of the coagulation mechanism result in the formation of a prothrombin activator or prothrombinase, which enzymatically converts prothrombin to thrombin. It is evident from the work of Magnusson, for example, that the conversion of prothrombin to thrombin is a proteolytic process.

In his earlier publication, Seegers (1964) claimed that the biological conversion of prothrombin is an autocatalytic process like the conversion of trypsinogen to trypsin, and that the thrombin is the catalysing enzyme.

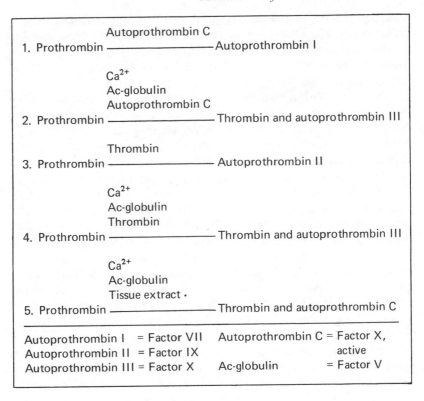

He postulated that in the conversion of prothrombin to thrombin inter-
mediary products are formed, which are called autoprothrombin I, II,
III and autoprothrombin C (Fig. 18). According to Seegers, prothrombin
derivative I has the same accelerating properties as those ascribed to
Factor VII; autoprothrombin II the same properties as those ascribed to
Factor IX; and autoprothrombin III the same properties as those ascribed
to Factor X. Autoprothrombin C is equivalent to active Factor X. Factor
VII, Factor IX and Factor X are thus only derivatives of prothrombin.
In recent years Seegers and coworkers (Seegers, et al., 1967, 1968; Seegers,
et al., 1970) have published a somewhat modified theory. The prothrombin
complex is still regarded as a source of prothrombin, Factor VII, Factor
IX and Factor X activity. On dissociation of the prothrombin complex
there forms an inhibitory product and autoprothrombins which he called
I, II, III and autoprothrombin C. Autoprothrombin III is converted
under the influence of Ca^{2+} and tissue factor or Factor VIII to autoprothrombin C, which in turn converts prothrombin to thrombin. This
reaction is accelerated by Factor V, Ca^{2+} and lipids.

Seegers' theories have several interesting aspects. In fact, they now
differ from the other theories mainly regarding the origin of the individual
clotting factors. It has not yet been possible to separate prothrombin,
Factor VII and Factor X without simultaneous loss of the other factors.
On isolation of Factor IX, Factor VII and Factor X these preparations

have been found to possess many of the chemical characteristics of prothrombin. These factors react also to vitamin K and dicoumarol in the same way as prothrombin. Neither has it been satisfactorily demonstrated that patients with Factor VII and Factor X deficiency ever have normal prothrombin.

Ganrot and Niléhn (Niléhn and Ganrot, 1968; Ganrot and Niléhn, 1968a, b, 1969) have devised an immunological method for determining prothrombin. Plasma from patients treated with dicoumarol has been found to have two prothrombin fractions, one fraction with a normal coagulation activity and one abnormal fraction that cannot be activated and cannot be adsorbed to $BaSO_4$. They also found that Ca^{2+} ions are bound to normal prothrombin but not to dicoumarol-induced prothrombin. In further experiments Ganrot and coworkers (Ganrot and Niléhn, 1969; Ganrot and Stenflo, 1970) have produced evidence suggesting that prothrombin is built up of thrombin and a 'non-thrombin' fragment. They isolated the 'non-thrombin' fragment from serum. On electrophoresis they could separate this fragment into two parts. These parts are described as having the same physical and chemical properties as those ascribed to Factor VII and Factor X. Ganrot feels that this finding supports Seegers theory that Factor VII and Factor X are derivatives of prothrombin.

Highly active prothrombin preparations contain about 3.000 Iowa-units of thrombin per mg. Complete activation of the prothrombin in one ml plasma results in the formation of 300 units of thrombin. According to this calculation, 100 ml plasma should contain 10–15 mg prothrombin (see Seegers, 1962).

Prothrombin forms in the liver and its formation requires the presence of vitamin K. Dicoumarol inhibits the formation of prothrombin. If dicoumarol is added to blood *in vitro*, it will not reduce the prothrombin. It was therefore formerly assumed that dicoumarol inhibits the synthesis of prothrombin. Since vitamin K is necessary, presumably as a coenzyme, for the synthesis of prothrombin in the liver, it was believed that dicoumarol probably serves as a competitive inhibitor, which prevents some of the enzymes in this synthesis from utilising the vitamin. As pointed out above, it has been shown that dicoumarol does not inhibit synthesis, but induces the formation of an abnormal prothrombin (Ganrot and Niléhn, 1968b). Stenflo (1972a, b) has prepared highly purified dicoumarol-induced bovine prothrombin and compared its structure with that of normal prothrombin. Quantitative amino acid and carbohydrate analysis gave identical results for both prothrombins, as did analysis of the NH_2-terminal and the COOH-terminal amino acids and determination of the molecular weights. Also peptide mapping gave identical results. Stenflo assumed that the difference in properties between the two prothrombins are due to a minor structural or conformational difference. Barnhardt (1960) has shown with the fluorescence antibody technique that only liver parenchymal cells, and thus not reticulo-endothelial cells, synthetise prothrombin.

The prothrombin is consumed during coagulation, and serum normally contains only small amounts of prothrombin.

The half-life of prothrombin has been determined by biological methods as 40–60 hours (Hjort, et al., 1961). Shapiro and Martinez (1969) have studied human prothrombin metabolism with ^{131}I-labelled human prothrombin. They found the half-life to be 2·8 days. The prothrombin content of plasma was determined by them as 0·15 mg per ml plasma, prothrombin catabolism as 43 per cent of the total plasma pool per day and the rate of synthesis as 2·4 mg per kg per day. Almost two thirds of the total prothrombin pool is found to be intravascular.

D. *Phase III—conversion of fibrinogen to fibrin*

In the last stage of the coagulation process the thrombin enzymatically converts fibrinogen to fibrin. Some data on fibrinogen and Factor XIII (FSF) are given below.

1. Fibrinogen

Fibrinogen constitutes only about one thirtieth of the plasma proteins, but when the fibrinogen is rendered insoluble by the effect of thrombin, it is sufficient to convert blood to a solid gel. Fibrinogen is one of the least soluble plasma proteins. We now have a fairly thorough knowledge of the chemical structure of fibrinogen. Excellent surveys of the chemistry and structure of fibrinogen as well as of the conversion of fibrinogen to fibrin have been published by B. Blombäck and M. Blombäck (Blombäck, B., 1967, 1969, 1971; Blombäck, B. and Blombäck, M., 1972) and by Laki (1968).

In Cohn's alcohol fractionation method about 50 per cent of fraction I consists of fibrinogen and can be precipitated by 8 per cent ethanol. With their glycine method, Birger and Margareta Blombäck (1956) have succeeded in purifying fibrinogen further from fraction I and obtained a stable fibrinogen preparation with coagulability as high as 98–99 per cent (Fig. 19). From fraction I-2-F, fibrinogen has been purified further by precipitation at low ionic strength. Despite the very high degree of purity achieved with this method and others, the product is not free from contaminants, which sometimes may prove troublesome when the fibrinogen is used for special purposes. The fibrinogen preparation thus contains plasminogen, and many attempts have been made to find a way of preventing this contamination. Using the glycine method, Mosesson (1962) precipitated the purified fibrinogen in the presence of aminocaproic acid, which maintained the plasminogen in solution. A similar procedure has been published by Bergström and Wallén (1961) in which lysine was used as a solvent for plasminogen. Also gel filtration on Sephadex G-200 has been described as producing good separation of plasminogen from fibrinogen (Berg and Korsan-Bengtsen, 1963). Other authors have used adsorption to charcoal or bentonite in order to obtain fibrinogen

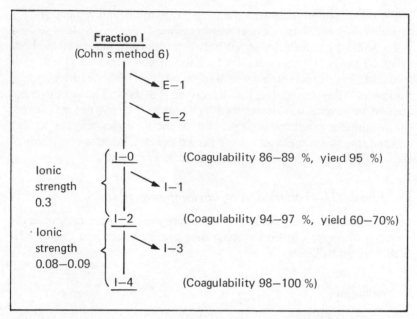

Fig 19. Preparatic
of fibrinogen from
Cohn's fraction I
(Blombäck, B. 195

free from plasminogen (Brakman, 1965). Ohlsson (1969) produced plasminogen-free fibrinogen by precipitating plasminogen with a specific antiserum.

Blombäck and coworkers have made praiseworthy contributions to our knowledge of the structure of fibrinogen. Fibrinogen has a molecular weight of about 340.000, which means that it is one of the largest proteins in the blood. The fibrinogen molecule is roughly 500 Å long. It is built up of two identical halves which are united to one another by at least three disulphide bridges (Fig. 20). Each half-molecule consists of three chains, the Aα-, Bβ- and γ-chain. The molecular weights of these chains have been given as 64.000, 57.000 and 48.000, respectively (Gaffney and Dobos, 1971; McDonagh, et al., 1972).

Fibrinogen does not contain any free sulphydryl groups. On the other hand, it has about twenty-nine disulphide bonds per molecule, which, however, are not available for reduction before denaturation with urea in high concentration at 50–60°C. Henschen has thoroughly studied the splitting of bovine fibrinogen and fibrin with sulphite under the influence of urea. She isolated three S-sulphopeptides (Henschen, 1964a, b). The molecular weight of each of these is roughly one sixth of that of fibrinogen. The N-terminals of the peptides agree with those found in intact fibrinogen.

Also the structure of the N-terminal disulphide, which constitutes roughly 16 per cent of the fibrinogen monomer, has now been clarified (Blombäck, B, and Blombäck, M., 1972). It consists of 185 amino acid esters and the amino acid sequence in the chains, the arrangement of the disulphide bridges and the positions of the prosthetic groups such as oligosaccharide fragments and phosphoric acid are now known (Fig 22).

Fig 20. Schematic model of the dimeric fibrinogen molecule with twofold rotation symmetry. Th: thrombin. Arrow indicates cleavage site of thrombin. The crosslinks in black are stable disulfides, and the lighter ones are labile disulfides (from Blombäck, B. and Blombäck, M.: *Ann. N. Y. Acad. Sci.* **202**, 78, 1972).

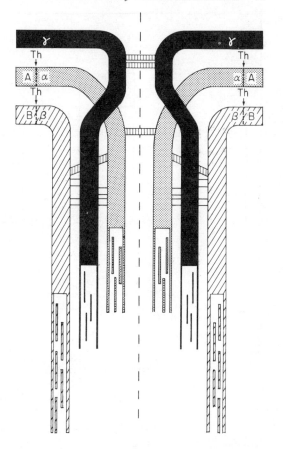

The chains have characteristic N-terminal sequences, tryptic peptide maps and immunological properties. They all have a free C-terminal residue (Blombäck, M., 1972). The disulphide bridges are unevenly distributed in the fibrinogen molecule. Roughly 40 per cent occur in a hydrophilic N-terminal portion (N-terminal disulphide knot, molecular weight 60.000), which, like the whole fibrinogen, is a dimer containing N-terminal portions of the three chains. Most of the remaining disulphide bridges are situated in three hydrophobic disulphide knots (Blombäck, M., 1972). One of these has been characterised by B. Blombäck and co-workers (Gårdlund, et al., 1972). They have found it to contain 4–6 disulphide bridges and to consist of at least two polypeptide chains with molecular weights of 17.000 and 7.500, respectively. One of the chains has immunochemically been found to have determinants common to those of fibrinogen. The other two hydrophobic disulphide knots have been partly purified by the same research group and have been shown to have molecular weights of less than 10.000. Together the hydrophilic and hydrophobic disulphide knots constitute about one third of the fibrinogen molecule.

It has long been known that the action of thrombin and fibrinogen

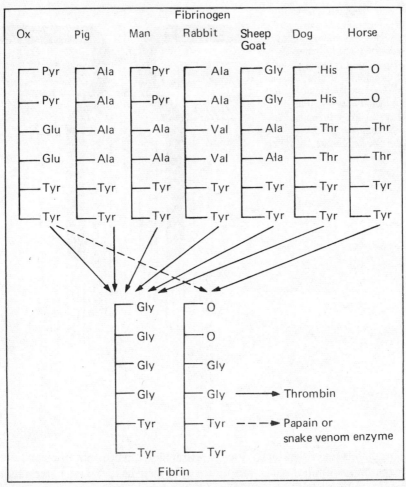

Fig 21. N-terminal
amino acids in fibri
nogen and fibrin. T
scheme is an extens
of that originally
presented by
Blombäck and
Yamashina (1958).
In the fibrin obtaine
from bovine fibri-
nogen with snake
venom enzyme or
papain, the circles a
most probably
identical with Pyr.
Pyr = pyroglutamyl
o = cyclic or blocke
chains.

results in the splitting off of two different peptides, so-called fibrinopeptides, which are called peptides A and B (Lorand, 1952; Bailey and
Bettelheim, 1955). Bailey and Bettelheim found that the N-terminal
amino acids in fibrinogen differ from those in fibrin. For example, tyrosine
and glutamic acid are N-terminals in bovine fibrinogen, while in bovine
fibrin the N-terminal glutamic acid fragment is not demonstrable and
has been replaced by N-terminal glycine. The N-terminals, also of
fibrinogen and fibrin from different animals, have since been investigated
by several workers. Blombäck (see Blombäck, B., 1967) used Edman's
phenyl-isothiocyanate method, which permits more exact quantitative
determinations. In human fibrinogen Blombäck found four N-terminal
amino acids per molecule, two of which consisted of tyrosine and two
of alanine. After activation with thrombin he found six N-terminals
per molecule; four glycine and two unchanged tyrosine molecules (Fig.
21). As far as human fibrinogen is concerned, then, thrombin splits off
four peptides, two A-peptides and two B-peptides, two of which have no

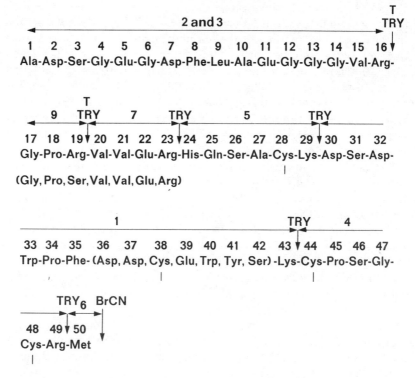

22. Amino acid sequence in N-terminal of human (A)- in. That part of the ide chain which has viating sequence in ents with fibrinogen roit is given in kets. After B. mbäck.

N-terminal amino acids. The N-terminal pattern differs from species to species. In all cases, however, the splitting occurs at an arginine glycine bond and the site of attack of the thrombin is thus specific for this bond.

Blombäck and coworkers (see Blombäck, B., 1967) have analysed the amino acid sequence in fibrin peptides A and B of fibrinogen from different species. Human A-peptide contains 16, and B-peptide 14, amino acids with a molecular weight of about 1600.

The fibrinogen molecule contains not only amino acids, but also carbohydrate made up of galactose, mannose, hexosamine and sialic acid. The carbohydrate part constitutes 4–5 per cent of the fibrinogen molecule. Some of the carbohydrate is released during coagulation and the carbohydrate part probably plays a role in the formation of the final clot, which is insoluble in urea.

The proteolytic enzyme thrombin activates fibrinogen by splitting the fibrinopeptides A and B from the N-terminal end of the Aα- and Bβ-chain in the disulphide knot, with exposure of reactive centres in the molecule as a result. When the fibrinogen molecule has lost its A and B peptides, it is called fibrin monomer. Activated fibrinogen molecules have an enormous capacity to react with one another. They first arrange themselves end-to-end to form thread-like structures. Then larger polymers are formed by side-to-side binding. When the aggregate has reached a certain size the fibrin fibres are precipitated. This process is reversible; the fibrin is thus soluble in strong solutions of urea. According to B,

Blombäck, the remarkable substrate specificity is due to the sequence of the amino acids in the Aα- and Bβ-chain close to the bonds, which are broken by thrombin. The splitting of the fibrinopeptides A and B by thrombin does not occur simultaneously. Thus, fibrinopeptide A is split off at a higher initial rate than fibrinopeptide B, which is not released until after the major part of the fibrinogen has already been converted to fibrin. The splitting off of both A- and B-peptides is, however, necessary for satisfactory formation of fibrin. If peptide A alone is separated off, which may occur on addition of a thrombin-like enzyme (Reptilase), obtained from a poison from a South American snake, only end-to-end polymerisation will occur. Such a Reptilase-clot is mechanically not so strong as a clot formed in the presence of thrombin, where both the A- and the B-peptides are split off. In congenital dysfibrinogenaemia (fibrinogen Detroit), where an amino acid substitution has occurred in the Aα-chain, M. Blombäck and coworkers (1968) have also found that the peptide A is split off at a normal rate, while the peptide B does not appear to be separated off (Fig. 22). The fibrin formation in this form of dysfibrinogenaemia is very slow and the affected persons have severe haemorrhagic symptoms. This clearly shows how critical the structure in and around the disulphide knot is for the function of fibrinogen.

After separation of the fibrinopeptides A and B from the fibrinogen molecule the urea soluble fibrin is stabilised to a urea insoluble fibrin under the influence of Ca^{2+} and a serum factor: fibrin stabilising factor (Factor XIII, FSF). At the same time the mechanical strength of the clot is increased.

The plasma fibrinogen has been shown to be heterogeneous in respect to solubility (see Blombäck, B., 1969, 1971). Recently Mosesson, et al. (1972a) showed that this is due to the presence of fibrinogen molecules of lower molecular weight and of more ready solubility. Using chromatography on CM-cellulose they have shown that fibrinogen molecules occur which are identical in the Bβ- and γ-chains, but differ from one another both quantitatively and qualitatively in the Aα-chains. After digestion with trypsin-L-1 tosylamido-2-phenylethyl chloromethyl ketone certain peptide spots were missing in the fibrinogen molecules of lower molecular weight. All the fibrinogen derivatives had 90 per cent clotting ability. The same research group also showed that the NH_2-terminal part of the Aα-chain was intact, for which reason the digestion of this chain must have occurred from the COOH-terminal part.

In another investigation Mosesson, et al. (1972b) showed the existence of two types of human fibrinogen, which could be separated by chromatography on DEAE-cellulose. Using chromatography on CM-cellulose they showed that the two forms differed in the composition of the γ-chains. One of these forms contained a heterogeneous γ-chain. All the γ-chains had the same molecular weight and the same cross-linking capacity. The two forms of γ-chains proved to contain different numbers of the amino acids histidine, glycine, isoleucine and tryptophan and they also differed in their content of sialic acid.

The concentration of fibrinogen in plasma is normally 0·24–0·32 g per 100 ml. Despite its high molecular weight, fibrinogen diffuses into the extravascular space. 70–80 per cent occurs intravascularly, 20–30 per cent extravascularly. The site of synthesis of fibrinogen has been widely discussed. It is, however, now widely assumed that it is formed in the liver. In perfusion experiments on rats' livers Miller and Bale (1954) produced evidence for the production of fibrinogen in the liver. Straub (1963) who used tissue culture, demonstrated fibrinogen formation by liver cells. With the aid of fluorescence-labelled antibodies, it has also been shown that it is formed in the parenchymal cells (Forman and Barnhardt, 1964). The production of fibrinogen has been estimated at 1·5–5 g per day (Macfarlane, et al., 1964). The turnover of fibrinogen has been thoroughly studied by Macfarlane, et al. (1964), who used fibrinogen labelled with radioactive iodine. Their experiments showed that the turnover of fibrinogen is largely proportional to the amount of circulating fibrinogen and that the turnover rate of fibrinogen is about 30 per cent per day and varies little between individuals. The turnover of fibrinogen has been studied by several investigators and the half-life has been estimated at 2–6·5 days (Adelson, et al., 1961; Macfarlane, et al., 1964; Blombäck, B., et al., 1966; Collen, et al., 1972a).

2. Fibrin stabilising factor (FSF, Factor XIII)

The last phase of coagulation is characterised by stabilisation and conversion of the fibrin clot to insoluble form (Fig. 23). This final reaction has been studied by Laki and coworkers (see Fibrinogen, edited by Laki, Marcel Dekker, Inc., New York 1968; Lorand, 1972). Laki and Lorand (1948) showed that this reaction requires the presence of an enzyme, called fibrin stabilising factor (FSF) and now known as Factor XIII. Characteristic of FSF is that its presence renders the fibrin clot insoluble in 5 M urea. It links together the fibrin molecules by covalent bonds and so to say vulcanises the clot. This action of Factor XIII requires the presence of Ca^{2+}. This reaction which, according to Lorand and others (see Lorand, 1970) consists of transamination or transpeptidation, requires the presence of intact carbohydrate. Fibrinogen, treated with sialidase does not react with Factor XIII. The carbohydrate part of the fibrinogen molecule thus plays a considerable role in the formation of the final stable clot. It is noteworthy that Buluk, et al. (1961) showed that thrombin converts FSF from an inactive precursor stage to an active form (active FSF, fibrinoligase). The transamination process which is catalysed by Factor XIII results in the formation of covalent bonds between lysine in ε-position in one fibrinogen molecule and glutamine in γ-position in the other fibrinogen molecule (Lorand, 1970). In their investigations on fibrinogen derivatives with Aα-chains that were digested to a varying extent from the COOH-terminal part, Mosesson and coworkers (1972a, b) showed that they had decreased cross-linking ability. This suggests that at least some of the cross-linking sites are situated in

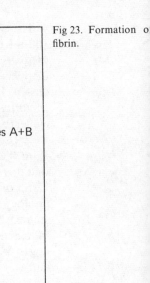

Fig 23. Formation of fibrin.

the Aα-chain. Several investigators (Pisano, et al., 1972; Ball, et al., 1972) have recently shown the formation of 6 mol cross-links/mol fibrin; four are contributed by the α-chains and two by the γ-chains (Doolittle, et al., 1972).

Loewy, et al. (1961) have purified Factor XIII from human plasma with the aid of $(NH_4)_2SO_4$ fractionation and chromatography on DEAE-cellulose. Lorand and Gotah (1970) purified it further by chromatography on DEAE-cellulose and elution with salt-gradient and sucrose density centrifugation. They concentrated the product about 8.000 times.

It has been shown that platelets contain a large amount of Factor XIII (McDonagh, et al., 1969). The platelet factor has been purified and crystallised by Bohn (1970). Its molecular weight is 150.000–200.000.

Investigations by Schwartz, et al. (1971, 1972) have revealed that plasma Factor XIII contains two forms of polypeptide chains (a and b) and that each molecule consists of two a-chains and two b-chains. On the other hand, platelet Factor XIII contains only two chains, both of a-type. The molecular weights of the a- and b-chains have been determined as 75.000 and 88.000, respectively. The molecular weight of plasma Factor XIII has been determined by the same research group as 320.000 and that of platelet Factor XIII as 146.000.

Duckert and coworkers (Duckert, et al., 1960) reported in 1960 a new type of haemorrhagic diathesis. They showed that it was due to a lack of fibrin stabilising factor.

In the determination of Factor XIII, use has usually been made of methods based on the determination of the solubility of the clot in 5 M urea or in monochloric acetic acid (Sigg and Duckert, 1963; Josso, et al.,

1964). Today also immunochemical methods are available (Bohn and Haupt, 1968). Lorand, et al. (1969) have shown that active FSF catalyses the incorporation of a fluorescent amine (monodansylcadaverine) into casein. This observation has been utilised in the development of a sensitive method for determining Factor XIII.

The half-life of Factor XIII has been given as 3–5 days (Ikkala, et al., 1964).

E. *Anticoagulating factors*

There is reason to assume that physiological inhibitors of the coagulation process are of importance in maintaining normal haemostasis. The inhibitors in the coagulation process have, however, received relatively little attention. The physiological inhibitors most probably act upon intermediate products in the coagulation process and not on the individual factors. In certain pathological conditions, on the other hand, there are inhibitors which are specifically directed against individual factors and which consist of abnormal proteins.

1. Heparin

The chemistry of heparin has been thoroughly investigated by Erik Jorpes and is described in his classical survey (Jorpes, 1962). Heparin is a strong anticoagulant, which inhibits all phases of the coagulation process.

Normally human blood does not contain free heparin in the form of a trisulphuric acid. In certain conditions, such as pepton shock, anaphylactic shock, and during radiation, free heparin can escape from the mast cells into the circulating blood and render it incoagulable. Investigations by Nilsson and Wenckert (1954) suggest that normal blood contains a less esterified, heparin-like anticoagulant in such quantities that it must surely serve some physiological purpose. Similar observations have been made by Engelberg (see Engelberg, 1963).

As pointed out previously, heparin interferes with the coagulation process in various ways. Given in a dose of 50 μg (5 units) per ml blood it will prolong the coagulation time from about 8 minutes to almost infinity. Heparin acts like an antithrombin, but it requires the presence of a cofactor occurring in the plasma. Heparin also acts as an antithromboplastin. It exerts a considerable anticoagulant effect by inhibiting the formation of intrinsic thromboplastin (see Nilsson and Wenckert, 1954; Shanberge, et al., 1959). Heparin in a dose of 1 μg per ml plasma is sufficient effectively to inhibit formation of plasma thromboplastin. It has been shown that heparin in association with a plasma cofactor is a potent inhibitor of activated Factor X (Factor Xa). In the presence of the plasma cofactor, heparin thus markedly accelerates the destruction of Factor Xa (Biggs, et al., 1970). The plasma cofactor and antithrombin III are believed to be identical. Heparin has no inhibiting effect on platelet adhesiveness (Hellem, 1960; Salzman, 1963; Cronberg, 1968). But it may partly block platelet aggregation by thrombin.

2. Antithromboplastin

Anticoagulants other than heparin have also been described. Tocantins, et al. (1948) reported a lipid inhibitor acting like an antithromboplastin. Though the existence of such an inhibitor does not sound unlikely, no attempts have been made to elucidate its nature.

3. Antithrombin

Even Morawitz spoke of an antithrombin. Howell and Holt (1918) showed that heparin plus a cofactor has an antithrombin effect. Since then several workers, particularly Astrup and coworkers (see Volkert, 1942) and Seegers and coworkers (see Seegers, 1962), have devoted much time to the investigation of antithrombin activity in the blood. Astrup's school claimed that there existed, besides heparin + cofactor (= 'immediate antithrombin'), a progressive antithrombin or 'natural antithrombin' which gradually inactivated thrombin, which was added to serum.

Seegers has shown that fibrin can adsorb large amounts of thrombin. Seegers' group also described an antithrombin, which they believed to develop in association with the activation of prothrombin to thrombin. Loeliger and Hers (1957) reported an antithrombin activity which was associated with pathological γ-globulins. Niewiarowski and Kowalski (1957) showed that thrombin is inactivated in plasmin-induced fibrinolysis. Seegers, Loeliger and Niewiarowski recommended the following symbols for antithrombin:

Antithrombin = AT	I	Fibrin
	II	Heparin + cofactor
	III	Progressive AT = the natural AT
	IV	AT-activity during prothrombin activation
	V	AT-activity of abnormal plasma globulins
	VI	AT-activity in association with fibrinolysis

It has now been shown that AT VI consists of fibrin/fibrinogen degradation products (Fletcher, et al., 1962). Our concept of other antithrombins has also been revised considerably in recent years. It has now been shown that α_2-macroglobulin (α_2M) is an inhibitor of thrombin (Lanchantin, et al., 1966; Steinbuch, et al., 1967; Ganrot and Niléhn, 1967). α_2M inhibits also the esterolytic effect of thrombin, but to a much less extent than the proteolytic effect (Lanchantin, et al., 1966). Steinbuch, et al. (1965, 1967) have shown that the maximum antithrombin inhibiting effect of α_2M occurs after 2 minutes. It has also been shown that α_2M has no heparin cofactor activity. Steinbuch used preparative ultracentrifugation and an immunochemical method by which they precipitated α_2M with the aid of anti-α_2M. The antithrombin activity in the supernatant was reduced, while the heparin cofactor activity was unchanged.

In recent years Abildgaard in Oslo has studied antithrombin activity (AT) in plasma and serum (Abildgaard, U., 1967a, b; 1968; 1969a, b).

He used heat-defibrinated plasma as a starting material. On gel filtration the antithrombin activity of the plasma separated into two fractions, a minor one (25 per cent) in the α_2M-region and a larger one (75 per cent) in the third protein peak. The latter fraction contained heparin cofactor activity. Further purification has shown that the macromolecular AT is associated with α_2M. With the aid of $BaSO_4$ adsorption, heat defibrination, Sephadex G-200 filtration and DEAE-Sephadex chromatography, Abildgaard has further purified that part of AT which has heparin cofactor activity and is of low molecular weight. The preparation thereby obtained has since been purified by repeated preparative disc gel electrophoresis. He obtained a highly active antithrombin preparation which on paper electrophoresis produced bands in the α_2-region and was homogeneous. Compared with the starting material, it was purified 700 times.

Yin, et al. (1971) also found that antithrombin III activity co-chromatographed with the heparin cofactor during purification on Sephadex G-200, DEAE-Sephadex and DEAE-cellulose columns. These authors also found the antithrombin III to be identical with the inhibitor of activated Factor X.

Instead of the above-mentioned six antithrombins, we need today to consider only the following three antithrombins.

1. Fibrin
2. α_2M
3. Antithrombin III (heparin cofactor)

4. Anti-factor Xa

As pointed out above, activated Factor X occupies a key position in the generation of thrombin. In the maintenance of the fluidity of the blood a prompt and effective removal of Factor Xa has been regarded as important as, or more important than, destruction of thrombin. In 1964 Seegers isolated from bovine plasma a protein fraction which corresponded to antithrombin III and rapidly inactivated autoprothrombin C (= Factor Xa). Biggs, et al. (1970) studied a natural inhibitor of Factor Xa and devised a method for measuring the inhibitory activity by addition of Factor Xa to diluted heated plasma and recording the amount of residual Factor Xa after incubation for 1 hour. They found that the activities of antithrombin III and anti-factor Xa were correlated. Yin, et al., (1971) produced evidence suggesting that biological activities, variously termed activated Factor X inhibitor, antithrombin III and heparin cofactor, are all ascribable to a single blood proteinase inhibitor with broad specificity. The inhibitor, a low molecular weight α_2-globulin, is most probably identical with the antithrombin III isolated by Abildgaard. Yin, et al. (1971) pointed out that the inactivation of Factor Xa by this inhibitor is profoundly enhanced by traces of heparin. Marciniak and Tsukamura (1972) recently reported the occurrence of two progressive inhibitors of Factor Xa in human blood. One of them, with a molecular size approximately equal to that of albumin, was probably identical with antithrombin III and heparin cofactor, and its effect was potentiated by heparin. The other Factor Xa inhibitor was discovered in the macroglobulin fraction. There were distinct dissimilarities between the inhibition of thrombin and Factor Xa by macroglobulin. The macromolecular inhibitor was unaffected by heparin. These authors pointed out that while the human component was a powerful antifactor to bovine Factor Xa it was only a weak inhibitor of human Factor Xa. It appears that inhibitors of Factor Xa may be of great importance in the maintenance of the haemostatic balance.

5. Pathological circulating anticoagulants

In certain diseases, particularly dysproteinaemia and immunising conditions, circulating anticoagulants, not normally occurring, may appear in the blood. In such cases the anticoagulant factors generally consist of pathological γ-globulins and may be directed against Factor VIII, Factor IX, Factors XI and XII, thromboplastin, Factor V and thrombin. These anticoagulants are treated in the clinical part of the book.

V. Fibrinolysis

See Fibrinolysis, thrombolysis and defibrination, page 111.

Haemorrhagic diseases

I. Diagnostic considerations

Pathogenetically, haemorrhagic conditions may be due to:
  Vascular abnormalities
  Platelet disorders
  Coagulation defects
  Disorders of the fibrinolytic system

Investigation of haemorrhagic disorders should include:
A. Determination of the type of bleeding.
B. Careful inquiry into the patient's history, especially regarding bleeding.
C. General physical examination.
D. Laboratory studies to ascertain the nature of the bleeding defect.

A. *Type of bleeding*

All the components of the mechanism of haemostasis take part in the arrest of bleeding, but their relative importance in a given case depends on the size of the vessels damaged. The platelets probably play the most important role in the arrest of bleeding from small vessels, while coagulation is a more important process in the checking of the flow of blood from larger vessels. The type of bleeding is therefore of diagnostic importance. In *vascular diseases,* purpura and petechiae appear spontaneously in the skin and mucosa, but profuse haemorrhage is rare. Purpura and diffusely scattered petechiae may occur also in *platelet disorders*. Primary platelet plugs fail to form at sites of injury; this results in oozing of blood from small vessels and prolongation of the bleeding. Mucosal haemorrhage is characteristic of platelet disorders. As a rule, spontaneous haemorrhage does not occur in *defective coagulation*. In vascular injury, platelet plugs are formed at the site of the injury, and the bleeding is therefore usually promptly arrested, i.e., the bleeding time is normal. On the other hand, the platelet plug will not be properly anchored if coagulation is defective. Proper anchorage requires not only aggregation of platelets by thrombin, but also the formation of a fibrin clot. The plugs will therefore be expelled after a while with recurrence of bleeding as a result. Such recurrent or secondary bleeding, which is very characteristic in patients with coagulation defects, was described as early as 1803 by Otto in his first report on haemophilia. Defective coagulation is also accompanied by ready bruising and excessive bleeding, especially into muscles, joints and tissues, following even relatively mild trauma.

B. *Medical history*

Careful inquiry into the patient's history is the first diagnostic step and is extremely important. In the investigation of suspected haemorrhagic diseases many physicians request determination of the patient's coagulation time and bleeding time. Also several surgeons wonder whether it might not be advisable to determine the coagulation and bleeding time of all patients before operation even in the absence of a history of suspected haemorrhagic diseases. As a screening procedure this is of no value since the coagulation time and the bleeding time according to Duke are both normal in mild haemorrhagic diseases, which are the most common. On the other hand, if the patient's history is properly considered, it will never, or at least hardly ever, give false information.

In the investigation of haemorrhagic disease it is important to find out when the symptoms first appeared, in order to ascertain whether the case examined is congenital or acquired. Inquiry should also be made into the patient's family history for heredity, because congenital bleeding diseases are transmitted in a characteristic way. When possible, a pedigree should be set up. A firm diagnosis of some conditions, e.g., in the mild form of von Willebrand's disease, may require examination of other members of the family.

The bleeding history should be detailed. The examiner should ask the patient whether he has ever had any petechiae and purpura, whether he bleeds readily from pinpricks, whether he has ever had nose-bleeding, gingival bleeding, or other mucosal bleedings. Females should be questioned concerning the menstrual flow. The time of the haemorrhage and its frequency, duration and severity should also be noted. In patients with a history of nose-bleeding, for example, one should ask whether the bleeding has ever required cauterisation in hospital, whether it has been followed by anaemia and whether it has necessitated blood transfusions. One should ask the patient whether he bruises readily and apparently spontaneously or only after injuries. Most patients with haemophilia always have bruises in various parts of the body and are, as a rule, unaware of the causal traumata. It is also important for the examiner to find out whether the haematomas are relatively small and superficial or whether they are usually widespread and painful, and whether they occur not only in the skin, but also in the muscles and other tissues. One should also ask the patient whether he has ever bled excessively after trivial injuries (shaving, tongue biting, cuts etc.), how long the bleeding lasted and how severe it was. It is also necessary to find out whether he has bled abnormally after any surgical intervention. One should, above all, also ask the patient whether he has ever bled abnormally after tooth extractions, since this question has proved very useful in the evaluation of the haemostatic process and much more informative than determination of the coagulation time. For instance, extraction of a wisdom tooth without abnormal bleeding weighs heavily against a congenital haemorrhagic disease. The examiner should, of course, also ask the patient about any joint bleeding, renal bleeding and gastro-intestinal bleeding.

C. *Physical examination*

General physical examination will often verify the type of bleeding and then the examiner may search for signs of previous bleeding, especially in the joints. The patient should also be examined for abnormal vessels. Telangiectasia of the fingers and mouth, for example, suggest Osler's disease.

The bleeding tendency is often secondary to some basal disease, such as leukaemia or liver cirrhosis. The general clinical examination is therefore important.

D. *Laboratory investigation of bleeding disorders*

After determination of the type of bleeding, analysis of the patient's history and general physical examination it is usually possible to decide whether the disease is congenital or acquired and to make a provisional differential diagnosis of the bleeding disease. This facilitates rational selection of the subsequent laboratory procedures.

The first step in the laboratory investigation is to obtain a general impression of the patient's status from some screening tests for platelet and coagulation disorders (see Methods page 209). The screening tests of choice are:

Platelet count
Bleeding time according to the method of Duke
Bleeding time according to the method of Ivy, if the bleeding time according to Duke is normal
Coagulation time in glass tubes and possibly also in plastic tubes
Cephalin time or activated partial thromboplastin time
One-stage prothrombin time (= thromboplastin time)
P&P-test (or thrombotest or Simplastin A-test)
Fibrinogen
Fibrinolysis (euglobulin clot lysis time)

These data will usually permit a qualitative diagnosis. It is thus possible, as a rule, to ascribe the bleeding defect to vascular injury, platelet disorder (thrombocytopenia or platelet defect) or coagulopathy. In most cases it is also possible to decide whether the patient has a defect in the first, second or third phase of coagulation. This investigation is, as a rule, sufficient for acquired defects, unless they are due to a circulating anticoagulant. As for the congenital defects, such an investigation is, as a rule, also sufficient for the choice of therapy in emergencies.

But a firm and quantitative diagnosis of cases of congenital defects requires the use of special procedures. The patient should therefore be referred to a coagulation laboratory.

The second step in the laboratory investigation is that performed at *special coagulation laboratories* where the defect can be both quantitatively and qualitatively appraised with special methods.

But coagulation laboratories have also another important purpose, *viz.*, planning and regulating treatment of the patients. Coagulation laboratories thus try various preparations for substitution therapy and find out the optimal doses. An important task is to give the patients and their families information about their disease, to recommend certain precautions, to see that they get special identity cards, social help, advice on education and occupation, and physical training etc. Further, coagulation laboratories should take care of patients with congenital bleeding diseases in the event of severe profuse haemorrhage and co-operate intimately with surgeons in association with operations on such patients.

II. Vascular bleeding disorders

Vascular bleeding disorders characterised by impairment of the permeability of the vessel walls or defective vasoconstriction, manifest themselves clinically as purpura. To these vascular diseases belong, for example, Henoch-Schönlein's purpura, Waldenström's purpura hyperglobulinaemia, purpura cryoglobulinaemia, Ehlers-Danlos syndrome and capillary telangiectasia. In these conditions the bleeding time, the platelet count and the coagulation mechanism are intact. But the capillary fragility test may often be positive. There is no known haemorrhagic disease due to impaired contractility of the large vessels.

Ehlers-Danlos syndrome (*cutis hyperelastica*) is a dominant hereditary disorder of the connective tissue and according to McKusick (1960), the characteristics of fully developed cases are:

1. hyperelasticity of the skin,
2. hyperextension of the joints, which are readily dislocated,
3. brittleness of the skin and the cutaneous vessels, which may result in superficial bleeding and skin injuries,
4. soft scars containing haematin and 'pseudotumours' at sites of repeated traumatisation.

Fully developed cases are rare. Only a few more than a hundred cases have been reported. The patients may also have severe bleeding after wounds, tooth extraction and surgical operations. Dissecting haemorrhage under the scalp is characteristic. Haemorrhage may occur in any organ. Gastro-intestinal haemorrhage and subarachnoid haemorrhage are the commonest causes of death.

Severe cases offer no diagnostic difficulties. The histological picture of biopsy specimens from the affected area is typical. There is severe oedema in the corium and numerous macrophages containing haemosiderin, as well as large blood vessels of almost angiomatous appearance. Sections stained for elastin reveal elastic tissue clumps in the deeper parts of the corium. It is assumed that the increased elasticity of the skin is due to an increased number of elastic fibres. Karaca, et al. (1972) studied the collagen fascia (the *musculus rectus abdominis*) from two patients with Ehlers-Danlos syndrome. They found this collagen to have a markedly decreased tendency to aggregate the platelets of both the patients and normals. The defect has since been found in five further patients with the syndrome (Nilsson, 1973). This abnormality of the collagen fibres might plausibly contribute to the bleeding tendency in Ehlers-Danlos syndrome.

III. Disorders of primary haemostasis
STIG CRONBERG

The bleeding tendency due to defective primary haemostasis is characterised by bruises, nose-bleeding and other mucosal bleedings, profuse menstrual bleedings and prolonged bleeding after minor incisions. The most important finding at examination is a prolonged bleeding time. For demonstrating minor abnormalities Ivy's method is more sensitive than Duke's (Cronberg, 1968). The abnormal primary haemostasis may be due to changes in the blood plasma, platelets or vessel walls.

A. *Thrombocytopenia*

Thrombocytopenia is by far the most common cause of a prolonged bleeding time (Bernard, et al., 1970). It may be secondary to many disorders that lead to diminished formation of new tissue in diseases such as leukaemia, aplastic anaemia, widespread bone marrow metastases and in patients treated with cytostatics. In the defibrination syndrome thrombocytopenia may occur owing to rapid consumption of the platelets.

Primary thrombocytopenia occurs in the relatively rare congenital forms as well as in the more common allergic-immunological forms. The former are due to impaired platelet formation with a relatively small number of megakaryocytes in the bone marrow (Myllylä, et al., 1967; Stavem, et al., 1969; Murphy, et al., 1972). In the latter the formation of platelets is increased but cannot compensate for their even more rapid destruction.

Congenital thrombocytopenia is usually inherited. Dominant inheritance is easiest to detect. This type is less severe than the recessively inherited types that may occur sporadically and therefore be more difficult to classify. Thrombocytopenia is often associated with qualitative changes in the function of the platelets. This is the case, for instance, in the giant platelet syndrome of Bernard and Soulier (1948) (Fig. 24). Other similar forms have been described and probably constitute a heterogenic group (Seip and Kjaerheim, 1965; Murphy, et al., 1972). Sometimes a remarkable cyclic form of thrombocytopenia is seen (Engström, et al., 1966; Wasastjerna, 1967). In the investigation of patients with thrombocytopenia estimation of platelet survival is clinically useful. A special disorder is Wiskott-Aldrich's syndrome. It occurs in boys and is characterised by severe thrombocytopenia, eczema and disturbances in the immunoglobulin synthesis (Gröttum, et al., 1969).

In allergic-immunological thrombocytopenia, platelet formation is markedly increased, but the destruction is rapid. The sequence varies—

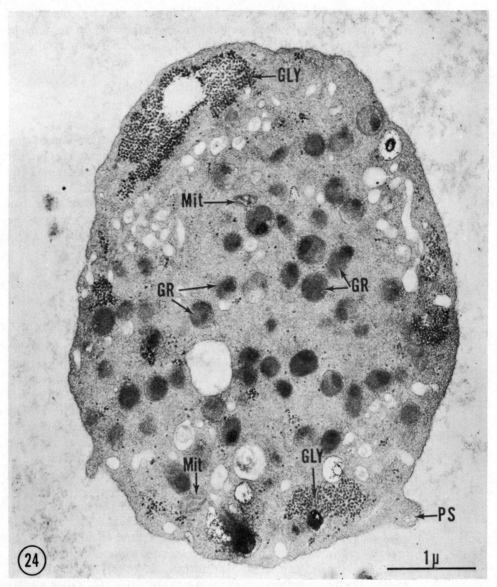

Fig 24. Platelet in macrothrombocytic thrombopathy. Symbols as in Fig 3, page 5
8 000 × . Photo T. Hovig (Hovig, T.: *Ser. Haemat.* **I,** 2 (1968) p 35).

the condition sometimes disappears spontaneously within one or more
weeks, sometimes it recurs and sometimes it becomes chronic. In some
cases the pathogenesis is obvious and may be due to hypersensitivity to
kinidin, diuretics, sedatives, sulphonamides, phenylbutazone, etc. and
in such cases it promptly regresses on withdrawal of the drug. In most
cases the cause is not known with certainty, and is then called idiopathic
thrombocytopenic purpura, ITP, but these cases are probably also of
immunological type.

Various methods have been devised for demonstrating antibodies, but the technique is difficult and the results vary from laboratory to laboratory. The use of such methods should still be reserved for laboratories with special interest in platelet and tissue immunology. In routine clinical work the examination is less important. Though the bleeding tendency does not always correspond to the platelet count, spontaneous purpura is seldom seen in patients with a platelet count of more than $30.000/\mu l$, and profuse bleeding is rare in patients with a platelet count above $60.000/\mu l$.

In the treatment of thrombocytopenia, corticosteroids should be tried first. Sometimes large doses may be given, and in some cases adrenocorticotropic hormone (ACTH) has a better effect. Usually the platelet count will increase, and then attempts are made to reduce the dosage and gradually to withdraw the drug completely. Should this not be possible, splenectomy might be considered. Such an operation often results in prompt improvement, which is permanent in about 75 per cent of cases. In selected cases cytostatics have proved to have a favourable effect. In patients with congenital thrombocytopenia the effect of splenectomy is rarely permanent. If the bleedings in patients with thrombocytopenia are heavy and possibly require surgical treatment, infusions of platelets might be given. Platelets may be administered in the form of fresh whole blood, platelet-rich plasma or platelet concentrate. Platelet concentrates should be prepared from blood collected in citrate solution with an addition of extra citric acid since the platelets are otherwise difficult to resuspend. Platelets prepared with EDTA have a short survival time *in vivo* (Aster and Jandl, 1964; Davey, 1966) and should not be used. If the bleeding is to be stopped, platelet concentrates prepared from several blood donors, as a rule 4–8, is necessary. Several platelet antigens have been described, partly identical with leukocyte antigens, but blood grouping of donors in this respect is in practice not possible. It is, however, recommended to infuse platelet concentrates which belong to the same blood ABO-group and Rh-system. Platelet concentrates should be given as soon as possible and within 6 hours. Up to 60 per cent of the platelets given may be recovered. In some cases antibodies exist or develop and make the infusion useless. The symptoms that might occur are largely the same as those of plasma incompatibility, i.e. febrile and allergic reactions, hepatitis and iso-immunisation. In platelet incompatibility the consequences are relatively moderate and not of the severe type seen after erythrocyte incompatibility.

Treatment of thrombocytopenia in pregnant women offers difficulties. The statistics have not shown any certain difference between surgically and medically treated patients. As a rule, splenectomy is recommended at the beginning of pregnancy because treatment with cortisone may then be regarded as unnecessary, and persistent thrombocytopenia may imply risks for both the mother and the child.

Apart from the treatment of thrombocytopenia, it should also be borne in mind that much can be done to prevent or reduce bleeding by measures of general and non-specific nature. Thus, trauma should be avoided, and if operation proves necessary, careful haemostasis is imperative. Injections and acetyl-salicylic acid should be avoided. AMCA and EACA prevent local fibrinolysis and thus have a certain haemostatic effect. Gestagens suppress serious menorrhagia.

B. *Qualitative platelet defects and plasma defects*

Much rarer than thrombocytopenia are qualitative platelet defects in association with a normal platelet count (Cronberg, 1968). The clinical pictures are similar and are dominated by mucosal bleeding, profuse menstrual bleeding and prolonged bleeding after even trivial cuts and other minor injuries.

1. von Willebrand's disease

The commonest condition is von Willebrand's disease, which is characterised by dominant inheritance, prolonged bleeding time, reduced content of Factor VIII as assayed both by biological and immunological methods and reduced platelet adhesiveness, as measured with Salzman's method. The disease may be mild or severe. It is treated with AHF preparations, which promptly raise Factor VIII content and shorten the bleeding time (see page 90).

2. Glanzmann's thrombasthenia

Of the true platelet defects, the type known as Glanzmann's thrombasthenia is the most serious. The disease is at present well defined, but has little in common with the condition originally described by Glanzmann. The disease is characterised by a prolonged bleeding time and lack of platelet aggregation even after large doses of ADP (Caen, et al., 1971). In addition, clot retraction is minimal. In most patients the fibrinogen content of the platelets is decreased. Electron microscopy has not revealed any pathognomonic morphological changes. Much suggests loss of affinity between platelets and fibrinogen-fibrin (Cronberg, 1971). The inheritance is recessive.

Treatment is symptomatic and in menorrhagia, AMCA and gestagens have proved to have a good effect.

3. Thrombopathia

In many families there is an increased bleeding tendency with reduced platelet adhesiveness, platelet aggregation and release reaction (Cronberg, 1968; Cronberg and Nilsson, 1968a, b; Hardisty and Hutton, 1967; O'Brien, 1967; Caen, et al., 1968; Weiss, et al., 1969; Sahud and Aggeler, 1969). Occasionally the total content of ADP is decreased (Holmsen and Weiss, 1970; Cronberg and Caen, 1971a, b). The inheritance is usually more or less clearly dominant. The bleeding time, as determined by the method of Ivy, is prolonged. In our most typical family with sixteen affected members, platelet adhesiveness was reduced, as measured by Hellem's or Salzman's methods, the bleeding time was prolonged and the release reaction was somewhat reduced. The inheritance was dominant and the bleeding tendency was similar to that in von Willebrand's disease. Factor VIII, on the other hand, was normal (Cronberg and Nilsson, 1968a). In the literature these conditions are referred to by different names. It has been proposed that thrombopathia characterised by a deficient storage pool of ADP should be called platelet storage pool disease. Cronberg (1972) retains the term thrombopathia and has proposed that the condition with a defective mechanism of release should be called 'dysliberation thrombopathia', and the condition with a low total amount of ADP should be called 'deficiency thrombopathia'.

Treatment is symptomatic. It is of theoretic interest that arteriosclerosis may occur in the presence of this congenital platelet disorder (Cronberg, et al., 1970).

4. Afibrinogenaemia

In afibrinogenaemia the bleeding time is moderately prolonged and the platelet aggregation and adhesion are decreased. These changes can be corrected by small amounts of fibrinogen (Inceman, et al., 1966). In hypofibrinogenaemia, platelet aggregation is normal (Nilsson, Niléhn, Cronberg and Nordén, 1966).

5. Acquired thrombopathia

Qualitative platelet defects occur also in acquired diseases, such as idiopathic thrombocythaemia. This is a myeloproliferative condition related to myelosclerosis, in which the number of platelets is markedly increased and usually exceeds $1.000.000/\mu l$. In the haemorrhagic type there is, strangely enough, an increased bleeding tendency. The bleeding time is often prolonged and platelet adhesiveness, aggregation and the release reaction are decreased (Cronberg, et al., 1965).

In Waldenström's macroglobulinaemia, the increased bleeding tendency is due to adsorption of macroglobulin to platelets with decreased adhesiveness and aggregation as a result (Cronberg, 1968). The platelet count and the coagulation factors may be reduced.

In uraemia there is also an increased bleeding tendency with reduced adhesiveness (Larsson, 1971 and others), aggregation and release reaction. The prothrombin consumption is often abnormal.

In scurvy, platelet aggregation is also reduced (Cetingel, et al., 1958) and the collagen is abnormal (Legrand, 1971).

6. Inhibitors of platelet function

Platelet adhesiveness and platelet aggregation are very susceptible to environmental factors such as pH, temperature, calcium concentration, and osmolarity. It is therefore not surprising that platelet function is susceptible to a wide variety of chemicals *in vitro*. In addition, it has been shown that metabolic reactions are necessary for which reason platelets, like other cells, are inhibited by a number of enzyme inhibitors. From a clinical point of view it is, above all, certain drugs that are of interest.

After administration of *acetyl-salicylic acid,* platelet aggregates formed in citrated platelet-rich plasma are rapidly and completely dispersed. The second wave of aggregation by ADP or adrenaline is inhibited, with the result that these substances do not induce release of ADP (O'Brien, 1968; Zucker and Peterson, 1968) (Figs. 8 and 9, page 11). Cronberg, et al., (1970) stressed that firm aggregates are necessary for this kind of release and suggested that the inhibition caused by the acetyl-salicylic acid is due to the rapid dispersal of the aggregates. The platelets are probably irreversibly injured. The profound effect of acetyl-salicylic acid explains why it is dangerous for haemophiliacs.

Dextran reduces platelet adhesiveness, as measured with Hellem's method (Cronberg, Robertson, Nilsson and Niléhn, 1966), which may explain why it is useful in the prophylaxis of thrombosis (Bygdeman, 1968).

The *prostaglandin* PGE_1 is a strong inhibitor of platelet aggregation (Kloeze, 1970).

Several other drugs affect platelet function *in vivo* and/or *in vitro* (for surveys see de Gaetano, et al., 1970; Mustard and Packham, 1970). Such drugs are pyrimido-pyrimidine derivatives, dipyramidole, analgetics such as phenylbutazone and indomethacin, amitryptiline, chlorpromazine, antihistaminics, local anaesthetics, etc. Reports on the value of such drugs in the prevention of thrombosis are both scanty and contradictory.

C. *Primary vascular abnormalities*

Many forms of purpura are ascribed to disorders in the walls of vessels, while platelet function, like the plasma factors, are normal. To these belong, for instance, the tendency to ready bruisability during long-term cortisone treatment and in advanced age. Some patients with a prolonged bleeding time of unknown cause have been found to have abnormal collagen, with impaired ability to aggregate platelets (Caen, et al., 1970; Karaca, et al., 1972).

Certain cases of purpura are due to inflammatory or allergic reactions such as Henoch-Schönlein's purpura, in which there is concomitant nephritis, joint symptoms and gastro-intestinal symptoms.

IV. Coagulation disorders

There are several known congenital or acquired coagulation defects. In patients with the former type there is, as a rule, a lack or deficiency of only one coagulation factor, compared with two or more in the latter. Coagulation defects are classified according to the phase of coagulation in which they occur.

A. *Defects in phase I—formation of plasma thromboplastin*

In patients with defects in the plasma thromboplastin formation, screening for bleeding disorders will show:

> a normal platelet count,
> normal or prolonged Duke and Ivy bleeding time,
> prolonged or normal coagulation time in glass tubes and in plastic tubes,
> prolonged cephalin time (partial thromboplastin time),
> prolonged activated partial thromboplastin time,
> normal one-stage prothrombin time, and a
> normal fibrinogen content (see chapter on Methods page 211)

Of other tests mention might be made of prothrombin consumption. An abnormal prothrombin consumption shows the presence of a platelet defect or a defect in plasma thromboplastin formation. Defects in this phase may also be studied with the aid of the thromboplastin generation test (see chapter on Methods). In the differential diagnosis of the different defects in phase I, special determinations must be made of Factors VIII, IX, XI and XII.

In phase I the following coagulation defects may be distinguished:

> AHF (Factor VIII) deficiency
> Factor IX deficiency
> Factor XI deficiency
> Factor XII deficiency
> Circulating anticoagulants.

1. Haemophilia A and B

Haemophilia has probably existed since prehistoric times. It was first described as a clinical entity in 1803 by the American, Otto. He described the disease as an inheritable bleeding disorder, occurring only in males, but added that though women in affected families were free from overt manifestations of the disease, they could transmit the disease to their children. He called the male patients 'bleeders'. The name of the disease, haemophilia, was originally coined by a German student, Friedrich Hopff (1828), a pupil of the well known German professor of medicine, Schönlein. Hopff called the disease 'Haemorrhapilia'. The name was afterwards abbreviated to haemophilia. In 1820 Nasse, a professor in Bonn, published a detailed description of the bleeding symptoms of haemophilia (see Brinkhous, 1965). The discovery that classical haemophilia was not a clinical entity but due to lack of either AHF (Factor VIII) or haemophilia B factor (Factor IX) was described earlier (page 25).

According to the classical definition, then, haemophilia is a recessive, sex-linked inheritable disease, which occurs only in males and which is transmitted by female carriers who are not themselves bleeders. The disease manifests itself early in childhood by an abnormal tendency to bleeding. This definition of haemophilia holds for both haemophilia A and haemophilia B, which have the same mode of inheritance and the same clinical picture, but are due to deficiency of two different factors.

1) VARIOUS TYPES OF HAEMOPHILIA A AND HAEMOPHILIA B

Haemophilia A as well as haemophilia B, may be severe, moderate, or mild. Assignment of a given case to one of these groups depends on the plasma content of AHF and B factor (Brinkhous and Graham, 1954; Nilsson, Blombäck and Ramgren, 1961). The affected members of a haemophilic family always have haemophilia of the same type and severity (Nilsson, Blombäck and Ramgren, 1961). In severe haemophilia the AHF or the B factor content of the plasma is less than 1 per cent of normal, the coagulation time is usually longer than 1 hour, and extremely severe bleeding symptoms and disabling joint bleedings are common (Table I). In moderate haemophilia the AHF or B factor content is 1–4 per cent of the normal and the clotting time is about 20–30 minutes; also these patients have severe bleeding symptoms, though not so pronounced as in severe haemophilia. Thus, in contrast with severe haemophilia, the bleeding in moderate haemophilia does not, as a rule, lead to complete disability. In mild haemophilia the AHF or the B factor content is 5–25 per cent of normal. The coagulation time is normal or only slightly prolonged. Severe spontaneous bleeding and joint bleeding are rare. But bleeding may be heavy in association with injury and surgery.

One might very well imagine that the different forms of haemophilia (severe, moderate and mild) are due to the inheritance of either different amounts of AHF or of B factor or of various malformations of the AHF or B molecule, so that it is a molecular disease, in analogy with the haemoglobin diseases. A genetic mutation may perhaps result in a decrease in the synthesis of a specific protein or in an abnormal amino acid sequence of the protein with partial or complete loss of its biological function. Thanks to the immunological technique, various genetic variants of haemophilia have been discovered. Human antibodies against AHF and B factor have been used as well as heterologous antisera raised by immunisation of animals with more or less pure concentrates of AHF and B factor.

Haemophilia A can be divided into two groups according to its ability to neutralise a human inhibitor of AHF. Hoyer and Breckenridge (1968) tested various haemophilia A plasmas for their ability to neutralise a potent IgG antibody to AHF prepared by Andersen and Troup (1968). They found that 30 out of 36 haemophilia plasmas could not neutralise the inhibitor, which suggested that the antigenic material was lacking in the larger group. But six patients had antigenic material that could neutralise the inhibitor. The antigenic AHF-like material had physico-

Table 1. Level of AHF and B factor in haemophilia A and B of varying severity.

		AHF %	B-factor %	Joint bleedings
Haemophilia A	severe	< 1	100	+ + +
	moderate	1–4	100	+(+)
	mild	5–25	100	(+)
Haemophilia B	severe	100	< 1	+ + +
	moderate	100	1–4	+(+)
	mild	100	5–25	(+)

chemical properties resembling those of normal AHF (Hoyer and Breckenridge, 1970). Denson, et al. (1969) found that 4 out of 48 haemophilia A patients could inactivate $Al(OH)_3$ adsorbed inhibitor plasma and they called these four haemophilia A^+ and the others haemophilia A^-. In a Swedish group Holmberg and Nilsson (1973a) found that 4 patients out of 39 could neutralise human antibodies. All four had mild haemophilia and all belonged to the same family.

If heterologous antiserum against Factor VIII is used, the results obtained will, however, be quite different. With the use of an antiserum against an impure preparation, Bennett and Huehns (1970) found 90 per cent cross reacting haemophiliacs. AHF can, however, now be prepared in highly purified form such as that found in an antiserum raised by Zimmerman, et al. (1971a, b) in rabbits. With Laurell's technique, the amount of antigenic material in ethanol concentrate from plasma was found to be the same in patients with haemophilia A and in normals. In patients with von Willebrand's disease the values were lower.

Stites, et al. (1971) obtained the same results using a haemagglutination inhibition test with rabbit antibodies. In a Swedish group Holmberg and Nilsson (1973a), who used a heterologous antiserum, found cross reacting material in all of 48 patients with haemophilia A, which was severe in 31, four of whom had also an anticoagulant, moderate in 9, and mild in 8. A protein with the same chromatographic properties as AHF but without AHF activity can also be directly demonstrated in haemophilia A (Hershgold, et al., 1967; van Mourik and Mochtar, 1970).

These findings were taken as evidence of a malformed AHF molecule in haemophilia A. The discrepancy between the findings with homologous and heterologous antisera, respectively, might then be due to the fact that homologous antiserum has a very narrow specificity for one or more antigenic sites on the AHF molecule, while heterologous precipitating antiserum may be directed against several antigenic sites. It is also possible that what is measured with heterologous antiserum is in reality the so-called von Willebrand factor (Bouma, et al., 1972). AHF may possibly be a very small molecule complexed with, or adsorbed to, the high molecular weight von Willebrand factor.

Different forms have also been reported in haemophilia B (Hougie and Twomey, 1967; Gray, et al., 1968; Roberts, et al., 1968; Denson, et al., 1968; Somer and Castaldi, 1970). Hougie and Twomey (1967) described the variant haemophilia B_M, which has a low B factor activity as well as a long prothrombin time, as measured with the use of thromboplastin prepared from ox brain. The prolonged prothrombin time was ascribed to a defective B molecule. Roberts, et al. (1968) reported that though they have no B factor activity, about 10 per cent of haemophilia B plasmas can inactivate a B factor inhibitor equally well as normal plasma. Another minor group of cases with mild to moderate haemophilia B have been found to have cross reacting material proportional to the clotting activity (Brown, et al., 1970). From a patient with haemophilia B but no B factor activity, Somer and Castaldi (1970), who used DEAE-cellulose, isolated a product with the same physio-chemical properties as normal B factor but without coagulation activity.

Veltkamp, et al. (1970) have described a genetic variant of haemophilia B, which is characterised by regression of the bleeding symptoms and a B factor content which increases with age.

2) OCCURRENCE AND INHERITANCE

All cases of inheritable coagulopathies in Sweden have been registered. We now know of 320 Swedish families with about 450 living haemophiliacs, which means 1 haemophiliac per 10.000 men. The incidence of haemophilia in Sweden is roughly the same as that given for other countries. Of the Swedish haemophilic families studied, 80 per cent have haemophilia A and 20 per cent haemophilia B. The ratio between haemophilia A and haemophilia B is the same in Sweden as in other countries, except in Switzerland, in which the number of cases of haemophilia B is relatively larger because of the large well known Tenna family with moderate haemophilia B (Nilsson, Blombäck and Ramgren, 1961). Half of the Swedish haemophilia A families examined has severe haemophilia, one fourth moderate, and one fourth mild. The corresponding distribution among haemophilia B families is roughly the same.

As previously mentioned, haemophilia is transmitted by a recessive sex-linked gene. The transmission of the disease is linked to the sex chromosome X. A bleeder thus has one affected X chromosome and one Y chromosome. A female carrier of haemophilia has one affected and one normal X chromosome. They do not develop haemophilia because they have a normal X chromosome, but they can transmit the affected X chromosome to their children. Fig. 25 shows that all daughters of a haemophilic male are carriers of haemophilia, while the sons do not develop haemophilia or any predisposition to haemophilia. As for children of a female carrier, half of the sons will be bleeders and half will be healthy without any predisposition to the disease. Likewise half of the daughters will be carriers and half will not. The transmission of the disease via male haemophiliacs, the classical maternal grandfather route, is not so common. In most families the disease has been transmitted through several generations by women.

Female haemophilia is very rare, and only 6 cases of homozygotes have

Fig 25. Mode of inheritance of haemophilia. The gene is linked to the sex chromosome X. Female carriers of the gene have one affected and one unaffected X chromosome. All daughters of a haemophilic man will be carriers of the haemophilia gene.

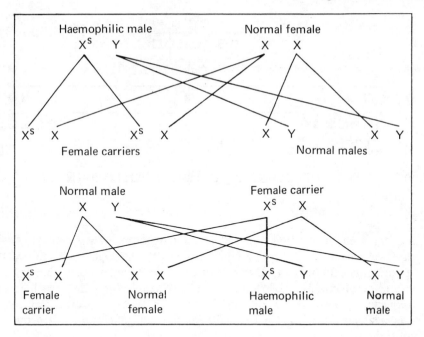

been reported in the literature (see de la Chapelle, et al., 1961; Mellman, et al., 1961). A female can get haemophilia, i.e. two affected X chromosomes, only if the mother is a carrier of haemophilia and the father a haemophiliac. The literature contains also some cases of female haemophilia, which from a point of view of inheritance, cannot be homozygotes (see Niléhn and Nilsson, 1962; Whissell, et al., 1965). The apparent exception from the classical sex-linked mode of inheritance in three cases could be explained by an abnormal chromosomal pattern. In a case of classical severe haemophilia A in a little 'girl', Nilsson, Bergman, Reitalu and Waldenström (1959) thus demonstrated a male chromosomal pattern and testicular feminisation. Gilchrist, et al. (1965) found XX XO mosaicism in a case of female haemophilia A. Bithell, et al. (1970) reported the lack of an X chromosome in a girl with Turner's syndrome and haemophilia B. In other cases of severe female haemophilia with no evidence of chromosomal deviations a mutation in the second X chromosome has been assumed, which would explain the occurrence of a homozygous female bleeder (Niléhn and Nilsson, 1962; Lusher, et al., 1969). It is very probable that some of these women believed to have mild haemophilia are in reality only carriers with an exceptionally low content of AHF (for references see Nilsson, Blombäck, Ramgren and v. Francken, 1962).

In the Swedish haemophilia series it has been possible to trace practically all the haemophilic families through four generations and to demonstrate positive heredity in 68 per cent of the haemophilia A families and in 74 per cent of the haemophilia B families. This is a higher percentage of positive heredity than that reported in other countries (for references

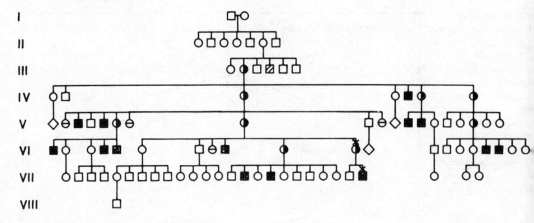

Fig 26. Pedigree of a Swedish family with severe haemophilia B.

Key:

○ Normal female

⊖ Normal female, childless

◑ Female carrier

◔ Female carrier, examined by coagulation tests

□ Normal male

■ Haemophiliac

◤ Haemophiliac, examined by coagulation tests

▨ Probable haemophiliac

◇ Offspring of no interest

see Ramgren, et al., 1962). In Canada, for instance, 67 per cent of all cases of haemophilia are sporadic. In view of the high frequency of sporadic haemophilia in other countries it has been assumed that the frequency of mutation of haemophilia is relatively high. But the high frequency of positive heredity in the Swedish series, however, clearly suggests that the mutation frequency in the last generation is, on the contrary, very low.

Twelve families with combined congenital deficiency of Factor VIII and Factor V are on record (see Saito, et al., 1969; Seligsohn and Ramot, 1969; Sibinga, et al., 1972). We have not been able to find any combined defects in the Swedish haemophilia series.

Fig. 26 gives the pedigree of a Swedish family (Fam. 44) with severe haemophilia B. The disease has been identified in five generations. Fig. 27 shows the pedigree of a Swedish family (Fam. 22) with severe haemophilia A. This family includes an example of maternal grandfather-grandchild inheritance.

3) FEMALE CARRIERS OF HAEMOPHILIA
During the last 50 years several attempts have been made to find out by coagulation studies whether a female is a carrier of haemophilia or not (see Veltkamp, et al., 1968a, b). During the last ten years endeavours have also been made to reveal carriers by determining the content of Factor VIII and Factor IX. Several reports have been published, but the results are often contradictory (for references see Nilsson, Blombäck, Thilén and v. Francken, 1959; Nilsson, Blombäck, Ramgren and v. Francken 1962; Nilsson, Blombäck and Ramgren, 1966; Veltkamp, et al., 1968a, b). Several authors (see Veltkamp, et al., 1968a, b) have found that carriers as a group have lower levels of Factor VIII and Factor IX than normals, but with considerable overlapping between carriers and normals, and it is not possible to draw any conclusion in a given case.

In Sweden we have examined a series of 61 definite carriers of haemophilia A, and 28 of haemophilia B (a woman who is a daughter of a haemophiliac or with one or more haemophilic sons and other relatives

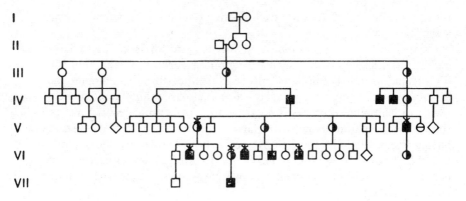

Fig 27. Pedigree of a
Swedish family with
severe haemophilia A.

with haemophilia) and 106 possible carriers of haemophilia A and 26
of haemophilia B (a woman without haemophilic sons, but with a 50
per cent or 25 per cent chance from a genetic point of view of being a
carrier). Factors VIII and IX were assayed by one-stage methods using
platelet-rich haemophilia A or haemophilia B plasma containing less
than 0·1 per cent of Factor VIII or Factor IX as a test base (see chapter
on Methods, page 221). We found a low Factor VIII content (15–60 per
cent) in 52 of the 61 definite carriers of haemophilia A. Of the 9 carriers
with normal Factor VIII, 8 were postmenopausal. Of the 106 possible
carriers of haemophilia A who, from a genetic point of view had a 50
per cent chance of being carriers, we found 58 with definitely decreased
Factor VIII content.

The possible carriers with normal AHF values have, since the assays,
given birth to 12 sons and 5 daughters. None of the boys have haemophilia.
The possible carriers with low AHF values have in the meantime produced
14 sons and 5 daughters. Six of the boys have haemophilia.

Of the 28 positive carriers of haemophilia B, 26 had definitely reduced
Factor IX values. Of the 26 possible carriers of haemophilia B, Factor IX
was reduced in 9.

Judging from our investigations, if repeated analysis shows low AHF
or B factor in a possible carrier in fertile age, she is almost certainly a
carrier of haemophilia. If repeated analysis shows normal AHF level in
a possible carrier of haemophilia A, she is, to 90 per cent probability,
not a carrier of haemophilia A. Normal B factor level does not exclude
the possibility of a person being a carrier.

According to Zimmerman, et al. (1971b) a carrier can be detected with
greater certainty by comparing the immunological determination of
AHF with the level of the biological AHF activity. An ethanol concentrate of the plasma was used for immunological determination. They found
the ratio of the activity to the antigen to range from 0·84 to 1·49, with a
mean of 1·11 in normal women, but from 0·13 to 1·03 with a mean of
0·52, in carriers. 92 per cent of the definite carriers could be identified.
Like others (Meyer, et al., 1972), we have found the method useful,

though a ratio of 1 : 1 does not exclude the possibility of a woman being a carrier.

Carriers of severe haemophilia in Sweden are advised not to have children and, if they wish, they can be granted sterilisation and abortion on eugenic grounds. But it is apparently impossible to eliminate the disease by such preventive measures. For there are many latent carriers owing to 'skipping' of genes through women in various generations. In the known Tenna family in Switzerland there are examples of the disease having skipped females through five generations before any haemophilic boy was born (Moor-Jankowski, et al., 1958). The sporadic cases of haemophilia can be largely explained by such skipping of the haemophilic gene.

We test suspected carriers of the haemophilic gene repeatedly, as a rule on ten occasions. It is important to check that patients are not pregnant and are not using P-pills, because pregnancy as well as the use of such pills causes an increase in Factor VIII content not only in normals, but also in carriers.

If a known carrier of severe haemophilia A cannot be dissuaded from having a child, we recommend determination of the sex of the foetus. If the foetus is a male, pregnancy may be interrupted. A daughter could be a carrier of the disease and she in turn must undergo the same procedure in the event of pregnancy.

A male haemophiliac may have sons. In such cases we also have the sex of the foetus determined. If it is a son, who will definitely not have the disease, pregnancy may continue. If the foetus is a female, abortion is recommended.

4) BLEEDING SYMPTOMS IN HAEMOPHILIA
Bleeding symptoms in severe and moderate haemophilia. As a rule, bleeding symptoms appear during the first year of life, but rarely during the neonatal period, unless the child is subjected to circumcision. The Swedish haemophilia series includes two cases in which intracranial bleeding occurred at birth. One of the children weighed 5 kg and was delivered with the aid of a vacuum extractor. The child was immediately given substitution therapy and afterwards developed in a normal way. The other became mentally subnormal. In another survey of 192 newborn haemophilic boys severe bleeding occurred in only two (Baehner and Strauss, 1966). Bleeding symptoms do not usually appear until the infants are 7–8 months of age. The haemorrhages manifest themselves in the form of haematoma, profuse bleeding after biting of the tongue and lip, and large haematomas in the forehead.

Patients with moderate or severe haemophilia often develop extensive subcutaneous haemorrhages and bleedings in the muscles after even trivial trauma, and often without any known trauma. These *tissue bleedings* may assume enormous dimensions because the blood in the haematomas is liquid and therefore diffuses freely through tissues and along fasciae. It may involve an entire arm, an entire leg, even half the body. Such a tissue bleeding may contain several litres of blood. They are extremely painful. These haemorrhages may cause not only a loss of blood, but also a variety of effects due to the pressure they exert. They may restrict the blood supply to limbs and abdominal organs with consequent necrosis and atrophy. Complications may occur in the form of injury to nerves with consequent paresis, contractures and impairment of sensibility. Injury to the sciatic nerve and ulnar nerve are the commonest complications. Extensive tissue bleeding can result in perforation of the skin with complicating infection and fistulation. In normals, heavy traumatic muscle bleeding results in the formation of a clot, which can generally be readily removed by incision. It is impossible to control tissue bleedings in haemophiliacs by incision. The tissues are diffusely saturated with liquid blood. If the tissue bleeding is extensive, the patient should be given substitution therapy. When the bleeding ceases, the pain generally stops and the blood is relatively quickly absorbed. Bleeding into tissues in the throat, oral cavity or mediastinum is a serious complication and may rapidly lead to death from suffocation. In these cases substitution therapy must be started immediately.

Bleeding in the iliopsoas muscle is not uncommon and is often misinterpreted as bleeding into the hip joint. The patients have severe pain in the groin, which is usually swollen. The hip joint as well as the knee is held in contracture. If the patients can walk, they do so with the hips and the knees bent. It is important that such bleedings be adequately treated, because they are believed to predispose to the development of iliac cysts.

A very serious sequela after deep tissue bleeding, especially in the region of the hip, is a progressive formation of blood cysts, which gradually assume enormous dimensions and erode the bone and may invade the entire pelvis and even destroy adjacent joints and muscles. Finally, they usually rupture and may then perforate the abdomen and intestine or form fistulae in the skin. Refractory bleedings and infections supervene. Such cysts are most common in the hips, but may develop anywhere in the body. They have sometimes been misinterpreted on X-ray photographs as sarcoma, with disastrous consequences. Such cysts are usually called pseudotumours. The formation of such cysts is generally regarded as a very serious complication, which sooner or later is fatal. This is one of the reasons why early and adequate treatment of such deep tissue bleeding is imperative.

In patients with severe haemophilia even *trivial injury,* such as a small cut, may cause obstinate bleeding which persists for weeks. Such bleeding was formerly often fatal. If a haemophiliac is operated upon without adequate precautions, he may bleed to death. Even minor surgery, such as tooth extractions, involves a considerable risk of abnormal bleeding. Several haemophiliacs have died from bleeding after tooth extractions.

Internal haemorrhage is not uncommon in haemophiliacs. Gastric bleeding in a haemophiliac is a serious complication. During such an attack the patient may vomit 1–4 litres of blood within a few minutes.

X-ray examination will rarely show signs of ulcer. Very intensive substitution therapy is indicated. Haemophiliacs may also have bleeding in the intestinal wall, which may produce symptoms resembling those in ileus. In all cases of acute abdominal pain in haemophiliacs, bleeding should therefore first be suspected. And then especially *retroperitoneal bleeding,* which is common in haemophiliacs and frequently offers considerable diagnostic problems. There are several reports of haemophiliacs who have been admitted to hospital because of suspected appendicitis or peritonitis but who, on closer examination, have been found to have retroperitoneal bleeding. Such patients may thus have right-sided abdominal pain and swelling in the right iliac fossa and, because of the bleeding, also leukocytosis. Adequate transfusion will usually soon control the symptoms. It is therefore wise to regard abdominal symptoms in haemophiliacs as manifestations of bleeding and give substitution therapy. If the abdominal symptoms increase despite treatment with AHF and if there are no further symptoms and signs suggesting that the pain is due to bleeding, operation under adequate protection against bleeding should, of course, be considered.

Haematuria is common in haemophilia. As a rule, the bleeding is renal. The patients may have severe gross haematuria for several days and even weeks. Pain in the region of the kidneys is common. The loss of blood is, as a rule, not heavy. The renal pelvis may sometimes be full of blood clots which results in urinary stasis, cessation of renal function and, on passage of the clot, pain resembling renal colic. In Sweden we have studied renal complications in haemophiliacs with isotope renography, which we have found to be a valuable method in the examination of such patients. Thus, some patients had pain and haematuria, but the renogram could exclude renal stasis. In other cases, the haematuria was painless, but the renogram showed renal stasis, which then required a very close follow-up. In some cases the pain was only unilateral, though the curves showed bilateral involvement. Stasis occurred equally as often in patients treated with inhibitors of fibrinolysis as in those who were treated with substitution therapy only. Of 20 personal patients with stasis, 18 recovered normal renal function within 2–3 months.

Prentice, et al. (1971) recently studied renal complications in 35 patients with haemophilia A and B. They found that 77 per cent had impairment of renal function, due most often to lesions in the upper urinary tract. As a rule, however, the renal lesions did not produce clinical symptoms. The incidence of complications was not higher among those who had been treated with EACA than among the others.

Intracranial haemorrhage requires special attention. It is clear from recent statistics that intracranial bleeding is the commonest cause of death of haemophiliacs (Ramgren, 1962a, b; Kerr, 1964; Biggs and MacFarlane, 1966; Blattner, 1967). The causal trauma is, as a rule, only trivial, but it is followed by a continuous oozing of blood, which gradually results in extensive intracranial haemorrhage. Head injury, though relatively trivial, is therefore a very strong indication for immediate

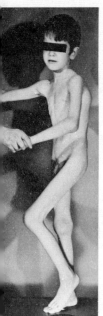

Fig 28. Boy with haemophilia with severe joint lesions.

preventative transfusions. Haemorrhages in the *peripheral nervous system* are also serious and may produce permanent injury.

Joint bleeding. The most characteristic feature of haemophilia is joint bleeding, which often occurs without any known preceding trauma. It usually appears when the child begins to learn to walk and it may affect any joint, though most often the knees, ankles and elbows. The affected joint swells markedly and is very painful, and stiff. Left untreated, such bleeding may last for weeks. Every attack of bleeding injures the joints, which may be gradually damaged more and more with consequent deformation. X-ray photographs reveal swollen epiphyses, the joint surfaces being irregular and rarefied. Incomplete reabsorption of the intra-articular blood is followed in turn by chronic synovitis with deposition of iron, thickening of the joint capsule, destruction of the joint cartilage and underlying bone with granulation tissue formation and eventually chronic osteoarthritis with irregular new bone formation, fibrous or even bony ankylosis or complete destruction of the joint. It has been shown that the hypertrophic haemophilic synovial membranes have a high fibrinolytic activity, and it has been suggested that local fibrinolysis might be involved in the pathogenesis of intra-articular haemorrhage in haemophilia (Pandolfi, et al., 1972). Previously damaged joints are most likely to be the site of further bleeding and then a vicious circle is set up. There is diffuse atrophy of bones and especially of muscles. The swelling of the joint is made more prominent by the wasting of the limb. In the knee joints severe contractures are common. The joints are usually severely deformed and, as a rule, there is outward bending and outward rotation of the joint. Defects of the epiphyses stimulate increased growth in length, and the affected leg is often longer than the other leg. Talus equinus is common and is often due to bleeding and consequent fibrositis of the calf muscle. In the elbow joint the head of the radius is often severely enlarged and pronation and supination are impaired or impossible. Bleeding in the shoulder joints is extremely painful. The joint changes in haemophilia have been described in detail by Ahlberg (1965). Owing to the joint bleeding the patients are, as a rule, severely disabled and patients with severe haemophilia were formerly obliged to use crutches or were confined to a wheelchair (Fig. 28). Patients with moderate haemophilia also have joint bleeding, but usually not so often or so profuse as those with severe haemophilia. In moderate haemophilia, disability is generally confined to a single joint.

Bleeding symptoms in mild haemophilia. Severe spontaneous bleeding and joint bleedings are relatively rare in mild haemophilia. Haematuria and gastro-intestinal bleeding, on the other hand, are not uncommon. The mildly affected patients bleed especially in association with injuries and surgical operations. Also in patients with mild haemophilia, life-threatening haemorrhage may occur after tooth extraction, for example. Mild haemophilia may remain concealed until adult age and then be detected in association with surgery or following trauma. Such patients create severe problems at operation because of unexpected heavy bleeding.

5) TREATMENT OF HAEMOPHILIA

Treatment of haemophilia consists of management of the patient in the acute situation, rehabilitation, and prophylaxis.

The main purpose of treatment of haemophiliacs is to normalise coagulation by administration of the missing factor.

α. Transfusions in haemophilia A

It is well known that in haemophilia A it is necessary to use fresh blood and fresh plasma in the treatment and for preparation of concentrates. For AHF (Factor VIII) is a labile substance. As much as 40–50 per cent of the AHF of citrated blood may be inactivated by 4–5 hours' storage at room temperature (Pool and Robinson, 1959). If fresh plasma is frozen, 20–30 per cent of its original AHF activity will be lost during thawing (Weaver and Langdell, 1966). AHF is also rapidly consumed *in vivo*. The half-life of AHF in the blood has been given as 9–18 hours. In the presence of bleeding and trauma and in fever and infections AHF is consumed much quicker, and practically all AHF administered may be consumed within less than 8–10 hours (see Nilsson, Blombäck and Ramgren, 1962; Abildgaard, Ch., et al., 1964).

In minor bleeding episodes the AHF content must be raised to 15–20 per cent of normal in order to secure haemostasis. In severe haemorrhagic conditions and if surgery is necessary, the AHF content must be raised to 40–60 per cent of normal (Brinkhous, et al., 1956; Nilsson, Blombäck and Ramgren, 1962; Biggs and Macfarlane, 1966). This cannot be achieved by infusion of blood and plasma alone. Moreover, administration of large volumes of plasma implies a severe risk of over-hydration. Severe haemorrhage and surgery therefore require the use of an AHF concentrate, which contains much more AHF per unit volume than does blood or plasma.

Several AHF concentrates are now available (see also page 18). Some of the most common preparations are given in Table 2.

I. Human fraction I-0 (AHF–KI; AHF-Kabi)

Since 1956 a human AHF concentrate has been available in Sweden, *viz* human fraction I-O prepared according to Blombäck and Blombäck's glycine method (Blombäck, B. and Blombäck, M., 1956; Blombäck, M. and Nilsson, 1958; Blombäck, M., et al., 1960; Nilsson, Blombäck and Ramgren, 1962; Jorpes, et al., 1962; Nilsson 1965) (see page 19 for preparation and properties). The preparation was originally made at Karolinska Institutet and each batch required 1400–1600 ml of fresh plasma, obtained from 8 blood donors. With this volume it was possible to prepare about 3 g of the concentrate of fraction I-O which was dissolved in two bottles each of 100 ml (100 ml = 1 dose of AHF). The activity of the preparation was 8 times that of normal plasma. The activity per milligram of protein in the preparation was about 20 times that of normal plasma. The AHF obtained in fraction I-O was 70–100 per cent

Table 2. Current AHF concentrates.

	AHF units per ml*	Number of times purified
Fraction I–0 (Blombäck's glycine method)		
a. (AHF–KI)	3–8	20–40
b. (AHF–Kabi)	2·5–4	7–15
Cryoprecipitate (Pool's method)	3–16	8–20
High potency glycine precipitated AHF = Hyland 4	35–105	100–400
American National Red Cross-AHF		
a. ANRC, intermediate purity	12	15–30
b. ANRC, high purity	100–300	> 200

* 1 unit AHF = the AHF activity in 1 ml of normal human fresh plasma.

of the AHF of the original plasma, but when larger batches were prepared from plasma from 16–32 donors the yield decreased. A good correlation was obtained between the *in vitro* and the *in vivo* yield.

Since 1967, A.B. Kabi has taken over the manufacture of AHF containing fraction I-O. Kabi uses about 25 litres of plasma (from about 125 donors) for each batch, from which they obtain 25 bottles each of 100 ml AHF concentrate. Kabi uses only frozen plasma as raw material. The use of larger batches, sterile filtration and deep freezing has resulted in a smaller yield. 100 ml of AHF concentrate (1 dose) has, as a rule, an activity corresponding to that of 250–300 ml fresh plasma. Since 1956 we have given fraction I-O because of haemorrhage or in association with surgical operations about 30.000 times to about 400 patients with AHF deficiency. Most of these patients have been treated repeatedly for 5–10 years. The therapeutic effect has proved very good. Major surgical operations and orthopaedic corrections have been performed without bleeding complications (Nilsson, Blombäck and Ramgren, 1962; Nilsson, 1965; Ahlberg, 1965; Österlind and Nilsson, 1968). The protein content of each 100 ml of AHF is 1·4–1·7 g, 85–90 per cent of which is fibrinogen. After administration of AHF the fibrinogen content increases. Levels of 1·4 g fibrinogen/100 ml. plasma have been recorded without any demonstrable side-effects.

In the 1960s the preparation of fraction I-O was started in Australia, France, Holland and Switzerland. AHF concentrates prepared according to modifications of the I-O-method have also been used (McMillan, et al., 1961; Newcomb and Watson, 1963; Ménaché, 1968).

II. Cryoprecipitate

Pool and Robinson (1959) reported formation of a precipitate when fresh frozen plasma was thawed slowly at + 4°C. This cryoprecipitate could be dissolved at + 37°C and was found to have a high content of AHF. In recent papers Pool and coworkers reported the successful use of this cryoprecipitate in the treatment of haemophilia A. They also gave a detailed description of its preparation and said that this method can be used with advantage for ordinary routine blood bank work (Pool, 1967, 1969; Pool and Shannon, 1965). Meyer, et al. (1967) have also given detailed descriptions of the preparation. Brown, et al. (1967) modified Pool and Shannon's method in that they thawed the plasma at $+ 8°C$ instead of $+ 4°C$. This accelerated the preparation of AHF, the thawing requiring only 90 minutes instead of the 20 hours previously required. They also obtained a higher AHF yield in the cryoprecipitate.

During the last six years a number of reports have appeared on the manufacture and clinical use of cryoprecipitate (Pool, 1969; Verstraete, et al., 1969; Simson, et al., 1967; Meyer, et al., 1967; Cooke, et al., 1968; Brown, et al., 1967; Brüster, et al., 1969; Bloom, et al., 1969; Rizza and Biggs, 1969; Forbes, et al., 1969; Mazza, et al., 1970; Ehrich, et al., 1971). Cryoprecipitate from 500 ml blood is usually dissolved in 5–20 ml saline, and this volume is generally called 1 unit of cryoprecipitate. The AHF activity in the cryoprecipitate may differ widely from one donor to another. Verstraete, for example, reported that the activity may vary from 40–430 AHF units per bag. One unit of cryoprecipitate has, on average, an AHF activity equal to that of 100–150 ml plasma. The differences in yield between different batches is a disadvantage and makes continual control of *in vivo* concentrations of the AHF necessary because it is not possible to calculate the exact amount of concentrate that should be given. To achieve a level high enough to produce a haemostatic effect, it is of course usually necessary to mix cryoprecipitate from several donors. For each recipient it is necessary to use cryoprecipitate prepared from ABO-compatible donors. One possibility of reducing the variation of the yield is to prepare AHF from larger pools of plasma.

Verstraete, et al. (1969) recommend an initial 'loading dose' of 1 cryoprecipitate unit per 3 kg bodyweight and then 1 unit per 6 kg bodyweight every 12th hour. Verstraete stated that this schema, will, as a rule, produce levels of 15–30 per cent AHF. Patients undergoing surgery require much larger doses. All authors have reported a very good therapeutic effect.

III. Glycine precipitated human AHF concentrate from cryoprecipitate
    (Hyland method 4)

Since 1967 human AHF preparations with a much higher AHF activity than that of previous preparations have been manufactured (Brinkhous, et al., 1968; Mazza, et al., 1970). Cryoprecipitate is used as starting material. Polyethylene glycol is added to the cryoprecipitate and the bulk of the fibrinogen is selectively precipitated. Afterwards the AHF is precipitated by addition of glycine. This results in a purification of 100–400 times. The AHF activity of the final solution for infusion is 35–100 times that of normal plasma. High AHF values have been achieved *in vivo* (20–140 per cent) and surgery has been possible on haemophiliacs without bleeding complications (Brinkhous, et al., 1968; Honig, et al., 1969).

Hyland's preparation 4 is prepared in essentially the same way as this method.

IV. American National Red Cross AHF preparation

Johnson, et al. (1969) described one method for the manufacture of human AHF preparation of 'intermediate purity' and another for the manufacture of 'high-purity AHF' (Table 2). In both methods the raw material consists of plasma, precipitated in the cold with 3 per cent ethanol. A cryoprecipitate is obtained which is slowly thawed, after which contaminating protein is precipitated by addition of 4–5 per cent polyethylene glycol. AHF is precipitated by increasing the polyethylene concentration to 12 per cent. The highly active preparation has been reported to contain 100–300 units per ml; the less active one, 12 units per ml. The clinical effect has been described as very good.

V. Side effects of substitution therapy

Hepatitis. The incidence of hepatitis has markedly increased among haemophiliacs. In 1968 the risk of patients with haemophilia A developing clinical hepatitis after substitution therapy was given as about 2 per cent. In recent years patients with haemophilia A have been examined more often for Au-antigen and Au-antibodies. Au-antigen has been demonstrated in 3–5 per cent of haemophiliacs who have received substitution therapy, while Au-antibodies have been found in as many as 29–40 per cent of such patients. Nordenfelt and Nilsson (1971) have discovered Au-antibodies in 39 per cent of Swedish patients treated with fraction I-O. No correlation was demonstrable between the incidence of Au-antibodies and clinical hepatitis or between the occurrence of Au-antibodies and intensity or duration of the substitution therapy.

To reduce the risk of hepatitis following transfusion, it is generally recommended to prepare the concentrate from plasma pools of specially selected donors. But this is hardly possible in the manufacture of commercial preparations. It has, however, been proposed that every donor of plasma for the manufacture of AHF concentrate should be examined for Au-antigen. Such a regulation would probably reduce the frequency of serum hepatitis. It is generally agreed that the risk of hepatitis does not preclude adequate transfusion of patients with severe haemophilia.

Anticoagulants. The most serious complication apt to occur during treatment with AHF is the development of an anticoagulant (see also section on circulating anticoagulants in haemophilia A and in haemophilia B, page 85). The reported frequencies of anticoagulants in haemophilia vary widely. In the United States (Strauss, 1969) it has been given as 20 per cent for severe haemophilia A, in England and France as 10 per cent. In Sweden anticoagulants have been found in 7 per cent of 112 patients with severe haemophilia A treated with fraction I-O.

Patients with anticoagulants are in a dilemma, because there is often no possibility to correct the coagulation defect. In such patients transfusion is followed, usually after 4–5 days, by a marked increase in the anticoagulant level, which makes continued transfusion impossible. It is therefore very important, both before and during transfusion, to examine the patients for circulating anticoagulants using sensitive tests (see Methods, page 227). Transfusion should not be started unless really necessary in patients with signs of even a weak anticoagulant.

A debatable question is whether the risk of anticoagulants varies with the type, intensity and duration of the transfusion given. Strauss (1969) and other authors (Ikkala and Simonen, 1971; Nilsson, 1971) have shown that the occurrence of anticoagulants is not related to the amount of the transfusion and that anticoagulants are often seen in patients who have received only one infusion. In addition, anticoagulants usually appear before the age of ten. According to Strauss, anticoagulants occur only in certain predisposed individuals, and in these a single infusion of blood, plasma or concentrate is sufficient to stimulate antibody formation. If, for example, a patient receives 90 AHF infusions and has not developed anticoagulants, he will, according to Strauss, not develop anticoagulants later either. These observations are in agreement with those made in the Swedish series of haemophiliacs. Mannucci and Ruggeri (1970) reported an interesting investigation in Italy. Before 1967 haemophiliacs in Italy had not been treated with concentrate and only rarely with plasma. In an investigation of a series of such patients (105) anticoagulants were found in 10 per cent. From 1967 on, cryoprecipitate and other concentrates have been given to this group of haemophiliacs immediately in the event of bleeding. Since then an anticoagulant has appeared in only one patient, a four-year old boy. Brinkhous, Roberts and Weiss (1972) made an international survey (14 haemophilia centres) to ascertain whether the incidence of anticoagulants in patients with haemophilia had risen since the wide use of plasma concentrates. They compared the frequency with which inhibitors had complicated haemophilia in 1964, when plasma concentrate transfusion was uncommon, with that in 1970, when intense concentrate transfusion was common. No difference was found in frequency. About half of the patients with inhibitors had received no such transfusion.

Some authors think prophylaxis unwise, and they even refrain from giving intense transfusions to patients with joint bleeding, for example, because of fear of the development of anticoagulants. In our opinion, such an attitude is indefensible for it may lead to disability and severe haemorrhagic complications.

Allergic reactions and serological reactions. Allergic reactions to infusions of cryoprecipitate have been described. Patients treated with fraction I-O have occasionally reacted with a mild rise in temperature, but otherwise no side effects have been observed. Cryoprecipitate contains blood group antigen. It is therefore imperative that any infusions given should always be ABO-compatible. Fraction I-O does not contain blood group antigen. As for the highly purified AHF preparations, it is not known with certainty whether they contain blood group antigen or not.

VI. Choice of AHF preparation

The choice of preparation naturally depends to some extent on those available in the country. A highly active preparation with as few side effects as possible is, of course, desirable. In most countries fresh frozen plasma and/or cryoprecipitate must be the preparations of choice. Treatment of patients with anticoagulants requires the use of more active preparations than cryoprecipitate or AHF-Kabi. Access to a very active preparation is also desirable at major operations as well as in the treatment of heavy bleeding. The new very active AHF preparations, especially Hyland method 4, have been used with success in such circumstances.

VII. Principles of treatment of haemophilia A

It might be convenient first to give a few general remarks on the treatment of patients with haemophilia.

In a leader in 1968, R. Biggs stressed that the doctor in charge of a patient with haemophilia should be well versed in the treatment of the condition and be able to judge the patient's situation. Since it is now possible for all hospitals with a blood bank to prepare AHF one might well imagine that more physicians will themselves take care of their patients with haemophilia. Such a practice would be indefensible. It is not only a question of injecting an acceptable AHF preparation into patients with haemorrhages and at operations. It is first of all very important that AHF be given in doses producing a sufficiently high AHF content for a sufficiently long time. It is extremely important to exclude the possibility of an anticoagulant. There are also many other important measures to be taken and facts to be considered in the care of haemophiliacs. The care of these patients needs special centres, where physicians with knowledge and experience of haemophilia may cooperate. One might take care of patients with minor haemorrhages at provincial hospitals and begin adequate treatment of acute cases. If the bleeding is severe, or if there are joint defects or if operation is necessary, a specialist should be consulted. The principles of treatment of different types of bleeding in haemophilia A are briefly outlined below (Table 3).

1. *Minor bleeding episodes.* In such conditions an AHF content of 10–20 per cent is sufficient to secure haemostasis. Such bleedings may consist of mild joint bleedings, intramuscular haematoma, large subcutaneous haematoma, nose-bleeds or minor traumatic haemorrhages. In such bleeding it is, as a rule, sufficient to give the patient 10–15 units of AHF/kg/24 hours. The AHF preparation may be fresh plasma, cryoprecipitate or AHF-Kabi (Table 3).

2. *Joint bleedings.* One of the most important aims of treatment of

Table 3.   Treatment recommended in different situations in haemophilia A.

	Desired F VIII level after infusion	Duration of treatment	Dose AHF per 24 hrs (U/kg b.w.)	Substitute
Minor bleeding episodes				
Superficial injuries Haematoma Nose bleeding Haematuria without stasis	10–20%	1–5 days	10–15	1) Cryoprecipitate (1 U/6 kg/12 hrs) 2) AHF-Kabi (100–200 ml/24 hrs) 3) Plasma: 15–20 ml plasma/kg/24 hrs
Joint bleedings				
Minor	10–20%	1–2 days	10–15	1) Cryoprecipitate 2) AHF-Kabi } see above 3) Plasma
Major	Day 1: 30% Days 2–5: 10–20%	3–5 days	Day 1: 20–25 Days 2–5: 10–15	1) Cryoprecipitate (1 U/3 kg/12 hrs + 1 U/6 kg/12 hrs) 2) AHF-Kabi 3) Highly active AHF (f.ex. Hyland 4)
Severe haemorrhagic conditions				
Large haematoma Renal haemorrhage with stasis Retroperitoneal haematoma Gastro-intestinal haemorrhage Head injury Intracranial haemorrhage Haemorrhage in pseudotumours Postoperative haemorrhage	First 30–50%, later 10–30% until bleeding controlled	7–14 days, treatment must be continued until condition healed	20–30	1) Cryoprecipitate (1 U/3 kg/12 hrs) 2) AHF-Kabi 3) Highly active AHF (f.ex. Hyland 4)
Prophylaxis				
In severe haemophilia it can be given to patients from 4–5 to about 18 years of age	30–50%		Dosage should be titrated by survival studies. AHF content should never fall below 1%	1) AHF-Kabi 100–200 m usually at 7–10 day intervals. Half-yearly follow up: joint function, circulating anticoagulants and AHF survival 2) Cryoprecipitate 3) Highly active AHF (Hyland 4) (?)
Major surgical operations				
Major operations Surgical orthopaedic correction	50–70% during op and first postop days 30–40% third to seventh postop day. Afterwards 10–20% until healing	2–4 weeks	40 U/kg just before op; afterwards 3 U/kg/hr continuously for first days, later about 1 U/kg/hr	1) Highly active AHF concentrate (f.ex. Hyland 4) 2) AHF-Kabi 3) Cryoprecipitate

able 3. (*contd.*)

	Desired F VIII level after infusion	Duration of treatment	Dose AHF per 24 hrs (U/kg b.w.)	Substitute
Minor surgical operations				
Puncture + aspiration in severe joint bleeding Incision Herniorrhaphy Appendectomy	20–40 % during op and first postop day, later 15–20 % until healing	6–10 days	First days 20–25 afterwards 10–15	1) Cryoprecipitate (1 U/3 kg/12 hrs initially, later 1 U/6 kg/12 hrs) 2) AHF-Kabi
Tooth extractions	50–100 % at op	1 day AHF + 6–8 days with Epsikapron® or Cyclokapron®	40–60 U/kg before op + Epsikapron® 50 mg/kg/6 hrs or Cyclokapron® 25 mg/kg/6 hrs for 6–8 days	1) Highly active AHF concentrate (f.ex. Hyland 4) 2) AHF-Kabi 3) Cryoprecipitate

s a rule, AHF concentrate should be given twice a day. Severe bleeding may require administration of
HF concentrate every 4–8 hours.

haemophilia is to control the joint bleedings and prevent the development of disabling lesions. It has been shown that joint changes can be prevented by immediate transfusion for *incipient joint symptoms* (pain and reduced mobility with or without swelling). Minor bleeding generally requires raising of the level of AHF to 10–20 per cent for 1–2 days. This in turn requires a dose of 10–15 units AHF/kg body weight/24 hours. Such treatment generally soon gives relief, after which the joint should be exercised without delay. It is important to start exercising the quadriceps muscle as soon as possible. Major bleedings with swelling of the joint and usually also severe pain require raising of the blood AHF content to about 30 per cent initially and then to maintain a level of 10–20 per cent until the bleeding has ceased. This requires a dose of 20–25 units /kg body weight initially. Physiotherapy should be started as soon as the pain has disappeared. Attempts should be made to attain the same range of motion of the joint as before the haemorrhage. If the bleeding of the joint is excessive, with much effusion, puncture may be indicated. AHF infusion should be started as soon as the joint is punctured, and the blood AHF should be raised to 30–50 per cent and afterwards maintained at 15–20 per cent until the bleeding has abated.

In haemophiliacs with recurrent involvement of a joint and signs of chronic synovitis Ahlberg (1971) tried treatment with intra-articular injection of radioactive [198]Au. This treatment usually produced good improvement.

In severe chronic arthropathy with recurrent bleeding in a joint, in e.g. the knee joint, synovectomy has been tried. These operations are performed under protection of AHF and simultaneous infusion of inhibitors of fibrinolysis (Epsikapron®, Cyclokapron®. The results have varied and the operation has, as a rule, led to reduced mobility. In Sweden we reserve such operations for patients with arthropathy combined with severe recurrent bleeding.

Contractures of the knee joints have been successfully treated with 2–3 weeks' balanced traction with increasing weights fixed to the limb via pulleys and afterwards with a Kreutz splint for 3–5 weeks. The blood AHF should be maintained at a level of 5–10 per cent (Ahlberg, 1965).

3. *Renal bleeding.* In the event of severe bleeding with urinary stasis or impairment of renal function, which should be detected by isotope renography done in the acute stage, the patient should be treated initially with AHF concentrate. The AHF level should be raised to 40–50 per cent until bleeding has been controlled, after which it should be maintained at 20–30 per cent for a further few days. In order not to impair dissolution of clots we now prefer not to give inhibitors of fibrinolysis in such cases. Patients with severe pain are given analgetics and are instructed to drink as much as possible.

In haematuria with a normal renogram it is sufficient to raise the AHF level to 10–20 per cent for 2–5 days. In these cases also, inhibitors of fibrinolysis may be given (Epsikapron®, Cyclokapron®), but we prefer not to do so. When inhibitors are given, the patient should drink ample amounts of fluid.

Active surgical measures are indicated only if both kidneys show signs of persistent urinary stasis and progressive renal insufficiency. We follow these patients with a renogram at every new attack of haematuria and, when possible, we repeat renography until renal function has become normal.

4. *Severe bleedings.* Severe haemorrhage, such as gastro-intestinal, retroperitoneal or intraperitoneal bleeding, head injury and intracranial bleeding, ruptured pseudotumours, iliopsoal bleeding, extensive tissue bleeding or joint bleeding, bleeding in the oral cavity, throat, post-operative bleeding, and heavy traumatic bleeding require AHF therapy (Table 3). Such patients should be given a dose of 20–30 units/kg body weight in order to raise the AHF level to 30–50 per cent. The blood AHF should be maintained at 20–30 per cent until the bleeding has stopped. Because of the rapid consumption of AHF in patients bleeding profusely, AHF should be given repeatedly at short intervals.

Intracranial haemorrhage requires special attention. Various recent statistics have shown that intracranial haemorrhage is the commonest cause of death in haemophilia. The causal trauma may be only trivial but nevertheless sufficient to initiate a continuous oozing of blood, which gradually results in a large haematoma. Therefore, head injury, no matter how trivial, requires prompt transfusion.

A very serious sequel after *bleeding in the deep tissues,* especially in the region of the iliopsoas, is a successive formation of *blood cysts,* pseudotumours, which gradually assume enormous dimensions and erode neighbouring bones, joints and muscles and finally often result in fatal perforation. It is therefore important to treat such haemorrhages adequately and in time in order to prevent such complications.

5. *Major surgical operations* may now be performed on haemophiliacs provided that the AHF is continuously maintained at a high level for 12 days–4 weeks. It is extremely important to exclude the presence of any anticoagulant before operation. Major surgery requires highly active AHF preparations and/or AHF-Kabi batches with a high activity. If cryoprecipitate is used, batches with a high activity should be selected. To secure an AHF level of at least 50 per cent the patient should initially be given 40–50 units AHF/kg body weight and afterwards 3 units/kg body weight per hour. Later bleeding, a week or so after operation, is common in all forms of haemophilia, for which reason it is important to continue treatment until the wound has healed completely. It has been recommended to give AHF continuously by infusion after operations, but it is not possible to use ordinary infusion pumps. We have therefore, as a rule, divided the dose into 3–6 doses per day. Major surgical operations should always be performed in the presence of a member of a coagulation laboratory and preferably by a surgeon experienced in the treatment of haemophilia. The indications for operations on patients with severe or moderate haemophilia A should always be considered more carefully than on patients without coagulation disorders.

6. *Orthopaedic correction,* such as supracondylar osteotomy, achillotenotomy, correction of foot deformities and synovectomy have been performed with increasing frequency in recent years (Ahlberg, 1965, 1971). These operations require AHF therapy to the same extent as other major operations. It has proved advantageous to give the AHF combined with Epsikapron® or Cyclokapron®, which reduces the risk of local postoperative bleeding. Such treatment has saved many a haemophiliac from spending the rest of his life on crutches or in a wheelchair.

7. *Minor surgical operations.* For such procedures as tooth extraction, joint puncture and operation for hernia, it is sufficient to maintain the AHF level at 20–40 per cent during the operation and around 15 per cent during the postoperative period, as a rule, 6–10 days. We have supervised a large number of minor operations, and nearly always without abnormal bleeding. Bleeding occurred in the postoperative course when the AHF content fell below 10 per cent or when treatment was stopped too early. A tendency to late local bleeding as late as one week or more after operation is common in haemophilia. *Treatment with AHF should therefore be continued even after the bleeding has stopped.*

A new method for the care of haemophiliacs undergoing *extraction of teeth* has recently been used at various centres (Webster, et al., 1971; Corrigan, 1972). According to this method the patient is given a single dose of AHF concentrate to raise the blood AHF to 50–100 per cent, and EACA in a dose of 50 mg/kg body weight. The patient receives no further doses of AHF but is given EACA in a dose of 50 mg/kg body weight every 6th hour for 6–8 days. We have used this procedure, but instead of EACA we have used AMCA by mouth in a dose of 25 mg/kg body weight every 6th hour (Björlin and Nilsson, 1973). No haemorrhagic complications have occurred. The patient should be kept under observation in hospital for about a week. Tavenner (1972) used only AMCA to control haemorrhage after extraction of teeth in haemophiliacs.

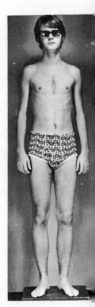

Fig 29. Boy, 18 yea with haemophilia and treated with AF concentrate sin 1959.

8. *Prophylaxis with AHF.* In moderate haemophilia A the AHF content is 1–4 per cent of normal. Joint bleedings occur, though not so often as in severe haemophilia. Ahlberg (1965) has also shown that patients with moderate haemophilia hardly ever have severe chronic joint deformities. This induced us to try to prevent the development of bleedings in patients with severe haemophilia A by raising the AHF content to a level at which severe spontaneous joint bleedings are rare, i.e. about 1–4 per cent. As early as 1958 we gave AHF prophylactically at fortnightly intervals to three boys with severe haemophilia A. After administration of 100 ml AHF the AHF content rose to 25–40 per cent. Though the AHF content fell rapidly to half its value within 10–12 hours, AHF was still demonstrable (as a rule 1–2 per cent) at the time of the next infusion. Such treatment apparently reduced severe haemophilia to moderate haemophilia.

We have now given 31 patients with haemophilia A AHF prophylaxis for 3–15 years (Nilsson, Blombäck and Ahlberg, 1970). The sizes of the doses and the intervals at which the doses were given were titrated by AHF survival studies. As a rule, the patients received 100–200 ml of AHF-Kabi at 7–10 day intervals. The patients were regularly followed up with examination of joint function and tests for circulating antibody and AHF survival. In most of the patients the AHF content was more than 1 per cent before the next infusion.

During the period of prophylaxis all patients except one have been in a good general condition. They have had bleeding episodes, which have, however, been much less severe and less frequent. The children have been able to lead a much more normal life than formerly. The number and duration of stays in hospital have been reduced and the patients have been able to attend school. Fourteen of the patients had had joint deformities of varying severity before the beginning of the prophylaxis. In four of these the changes in the already affected joints progressed slightly, but no new joint deformities occurred. The others had no changes at the beginning of prophylaxis and no such changes have developed in the joints.

The number of doses of AHF concentrate given during the period of prophylaxis was roughly the same as that before. In recent years several other haemophilia centres have also begun to use prophylactic treatment with AHF. Most of them have given highly active AHF concentrates or cryoprecipitates at very short intervals, such as 48–72 hours (Shanbrom and Thelin, 1969; Kasper, et al., 1970; van Creveld, 1971). The results have been good and joint haemorrhages have been prevented.

9. *Domiciliary transfusion*. In regions where systematic prophylaxis has not been possible, domiciliary therapy with AHF has proved very useful. The preparation was given intravenously at the very slightest sign of bleeding. Rabiner, et al. (1972) found such treatment to reduce absence from school and work and, in practice, to prevent the development of chronic joint lesions. Also Smith, et al. (1972) and Lazerson (1972) found that a home transfusion programme improved school attendance.

β Transfusions in haemophilia B

It has been the rule to treat patients with haemophilia B with blood or plasma transfusions. In haemophilia B, on the other hand, it is not necessary to give fresh blood or fresh plasma since the B factor is relatively stable. Geratz and Graham (1960) have thus shown that blood stored for 3 weeks at + 4°C still has 95 per cent of its Factor IX activity. The half-life of Factor IX *in vivo* has been given as 18–40 hours (Loeliger and Hensen, 1961b; Biggs and Denson, 1963) and is thus much longer than that of AHF. Various authors have shown that the *in vivo* yield of Factor IX after infusion of both plasma and concentrate is much lower than that of Factor VIII and corresponds to only 20–40 per cent of the Factor IX activity of the plasma or the concentrate administered (Loeliger, et al., 1967; Gilchrist, et al., 1969; Hoag, et al., 1969; Biggs, 1970; Nilsson, Ahlberg and Björlin, 1971). The lowness of this yield has been ascribed to the fact that Factor IX is distributed both intravascularly and extravascularly.

To achieve haemostasis the Factor IX content should be raised to a level recommended for AHF in different bleeding episodes and operations.

In recent years B factor concentrates have become available for clinical use (Table 4).

I. Fraction PPSB

Soulier and coworkers in Paris (Soulier, et al., 1964; Soulier, et al., 1969; Josso, et al., 1970) have prepared concentrates of Factors II, VII, X and IX (fraction PPSB). Their concentrations are 20–30 times those in normal plasma. Fraction PPSB is prepared from fresh human EDTA-plasma. The coagulation components are adsorbed to tricalcium phosphate, then eluted with citrate and precipitated with 25 per cent ethanol at − 5°C. Fraction PPSB has been given to a number of patients with haemophilia B during bleeding episodes and in association with surgery. The Factor IX content has increased to levels corresponding to about 40 per cent of the *in vitro* activity. The therapeutic effect has been good and no side-effects have been reported (Ahlberg, 1965; Loeliger, et al., 1967; Soulier, et al., 1969).

	F IX units per ml*	*Table 4. Current B factor concentrates.*
Fraction PPSB (Soulier)	30–40	
Oxford 'routine' (Bidwell)	6–15	
Oxford-DE (Dike, Bidwell)	30–60	
Konyne (Cutter)	10–60	
B-factor concentrate (Kabi)	20–30	

* 1 unit F IX = the F IX activity present in 1 ml of normal human fresh plasma.

In recent years various investigators have produced B factor concentrate according to modifications of Soulier's method. Bruning, et al. (1970) in Holland used ACD-plasma and aluminium hydroxide for preparing Factor IX concentrate on a small scale. Shanbrom (1970) used fraction III as starting material and then applied a method similar to Soulier's. Gilchrist, et al. (1969) have given this fraction to four patients with haemophilia B with good effect. The *in vivo* yield was 20–30 per cent of the activity *in vitro*.

II. Factor IX concentrate according to Bidwell

Bidwell and coworkers (Bidwell, et al., 1967; Biggs, 1970) in England have devised a method for enriching Factor IX from the supernatant fluid obtained on alcohol fractionation of plasma. This concentrate (Oxford 'routine') has been described as containing 6–15 units of Factor IX per ml. The therapeutic effect has been reported as good.

Bidwell and her coworkers (Dike, Bidwell and Rizza, 1972) have recently worked out a new method for preparing a concentrate of Factors IX, II and X for therapeutic use. The method is based on adsorption of the factors on DEAE-cellulose from plasma or from the supernatant after removal of Factor VIII. The yield of Factor IX *in vitro* is about 50–75 per cent and its purification about 300-fold. Their concentrate contained 30–60 units of Factor IX per ml. The preparation was given to 29 patients with haemophilia and with good effect. The *in vivo* yield was about 25 per cent of the activity *in vitro*.

III. Konyne

Tullis and coworkers (1965) in America have worked out a method for the preparation of Factor IX concentrate with the use of DEAE-Sephadex. This preparation has been described as containing 10–70 units of Factor IX per ml (Tullis, et al., 1965; Tullis, 1970). Breen and Tullis (1969) have reported the clinical use of this preparation in 14 patients, including 5 with haemophilia B. Cutter Laboratories now produce a Factor IX concentrate, called Konyne, according to a modification of Tullis' method. They use the supernatant fluid from fraction I, which is adsorbed to DEAE-Sephadex. Konyne contains 10–60 units of Factor IX per ml. Hoag, et al. (1969) have studied the effect of this preparation in nine patients with haemophilia B. The *in vivo* yield was about 40 per cent.

IV. B factor concentrate Kabi

A.B. Kabi has now begun to produce a B factor concentrate according to a modification of Tullis' method. The supernatant fluid from fraction I-0 is used as starting material. This preparation contains about 20 units of Factor IX per ml. The purification per mg protein of Factor IX compared with that of the starting plasma is about 70 times. The fraction has roughly the same activity of Factors II, VII and X. Nilsson, Ahlberg and Björlin (1971) used this preparation during acute bleeding and surgical operations of 18 patients with severe haemophilia B. The patients' Factor IX content rose to values corresponding to about 40 per cent of the activity of the preparation *in vitro*. Good haemostasis was noted. The operations could be performed without any bleeding complications. Three of the patients afterwards had hepatitis. No other side-effects were observed.

V. Principles of treatment of haemophilia B

The principles of treatment of haemophilia B are essentially the same as those recommended for the treatment of haemophilia A. As pointed out, in different bleeding episodes and in association with different operations, the Factor IX content should be raised to a level corresponding to that of AHF. Since the *in vivo* yield by infusion of plasma and B factor concentrate is only 20–40 per cent of the *in vitro* activity of Factor IX administered, and since the half-life of Factor IX is longer than that of AHF, *viz.,* about 20 hours, the dosage of plasma and concentrate must be planned differently than for haemophilia A. As in haemophilia A, the Factor IX content must be continuously checked at operations and during heavy bleeding. As a rule, haemophilia B requires only daily infusions of plasma or concentrate. On the basis of our experience some principles of treatment of different types of bleeding in haemophilia B are given in Table 5.

As in haemophilia A, treatment of haemophilia B involves the risk of hepatitis and of the appearance of circulating anticoagulants.

6) OCCURRENCE AND TREATMENT OF CIRCULATING ANTICOAGULANTS IN HAEMOPHILIA A AND HAEMOPHILIA B

Haemophilia A and haemophilia B may be complicated by circulating anticoagulants (see page 75). Several instances of such anticoagulants in haemophiliacs are on record (for references, see Margolius, et al., 1961; Hardisty, 1962; Biggs and Macfarlane, 1966; Strauss and Merler, 1967; Bidwell, et al., 1966; Nilsson, Blombäck and Ramgren, 1961; Shapiro, 1967; Strauss, 1969; Brinkhous, et al., 1972). These anticoagulants are antibodies and are directed against Factor VIII or Factor IX. The antibodies have been analysed in several cases and found to belong to the IgG-class of immunoglobulins (Shapiro, 1967; Andersen and Troup, 1967; Andersen and Terry, 1968; Shapiro and Carroll, 1968; Bidwell, 1969; Lusher, et al., 1968; Feinstein, et al., 1969).

Table 5.   *Treatment recommended in different situations in haemophilia B.*

	Desired F IX level after infusion	Duration of treatment	Dose F IX per 24 hrs (U/kg b.w.)	Substitute
Major surgical operations				
Major operation	40–70% during op and first postop days, 30–40% till about seventh postop day, later 10–15% until healing	10–20 days	Day 1: 50–60 Days 2–3: 30–40 Days 4–10: 10–16 Days 11–20: 10/48 h	B factor concentrate
Surgical orthopaedic correction				
Minor surgical operations				
Tooth extraction	20–40% during op, later about 15% for 6–8 days	6–8 days	Day 1: 20–30 Days 2–8: 10–16	1) B factor concentrate 2) Plasma
Aspiration in heavy joint bleeding				
Incision				
Herniorrhaphy				
Appendectomy				
Severe haemorrhagic conditions				
Large haematoma	20–50%	As a rule 7–14 days; treatment must be continued until healing	Days 1–3: 20–30 Days > 3: 10–16	1) B factor concentrate 2) Plasma
Renal haemorrhage with stasis				
Retroperitoneal haematoma				
Gastro-intestinal haemorrhage				
Head injury				
Intracranial haemorrhage				
Haemorrhage in pseudotumour				
Joint bleeding (severe)				
Postop bleeding				
Minor haemorrhagic conditions				
Superficial injuries	10–20%	2–5 days	10–16	1) B factor concentrate 2) Plasma
Haematoma				
Joint bleeding (mild)				
Haematuria without stasis				
Nose bleeding				

The antibody level may vary considerably from case to case and even from one occasion to another in one and the same patient. Transfusions usually produce a marked rise of the anticoagulant level after 4–5 days. It usually takes 4–8 months before it falls to its original level (Strauss, 1969; Nilsson, et al., 1973a, b). If the patient has a circulating anticoagulant, a conventional transfusion will not demonstrably raise the content of AHF or Factor IX. If the patient is resistant to transfusion, an anticoagulant should be suspected. The presence of such anticoagulants can be demonstrated by special laboratory tests (see Macfarlane and Biggs, 1966; Strauss and Merler, 1967; and Methods, page 227).

The figures available on the frequency of anticoagulants in haemophilia vary widely. Margolius, et al. (1961) reported that 21 per cent of 84 haemophiliacs studied in Baltimore and Cleveland had anticoagulants. In England and France anticoagulants have been found in about 10 per cent of patients with severe haemophilia. Strauss (1969) claimed that in America the frequency of circulating antibodies is now high. He estimates that 20 per cent of all severe haemophiliacs have anticoagulants. In Sweden we have examined 132 patients with haemophilia A and found circulating anticoagulants in 12 with severe haemophilia A. Among 60 patients with haemophilia B, we found anticoagulants in 4 with severe haemophilia B. In only a few cases have anticoagulants been found in mild haemophilia (Beck, et al., 1969).

Patients with anticoagulants are in a very precarious situation because it is not possible to control the abnormality. If an anticoagulant is discovered, all transfusion and substitution therapy should be stopped in the hope that the level will fall.

One should try to control the bleeding by immobilisation and local compression. One may also try to give the patient an inhibitor of fibrinolysis (EACA or AMCA). If a bleeding episode is severe, the patient may be given much larger doses of AHF and Factor IX concentrate than is usually given to haemophiliacs. Preparations used for this purpose must be highly concentrated. The amount of AHF and B factor to be given in such situations should be calculated from the number of inhibitor units per ml in the patient's plasma. Neutralisation of the anticoagulant for 4–5 days may be achieved and this time must be utilised for any absolutely necessary operations. This time is followed by a considerable rise in the anticoagulant level.

Josso, et al. (1969) have treated patients with anticoagulants by giving various animal preparations and have thereby been able to prolong the effect.

To replace the blood loss, patients with anticoagulants should be given suspensions of washed erythrocytes. Exchange transfusions combined with substitution therapy has been tried in the treatment of life-threatening haemorrhage (Hall, 1961; Roberts, et al., 1965). Another method used for controlling the antibodies is long-term treatment with corticosteroids or immunosuppressives (Bidwell, 1969; Sherman, et al., 1969; Green, 1971b). We tried long-term steroid therapy in small doses in four of our patients with anticoagulants. The anticoagulant level fell in all of them. But most investigators have found steroids to have an uncertain effect. Results of treatment with immunosuppressives alone have not been convincing either.

Green (1971b) described a patient who had an anticoagulant against AHF and in whom the inhibitor was suppressed by simultaneous administration of an intravenous dose of cyclophosphamide and a large dose of AHF. Lusher, et al. (1971) described two patients who had haemophilia

A and antibodies against AHF and in whom a single dose of AHF concentrate and cyclophosphamide suppressed AHF antibody production. Lechner, et al. (1972) treated two patients with haemophilia A with AHF concentrate and azathioprine, but they were not able to prevent a rise in the inhibitor level. Nilsson, et al. (1973a) treated four patients with severe haemophilia A and an anticoagulant with a large dose of AHF (4.000–8.000 units) and cyclophosphamide during bleeding episodes. Cyclophosphamide was first given as an intravenous injection in a dose of 250–1.000 mg and later orally in a dose of 3 mg/kg body weight per day for at least 8 days. In three of the patients the treatment had a good haemostatic effect and immediately raised the AHF to 50 per cent. The antibody level was zero for 5–10 days, after which it gradually rose to its original level. In the fourth patient the AHF rose to only 8 per cent, and after some time the antibody titer rose markedly. Good results have also been obtained by such treatment in two patients with haemophilia B and anticoagulants (Nilsson, et al., 1973b). Effective substitution therapy can thus now be offered to such patients temporarily during severe bleeding episodes and surgery, provided that highly concentrated AHF (e.g. Hyland 4) and B factor concentrate are available. If the patient has a very high anticoagulant level (> 5 units per ml plasma) it is probably necessary first to lower the anticoagulant level by repeated plasmapheresis.

7) GENERAL RECOMMENDATIONS FOR THE TREATMENT OF
   HAEMOPHILIA

In Sweden and most countries patients with haemophilia and other haemorrhagic diseases are now provided with a special identity card containing information on their blood group, coagulation defect and its treatment and the names and addresses of physicians who should be contacted in the event of bleeding or surgery.

Patients with haemophilia are delicate and the risks attending the increased bleeding tendency must always be borne in mind. One should listen to the patients, for they understand their disease and know what they can tolerate. As previously pointed out, all surgical operations, even minor surgery, can never be performed without adequate protection against increased bleeding.

Venepuncture should be performed very carefully and by well trained personnel. A needle should never be inserted more than once. Several patients have developed haematomas which have involved the entire arm and trunk after punctures. The femoral vein should never be punctured. If angiography is to be done, the patient must be prepared as for an operation with substitution therapy.

Cutting down of veins in haemophiliacs should be strictly forbidden. These patients need their veins, and we have had great difficulties in the treatment of several haemophiliacs who have since childhood been subjected to repeated surgical exposure of veins. Intramuscular injections are to be avoided unless preceded by substitution therapy. They may cause enormous haematomas, which may in turn lead to necrosis and circulatory disorders. Haemophilia does not, of course, preclude vaccination, provided the vaccine can be given subcutaneously.

Preparations containing salicylic acid, phenylbutazone and analogues, and possibly also indometacin, inhibit platelet aggregation and are not suitable for the treatment of patients with haemophilia because they increase the tendency to bleeding. We consider the use of acetyl-salicylic acid absolutely forbidden. Tissue bleeding, renal bleeding, abdominal bleeding, joint bleeding and various other haemorrhages can be very painful in patients with haemophilia and they then require large doses of morphine or its derivatives. Otherwise one should, if possible, refrain from using morphine preparations. Several haemophiliacs have become drug addicts.

Patients with *mild haemophilia* can lead a practically normal life provided they are aware of their disease and can obtain proper treatment in the event of bleeding episodes and provided that operations, if necessary, are performed with the necessary precautions. In Sweden haemophiliacs are exempted from military service. They should avoid an occupation with too high a risk of accidents. We do not generally dissuade patients with mild haemophilia or female carriers of mild haemophilia from having children.

Patients with *severe or moderate haemophilia* cannot lead a normal life. They are delicate and must be handled with care from early childhood. We advise the use of foam-rubber mattresses for small children with haemophilia. For small children we also recommend foam-rubber lined long trousers and a helmet, also lined with foam-rubber. Suitably designed knee and ankle pads offer good protection.

For all patients with haemophilia, riding on mopeds and motorcycles is absolutely forbidden, for even relatively slight accidents may have serious consequences in haemophiliacs. Special precautions should be taken at school, and the teacher should be informed about the disease. Children with haemophilia should, of course, not take part in gymnastics or woodwork at school. Football is not allowed either. On the other hand, it is important for haemophiliacs to keep themselves physically fit and to exercise their muscles. Muscle training increases the resistance to joint bleeding. It has become increasingly obvious that physical training is an important part of treatment. A very suitable sport for haemophiliacs is swimming, which exercises all the muscles without involving any risk of bleeding. Cycling is also a useful exercise but must, of course, be practised with caution to avoid accidents. Table tennis is another sport which may be regarded as suitable for haemophiliacs. There is now a tendency to persuade haemophiliacs to do a number of certain specially designed exercises every day at home. It is also important that haemophiliacs should not be overweight, because it places an unnecessary strain on the joints.

Dental care has offered serious problems in haemophilia. Several patients need treatment of the entire dentition. It is therefore urgent that the patients have their teeth looked after with greatest care from early childhood. We recommend all patients to see their dentist regularly three times a year, so that all cavities may be detected in time and dental surgical intervention thereby be avoided. Fluoridation of the teeth is probably useful. We also recommend children not to eat sweets.

A good school education is of utmost importance for haemophiliacs, even though it may require an extra year or so because of absence due to the disease. Choice of occupation is also important, and in most countries the patient is given expert advice in the planning and choice of occupational training. A haemophiliac can manage intellectual and light manual work just as well as a healthy man.

In most countries there are haemophilia associations which are members of the World Federation of Haemophilia. These associations give the patient socio-medical advice and any information they may desire.

Haemophiliacs constitute a relatively small group of patients but require a considerable amount of medical attention. Thanks to modern methods of rehabilitation such patients can now lead a useful life, whereas formerly they were largely bound to wheelchairs.

2. von Willebrand's disease

von Willebrand (1926) of Helsingfors described a congenital haemorrhagic diathesis which he had observed in several members of a family from Föglö on Åland. He found 23 cases among 66 family members. The disease manifested itself as cutaneous and severe mucosal haemorrhages and occurred in both men and women. Several children had died early in life from intestinal bleeding and profuse bleeding after trauma of varying severity. One girl was described as having bled to death from a gnat bite. von Willebrand found that the patients had a prolonged bleeding time, normal coagulation time and normal platelet count. The platelets were morphologically normal. von Willebrand therefore claimed that the disease was clearly distinguished from that described by Glanzmann as thrombasthenia (1918). Because of its similarity to haemophilia von Willebrand first called the disease 'pseudohaemophilia' (von Willebrand, 1931). In 1933 von Willebrand began to collaborate with a German physician, Rudolf Jürgens, who was to investigate the cause of the abnormal haemostasis. In the following years Jürgens repeatedly visited Åland and tried out every new available coagulation method on these patients (for references, see Blombäck, Jorpes and Nilsson, 1963). Unfortunately these investigations did not result in any clarification of the disease. Jürgens therefore ultimately felt that the bleeding tendency in this disease was due to some impairment of platelet function, including platelet factor 3 deficiency. This resulted in the disease being called von Willebrand-Jürgens thrombopathy. Further cases were discovered in Åland. Genetic studies (Lehmann, 1959; Eriksson, 1961) have shown that practically all the cases in Åland can be traced to von Willebrand's original Föglö family and that it is inherited as an autosomal dominant characteristic. In the last five generations of this family 132 members have been known to be affected.

Alexander and Goldstein (1953) of Boston reported some cases of haemorrhagic diathesis with a reduced content of antihaemophilic globulin and a prolonged bleeding time. The bleeding symptoms in these patients resembled those seen in the Åland's disease, but the disease was thought to differ from the Åland's disease because the platelet function in these patients appeared normal. Singer and Ramot (1956) published a survey of nineteen literature cases with a prolonged bleeding time and AHF deficiency. They called this syndrome pseudohaemophilia B. But no satisfactory explanation could be offered for the prolonged bleeding time in this syndrome. Most authors, however, thought that the prolonged bleeding time was due to some defect in the vessel wall. Schulman, et al. (1955), who described such cases, therefore called this bleeding syndrome vascular haemophilia, a term which has caused much confusion.

In 1956 and 1957 we described 13 members of 10 families in Sweden who had a congenital haemorrhagic diathesis characterised by AHF deficiency and prolonged bleeding time (Nilsson, et al., 1956; Nilsson, 1957; Nilsson, Blombäck and v. Francken, 1957). Genetic studies showed that the gene which caused AHF deficiency was autosomal and dominant, but with varying expression. All of these cases had previously been regarded as instances of thrombopathy. At that time Birger and Margareta Blombäck in Stockholm were working on a method for the purification of fibrinogen by treatment of Cohn's fraction I with 1 M glycine solution (see page 19). Since we found that the AHF activity of the starting plasma could be practically quantitatively recovered in fraction I-O, this fraction was prepared under sterile conditions and its effect was tried on patients with this bleeding disease. After the injection of fraction I-O, bleeding stopped and the AHF deficiency disappeared, as did the prolongation of the bleeding time. This was of interest in that it argued against a disorder of the capillary wall as the cause of the prolonged bleeding time, and suggested that it was due to a deficiency of a plasma factor that could be recovered in fraction I-O from normal plasma.

The clinical symptoms and the mode of inheritance of our cases closely resembled those in von Willebrand's disease, but not the laboratory findings. Jürgens in his investigation of von Willebrand's disease on Åland found a normal AHF content, but an abnormal platelet function, which could not be demonstrated in our patients (Jürgens and Deutsch, 1955).

In June 1957 we visited Åland and examined 15 patients with von Willebrand's disease; some of them belonged to von Willebrand's original group (Nilsson, Blombäck, Jorpes, Blombäck and Johansson 1957). We found the AHF to be deficient and platelet function as well as platelet factor 3 to be normal. One of the patients in Aland was treated with fraction I-O, which normalised the AHF level and the bleeding time. On the basis of these findings it was concluded that the *inherited bleeding*

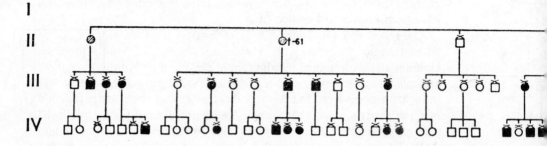

disease with AHF deficiency and prolonged bleeding time was identical with von Willebrand's disease.

We feel that the disease should be called von Willebrand's disease and not von Willebrand-Jürgens' disease. It was von Willebrand who first described the disease.

Fig 30. Pedigree of the largest family in Sweden with von Willebrand's disease For other symbols se Fig 26 page 66.

1) INCIDENCE

Judging from recent literature, von Willebrand's disease is one of the commonest of the known inheritable haemorrhagic diatheses (Quick, 1967; Aggeler, 1969; Jürgens, 1969), but so far no investigation of the incidence has been made in a well defined population. In 1970 there were 500 known cases of von Willebrand's disease in Sweden. This means an incidence of 1 in 16.000 inhabitants. The corresponding figure for haemophilia in Sweden is 1 in 10.000 men, i.e. barely 1 in 20.000 of the population as a whole. Many mild cases, however, probably never produce manifest symptoms. It is therefore very probable that von Willebrand's disease is the commonest haemorrhagic disease in this country.

Key:

◯ Normal female

☐ Normal man

● Affected with von Willebrand's disease, examined by coagulation tests

◕ With bleeding symptoms, not examined

◯ Normal, examined by coagulation test

2) HEREDITY

Most authors agree that the disease is inherited as an autosomal dominant character (Nilsson, Blombäck and v. Francken, 1957; Achenbach, 1960; Silwer, 1973). Its penetrance and expression have been found to vary. Silwer (1973) has recently surveyed all known cases of von Willebrand's disease in Sweden. He found the disease in relatives of probands in 88 per cent of the families examined. The penetrance, as judged from examination of the parents, was 73–90 per cent. The expression varied widely, often within the same family. But analysis of variance showed that the expression regarding the AHF content was much more uniform in the sibships than between unrelated patients. Like other authors, Silwer found the disease to be much more common among females than among males. He found the risk of the child of a person with von Willebrand's disease developing a clinically manifest haemorrhagic diathesis, to be 40 per cent. The probability of severe bleeding disease was much lower, namely barely 4 per cent, whether the affected parent had the severe or mild form of the disease.

Figure 30 gives a pedigree of the largest family in Sweden with von

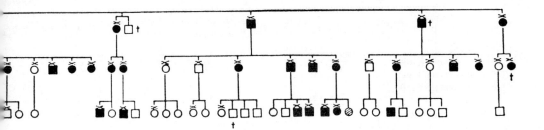

Willebrand's disease (Silwer and Nilsson, 1964). This family has 51 affected members. The family consists of 123 members belonging to four generations. Of the 41 members in generation III, 24 had a prolonged Ivy bleeding time and low AHF values. Of the 71 members in generation IV the disease has been diagnosed in 19.

3) PATHOGENESIS

The finding that it was possible to correct the prolonged bleeding time in von Willebrand's disease by injection of human fraction I-O opened up a new approach to the investigation of the pathogenesis. Table 6 shows the effect of administration of different preparations on patients with von Willebrand's disease (Nilsson, Blombäck and v. Francken, 1957; Nilsson, Blombäck and Blombäck, 1959; Nilsson and Blombäck, 1963). Fraction I-O prepared from fresh normal plasma raised the AHF content and normalised the bleeding time. The AHF content successively increased during the first 24 hours after the injection of fraction I-O. The fraction thus appeared to stimulate the production of AHF. Fraction I-O has a high content of fibrinogen. Yet the infusion of highly purified fibrinogen had no effect on the bleeding time or the AHF content. Fraction I-O prepared from plasma from patients with severe haemophilia A completely controlled the bleeding time. After injection of this haemophilic fraction, which contained no AHF activity, the patient's AHF activity began to rise after about 2 hours, and within 10 hours it had risen by about 30 per cent. Cornu, et al. (1961) of Paris and van Creveld and Mochtar (1960) of Amsterdam have since confirmed these findings. Barrow and Graham (1964) have reported that the AHF produced in a person with von Willebrand's disease after injection of haemophilia A plasma behaves in the same way as normal AHF when heated, on change of pH and in the thromboplastin generation test. Fraction I-O prepared from plasma from patients with von Willebrand's disease had, in contrast with the haemophilic fraction, no effect on the bleeding time or the AHF content.

Normal fraction I-O had the same effect on the bleeding time whether it was prepared from platelet-rich or platelet-poor plasma. Transfusion of platelets had no effect. Infusion of fresh plasma prepared from blood collected in siliconised tubes, of volume 400–1.000 ml, increased the

Preparation	Effect of preparation		
	Increase in AHF content	Normalisation of bleeding time	Increase in fibrinogen content
I–0 from normal plasma	+	+	+
I–0 from haemophilia A plasma	+	+	+
I–1–A (AHF separated from I–0)	+	+	+
I–2–F (fibrinogen separated from normal I–0)	—	—	—
Purified fibrinogen from bank blood	—	—	+
Platelet suspension	—	—	—
Fresh plasma (silicone-technique)	+	+	—

Table 6. Effect various preparatio on patients with v Willebrand's disease.

AHF content and normalised the bleeding time. Injection of corresponding volumes of serum or stored plasma had no effect on the AHF content or bleeding time. Albumin had no effect.

Administration of progesterone, ACTH, and cortisone had no effect on the bleeding time or the haemorrhages in von Willebrand's disease.

The nature of the factor missing in von Willebrand's disease, its mode of action and its relation to the AHF deficiency have attracted extensive attention. Some authors (Biggs and Matthews, 1963; Egeberg, 1963; Meili, et al., 1969) believe that the factor that normalises the bleeding time and the factor that stimulates AHF formation in patients with von Willebrand's disease are not identical. We have found a good correlation between AHF deficiency and prolonged bleeding time (Silwer, 1973).

It has often been suggested that von Willebrand's disease is characterised by impairment of aggregation or adhesiveness of the platelets (Zucker, 1963; Salzman, 1963; Ödegaard, Skålhegg and Hellem, 1964; Strauss and Bloom, 1965; Meyer, et al., 1967b). In von Willebrand's disease the platelets are normal with regard to their content of various platelet factors (Nilsson, Blombäck and v. Francken, 1957; Nilsson, Blombäck, Jorpes, Blombäck and Johansson, 1957; Larrieu, et al., 1968). Platelet adhesiveness determined with Hellem's original method is normal in von Willebrand's disease (Cronberg, Nilsson and Silwer, 1966). Salzman (1963), who determined the platelet adhesiveness according to the method devised by him, found the values to be low in most cases of von Willebrand's disease. Similar results have now been reported by several other authors using Salzman's method or modifications of it (Perkins, 1967; Meyer, et al., 1967b; Cronberg, 1968). It is, however, obvious that several normal persons may have low values as measured by Salzman's method, while some patients with von Willebrand's disease may have normal values. In addition there is a relatively poor correlation between the decrease in platelet adhesiveness and the severity of the symptoms. On determination of platelet adhesiveness with Salzman's method in 235 Swedish patients with von Willebrand's disease, we found the values to be clearly decreased in 60 per cent of cases. Certain authors (Lemoyne and Larrieu, 1967) have normalised the platelet adhesiveness according to Salzman, by administration of fresh plasma and AHF-rich plasma concentrate. Bowie, et al. (1969) have also described a further glass bead test for determining platelet adhesiveness. They use heparinised plasma and relatively long glass bead tubes and claim that the method can distinguish between normals and patients with von Willebrand's disease with a high degree of reliability. Other laboratories have, however, found a wide variation with the method (Coller and Zucker, 1971; Rossi and Green, 1972).

In recent years interesting findings have been made in von Willebrand's disease with the aid of the immunoelectrophoretic technique. Zimmerman, et al. (1971a) raised a rabbit antiserum specific to AHF. Immunological analysis showed that in patients with von Willebrand's disease the plasma content of this protein was abnormally small. The content of immunological material in these patients corresponded to the AHF activity. Similar results have been reported by others (Stites, et al., 1971; Holmberg and Nilsson, 1972) also in tests directly on plasma. In von Willebrand's disease the material normally eluted with the void volume on Sepharose is missing (Bouma, et al., 1972). In contrast to the AHF activity, the amount of AHF related antigen in von Willebrand's disease does not increase progressively after infusion of AHF concentrate (Bennett and Ratnoff, 1972; Holmberg and Nilsson, 1973b). The AHF activity may still be high when the antigen has fallen to low levels. The protein which is missing in von Willebrand's disease and which can be determined immunologically should therefore perhaps be called the von Willebrand factor. AHF may be bound to this protein but may also occur in some other form in the plasma.

The von Willebrand factor-AHF-molecule which can be isolated by agarose gel filtration has proved to be able to normalise abnormal platelet adhesiveness in von Willebrand's disease in tests with tubes containing glass beads (Bouma, et al., 1972). It is probable that this molecule is necessary *in vivo* for quick adhesion of platelets to an injured vessel wall. If the content of the substance is low, formation of a platelet plug will be defective and the bleeding time prolonged.

4) CRITERIA FOR DIAGNOSIS OF VON WILLEBRAND'S DISEASE
In order to establish a firm diagnosis of von Willebrand's disease the patient should have:
1. Positive history of bleeding
2. Positive heredity (autosomal dominant inheritance)
3. Prolonged bleeding time according to Ivy and, as a rule, also according to Duke
4. AHF deficiency: < 60 per cent
5. Decreased platelet adhesiveness according to Salzman and/or Bowie.

In our opinion a diagnosis of von Willebrand's disease is also warranted under the following conditions:

A. Relatives not available for examination, but the patient fills the above requirements 1 and 3–5.

B. Typical disease in the family, but the patient need not satisfy all the requirements 3–5.

All persons in whom abnormal values have been found at any of the examinations enumerated above under 3–5 should be re-examined on one or more occasions. If the diagnosis is then still uncertain, fraction I-O or some other AHF concentrate containing von Willebrand factor should be given, to ascertain whether the patient responds with normalisation of the bleeding time and a progressive rise of AHF characteristic of von Willebrand's disease. From a differential-diagnostic point of view von Willebrand's disease must be distinguished from, above all, mild haemophilia A and from the carrier state of haemophilia A in females, where the decrease of AHF is the most dominant abnormal finding under points 3–5, and from primary platelet defect in those cases where the prolongation of the bleeding time and/or decreased platelet adhesiveness according to Salzman are the dominating findings. The best way to distinguish mild haemophilia A from von Willebrand's disease is to study the AHF response after infusion of AHF concentrate. By special examination of platelet adhesiveness and aggregation it is generally easy to distinguish von Willebrand's disease from platelet defects.

Two methods are available for determining the bleeding time, *viz.,* Duke's method and Ivy's method. In Duke's method the tip of the ear is pricked with a lancet and the interval between the incision and the cessation of bleeding is determined (see Methods). In Ivy's method as modified by Borchgrevink and Waaler the veins of the lower arm are occluded and three transverse incisions, 1 mm deep and 10–14 mm long, are made on the lower arm with a surgical blade and the mean bleeding time of these three incisions is used (Borchgrevink and Waaler, 1958; Nilsson, Magnusson and Borchgrevink, 1963). Comparison between Ivy's and Duke's method has shown that Ivy's method is much more sensitive (Nilsson, Magnusson and Borchgrevink, 1963; Abildgaard, Ch.,et al., 1968). In cases of von Willebrand's disease with mild bleeding symptoms as well as in other cases of haemorrhagic diathesis with a prolonged bleeding time the Duke bleeding time may be normal or only slightly prolonged, while the Ivy bleeding time is always clearly prolonged. In cases of von Willebrand's disease with severe bleeding symptoms, both the Duke and Ivy bleeding times are usually prolonged. In the investigation of patients with suspected von Willebrand's disease it is therefore recommended to use Duke's method first. If the bleeding time according to this method is normal or only slightly prolonged, the bleeding time is determined according to Ivy's method. If the Duke bleeding time is markedly prolonged, there is no reason to perform the test according to the method of Ivy. The bleeding time in von Willebrand's disease tends to be shorter with advancing age.

The normal AHF level, as measured by different methods, lies between 60 and 140 per cent. In patients with severe von Willebrand's disease the value may be below 15 per cent and occasionally as low as in cases of moderate haemophilia A, i.e. 1–4 per cent. In less severe cases of von Willebrand's disease the level may vary from 15–20 per cent up to almost the lower limit of the normal range. In the evaluation of the AHF value it should be borne in mind that in women with von Willebrand's disease the value is increased if they use P-pills, if they are pregnant, or if they are in the menopause. In von Willebrand's disease the level of the AHF is not so stable as in haemophilia. In patients with von Willebrand's disease the AHF rises also during reactive processes. The AHF content is also higher in elderly affected patients than in younger ones with an initially equally severe form of the disease.

Platelet adhesiveness, as measured by the method of Salzman, gives values above 20 per cent in normals, and in von Willebrand's disease lower values, often down to 0 per cent. The method has several sources of error and in our hands it gives false positive results or false negative results more often than does the bleeding time. This method, when compared with the bleeding time and AHF, also has the disadvantage that it does not allow such clear grading of the severity of the disease.

Patients with von Willebrand's disease can be classified as severe or mild according to the following characteristics:

Severe von Willebrand's disease
    Severe bleeding symptoms
    Markedly prolonged Duke bleeding time (as a rule >20 minutes)
    Ivy bleeding time >30 minutes
    AHF content of 1–20 per cent

Mild von Willebrand's disease
    As a rule only mild bleeding symptoms
    Duke bleeding time normal or slightly prolonged (< 20 minutes)
    Ivy bleeding time prolonged
    AHF content 20–60 per cent

5) SYMPTOMS

The clinical picture of von Willebrand's disease has been described in detail by von Willebrand himself and since then by several other authors. Silwer (1973) in his monograph of Swedish cases has given a detailed description as well as the frequency of the bleeding symptoms in severe and mild von Willebrand's disease.

In our patients with *severe von Willebrand's disease* the bleeding symptoms usually appeared within the first year of life. The severe cases thus had a haemorrhagic diathesis from infancy, manifest in the form of bruises, bleeding from the gums, nose-bleeding and abnormal bleeding after trauma and cuts. Further, the patients have had gastro-intestinal bleeding, haematuria, intraabdominal bleeding, as a rule owing to ruptured ovarian cysts, and profuse menstrual flow. Tooth extraction and surgical operations, even minor operations, have caused severe bleeding in all patients. Joint bleeding has occurred in half of the cases. These patients had AHF values of 1–4 per cent. In several cases permanent impairment of the range of movement of single joints have occurred, though not complete disability. X-ray examination has shown skeletal and joint changes of the same type as in haemophilia. The profuse menstrual bleeding has been a troublesome problem. One patient has died, and in three it was necessary to perform hysterectomy or X-ray sterilisation before the age of 16 years. Ovarian bleeding has been demonstrated in several of the women. In addition, several women have been operated upon because of ovarian cysts which have probably formed as a consequence of follicular bleeding. Women with severe von Willebrand's disease gave birth successfully only under treatment with fraction I-O. A special group of traumatic haemorrhages is intracranial bleeding, which in two of our cases proved fatal. These patients had AHF values between 1–2 per cent. These cases may be compared with haemophilia where intracranial haemorrhage is now the commonest cause of death. Gastrointestinal bleeding, in contrast with what is seen in the majority of other types of bleeding, occurred mainly in adult age. It has been extremely serious and sometimes fatal. Only in one fatal case has an X-ray demonstrated a peptic ulcer. The symptom which usually resulted in discovery of the disease in children was persistent bleeding after biting of the tongue or lip. It is remarkable that the severity of the bleeding decreases with increasing age. The bleeding symptoms in severe von Willebrand's disease are not so serious as in severe haemophilia A and the prognosis for the patients is therefore much better, especially with modern therapeutic methods.

Patients with *mild von Willebrand's disease* have only mild spontaneous bleeding, mainly nose-bleeding, gingival bleeding, bruises and profuse menstruations. Yet occasionally gastro-intestinal bleeding and haematuria have been the predominant symptoms. Even in these mild cases the gastro-intestinal bleeding has been severe and occasionally even fatal. Also in these mild cases the tendency to bleeding has been markedly increased during tooth extraction, surgery and major trauma. Several cases of mild von Willebrand's disease have been discovered by bleeding complications at tooth extraction and operations on the ear, nose or throat. In half of the women with mild von Willebrand's disease the menstrual flow is profuse. In our series 11 per cent of pregnant women required blood transfusions at delivery. The reason why abnormal bleeding at delivery was relatively uncommon is probably that the AHF level and the bleeding time tend to approach normal levels during pregnancy. When abnormal bleeding occurred it often did so about one week or more after delivery. Also in patients with mild von Willebrand's disease the bleeding symptoms are most troublesome during childhood and adolescence. The patients with mild von Willebrand's disease have been able to lead a normal life and have even been able to manage heavy manual labour.

6) TREATMENT

The discovery of AHF deficiency and lack of a bleeding factor (von Willebrand factor) in the plasma has, since 1956, made it possible to give specific therapeutic and prophylactic treatment of the bleeding in von Willebrand's disease. As pointed out previously, fraction I-O, which contains both AHF and von Willebrand factor, can be used for specific therapy. It has now been shown (Bennett and Dormandy, 1966; Perkins, 1967; Meili, et al., 1969; Owen, et al., 1970) that cryoprecipitate also normalises the bleeding time in von Willebrand's disease and can be used to advantage in the treatment of the disease. Fresh plasma can also be used in those cases not requiring more intensive substitution therapy.

Patients with von Willebrand's disease should be treated essentially in the same way as patients with haemophilia A. To achieve effective haemostasis, transfusion should be given in such quantities that the Duke bleeding time is kept normal throughout. On the other hand, it is not necessary to normalise the Ivy bleeding time (Nilsson, Magnusson and Borchgrevink, 1963). During bleeding episodes and surgical operations the AHF content should be raised to the same level as in haemophilia A. The interval between the doses in von Willebrand's disease may be longer than in haemophilia A because of the progressive increase in AHF obtained in these patients. Table 7 gives suggestions for the treatment of various bleedings in von Willebrand's disease.

It should be observed that menorrhagia in patients with von Willebrand's disease can be treated with a good effect with EACA or AMCA (Nilsson and Björkman, 1965). In menorrhagia also P-pills of combined type have proved useful.

3. Haemorrhagic disorder resembling both haemophilia A and von Willebrand's disease

In an immunological investigation of the Swedish patients with von Willebrand's disease, Holmberg and Nilsson (1972, 1973b) found some families where the affected members had a normal content of AHF related protein despite a low AHF activity and a prolonged bleeding time. The disease appeared to be transmitted by the X-chromosome and in some respects it therefore resembled haemophilia A. But females in these families had much more troublesome bleedings than carriers of haemophilia. A similar family has also been described by Egeberg (1965b).

4. Haemophilia C

Haemophilia C (Factor XI deficiency, PTA deficiency, was first described by Rosenthal, Dreskin and Rosenthal, 1953) in a report of an investigation of a family with bleeders. Two siblings and their maternal uncle had a mild bleeding disease, which Rosenthal, et al., showed to be due to deficiency of a previously unknown plasma factor for which they coined the term 'plasma thromboplastin antecedent' or PTA. Since then more

Table 7.   Treatment recommended in different situations in von Willebrand's disease.

	Desired lab. values for			Severe cases		Mild cases	
	AHF	Duke (min)	Duration of treatment	Dose AHF/ 24 hrs (U/kg b.w.)	Substitute	Dose AHF/ 24 hrs (U/kg b.w.)	Substitute
Major surgical operations							
Tonsillectomy Gastrectomy Cholecystectomy Hysterectomy	40–70% during op and first postop days, 30–40% till about seventh day, afterwards 10–15% till healed	≦5	2–3 weeks	Days 1–2: 20–40 Days 3–8: 10–20 Days >8: 5–10	1) Cryopre- cipitate, possibly with plasma 2) AHF- Kabi possibly with plasma	Days 1–2: 15–30 Days 3–8: 5–15	1) Plasma 2) Cryopreci pitate 3) AHF- Kabi
Minor surgical operations							
Tooth extraction Appendectomy Herniorrhaphy	20–50% during op, later about 15% for 6–8 days	≦5	6–8 days	Day 1: 15–20 Days 2–8: 5–10	1) Cryopre- cipitate, possibly with plasma 2) AHF- Kabi, possibly with plasma 3) Plasma	Day 1: 5–15 Days 2–8: 5	1) Plasma 2) Cryoprec pitate 3) AHF- Kabi
Delivery	As for major surgery		2–4 weeks	As for major surgery		As for minor surgery	
Severe haemorrhagic conditions							
Gastro-intestinal bleeding Severe menorrhagia Head injury Intracranial haemorrhage Postop haemorrhage	20–50%	≦5	About 7 days	15–20	1) Cryopre- cipitate, possibly with plasma 2) AHF- Kabi, possibly with plasma 3) Plasma	5–15	1) Cryoprec pitate 2) AHF- Kabi 3) Plasma
Minor bleeding episodes							
Superficial injuries Nose bleeding Haematuria	15–20%	≦10	2–5 days	5–10	1) Cryopre- cipitate 2) AHF- Kabi 3) Plasma	0–5	Possibly plasma

than 200 cases of PTA deficiency have been described. It is a rare congenital disease. It occurs in both males and females and manifests itself as a mild haemorrhagic diathesis. The condition has been described as being more common among women than among men. It is also said to be relatively common among Jews. The symptoms may be nose-bleeding, profuse bleeding after trauma, menorrhagia and abnormal bleeding after tooth extraction and surgical operations. Spontaneous bleeding is rare. Several authors (Rapaport, et al., 1961; Egeberg, 1962a; Todd and Wright, 1964; Edson, et al., 1967) have, however, reported cases in which laboratory tests have shown PTA deficiency in persons with no abnormal bleeding tendency. Rosenthal, et al. (1953), who first described the disease, claimed that it is inherited as an autosomal dominant character. On the basis of investigations of some families with haemophilia C, Rapaport, et al. (1961) claim that the disease is transmitted as a recessive autosomal character and that only homozygotes have clinical symptoms.

The frequency of the disease is not known with certainty. Rosenthal (1961) observed as many cases of haemophilia C as of classical haemophilia. Biggs and Macfarlane (1966) had diagnosed only three cases. Ratnoff (1960a) reported that he had not seen any cases at all. In Sweden we know of 32 patients belonging to 17 families who, according to our tests, have haemophilia C. Conrad, et al. (1965) from Texas reports that he has found haemophilia C substantially more often than haemophilia A and B. This variation in the distribution might be explained in part by diagnostic problems, as pointed out by several authors (de Vries and Braat-van Straaten, 1964; Edson, et al., 1967 and others).

The diagnosis of haemophilia C is difficult to establish. The bleeding disease is said to be characterised by normal or mildly prolonged coagulation time in glass tubes, normal or prolonged coagulation in siliconised tubes, abnormal prothrombin consumption, which, however, need not always be demonstrable in a given patient, abnormal thromboplastin generation test if this test is performed with both adsorbed plasma and with serum from the patient. The partial thromboplastin time may be normal or slightly prolonged. The platelet count and other coagulation factors have been described as normal. The one-stage prothrombin time is also normal. It should be observed that in several cases the bleeding time has been described as prolonged (White, et al., 1963; Conrad, et al., 1965). Karaca and Nilsson (1972) recently described a case of severe PTA deficiency and prolonged bleeding time. In that case the patient showed a defective release of ADP and of PF-3 as well as a rapid disaggregation of the platelets. Transfusion studies in this case argued against the Factor XI deficiency being related to the platelet defect.

For quantitative determination of Factor XI, one-stage methods have been described with the use of a test base in which Factor XI has been removed by adsorption with Celite, kaolin or glass (see Waaler, 1959; Soulier, et al., 1959; Horowitz, et al., 1963; Nossel, 1964). The test base most often used is 'Celite exhausted plasma'. But it is not possible to produce a test base absolutely free from Factor XI by adsorption with

Celite or kaolin without at the same time adsorbing Factor XII. Further, the Factor XI defect may be normalised by freezing of plasma (Rosenthal, 1955). If Factor XI deficiency plasma is available, however, only small amounts of Celite can be added to obtain 'exhausted plasma'. To distinguish between haemophilia C and Hageman trait by these one-stage methods it is necessary to have Hageman deficiency plasma available and to determine the content of Hageman factor in a separate test system. Biggs and Macfarlane (1966) used the thromboplastin generation test to demonstrate Factor XI deficiency. It has been pointed out by Horowitz, et al. (1963) (and we have made the same observation) that the coagulation defect in a given patient may vary considerably from one occasion to another. In haemophilia A and B the coagulation defect is always stable.

No specific treatment is available for haemophilia C. In the event of bleeding the patient should be treated with blood and plasma transfusions. It is not necessary to use fresh blood. According to Rosenthal and Sloan (1965), the half-life of Factor XI after infusion of plasma is 40–84 hours. All operations should be performed under the protection of plasma.

5. Hageman Trait

The value of genetic studies in the investigation of the normal coagulation mechanism has been clearly exemplified in the peculiar syndrome, Hageman's disease, or more correctly, Hageman trait. As pointed out earlier, Ratnoff (1954) was the first to describe this defect. The disorder is characterised by a markedly prolonged coagulation time in glass tubes and siliconised tubes, though the patients themselves show no signs of an increased bleeding tendency. The prolonged coagulation time is due to deficiency of a specific coagulation promoting substance, Hageman factor or Factor XII. Hageman factor is necessary for coagulation to occur at a normal rate in a test tube, but its effect *in vivo* is not known. At any rate, its deficiency or absence causes no haemostatic disorders. As in PTA deficiency, the patients have an abnormal prothrombin consumption and abnormal thromboplastin generation test if the test is performed with both adsorbed plasma and serum from the patients. All other coagulation factors are normal (see Ratnoff, 1965). Walsh (1970) has found platelet adhesiveness as estimated by Salzman's method to be decreased in patients with the Hageman trait. Platelet studies, however, produce no evidence for defective aggregation.

Loeliger and Hensen (1961a) and Haanen, et al. (1960) advanced the hypothesis that in patients with the Hageman trait there is no deficiency of Factor XII but instead an abnormal Hageman-protein, which cannot be activated by glass. Smink, et al. (1967) have, however, stated that with the immunologic technique they were unable to demonstrate any antigen identical with the Hageman factor in patients with the Hageman trait.

If Hageman deficient plasma is available as a test base, it is possible to determine the Factor XII content in a one-stage system.

No studies are available on the frequency of the Hageman trait. Such cases are discovered only incidentally for they produce no bleeding symptoms. Ratnoff (1965) feels that the disorder is rare. About 140 cases equally distributed among males and females have been identified with certainty (Ratnoff, 1965; Baumann and Straub, 1968). In Sweden we know of six cases of Hageman trait. It is a hereditary coagulation defect and transmitted as an autosomal recessive character (Ratnoff, 1965; Baumann and Straub, 1968).

Operations have been performed on Hageman patients without any special prophylactic measures against bleeding and without signs of abnormal bleeding. Cases of myocardial infarction have also been observed in patients with Hageman factor deficiency (Hoak, et al., 1966). Mr Hageman died in 1968 from pulmonary embolism (Ratnoff, Busse and Sheon 1968).

B. *Defects in phase II—conversion of prothrombin to thrombin*

Defects in phase II can be recognised in screening tests by the following characteristics:

Normal platelet count
Normal Duke and Ivy bleeding time
Prolonged or normal coagulation time in glass tubes and plastic tubes
Prolonged cephalin time or partial thromboplastin time
Prolonged activated partial thromboplastin time
Prolonged one-stage prothrombin time
Normal fibrinogen content
Decreased P&P-test (Prothrombin-Proconvertin test) or normotest or thrombotest in deficiency of Factors II, VII and X.

Of other methods useful for distinguishing defects in phase II, mention might be made of the Stypven time. As pointed out earlier, Stypven plus phospholipids have an effect corresponding to that of tissue thromboplastin plus Factor VII. The Stypven time is thus normal in the presence of Factor VII deficiency, but prolonged in other defects in phase II. Special methods are available for separate testing of the different factors in phase II (see Methods).

In phase II the following hereditary coagulation defects may be distinguished:

Prothrombin deficiency
Factor V deficiency
Factor VII deficiency
Factor X deficiency

These hereditary deficiencies are rare and of less clinical importance than the congenital deficiencies in phase I. The commonest causes of a decreased content of the factors in phase II are acquired deficiencies, e.g. dicoumarol therapy and liver diseases. The acquired defects are discussed in the chapter on acquired deficiencies (page 201).

1. Congenital prothrombin deficiency

Isolated prothrombin deficiency is extremely rare. In most published cases further analysis has shown that the symptoms were due to Factor VII or Factor X deficiency instead. About 15 cases are on record in which there was evidence of congenital prothrombin deficiency (see Girolami, et al., 1970a). In these cases, however, prothrombin was not completely lacking, but was decreased to about 10 per cent of normal. These patients had moderate bleeding symptoms consisting of haematuria, haematoma and increased bleeding tendency after trauma and surgical operations. Data about the published cases suggest that the gene causing prothrombin deficiency is recessive and not sex-linked.

2. Congenital Factor VII and Factor X deficiency

Several cases of what was believed to be hereditary prothrombin deficiency were published in the 1940s. In several of these, however, the prolonged one-state prothrombin time (Quick-time) could be normalised by addition of serum, which does not contain prothrombin. Alexander, et al. (1949) and Owren (1952), who had patients with a markedly prolonged one-stage prothrombin time, which was normalised after addition of serum, stated, however, that the deficiency in these cases was not due to lack of prothrombin but to some other factor, *viz.,* Factor VII or proconvertin.

Several cases of congenital bleeding defects characterised by prolonged one-stage prothrombin time, which was normalised after addition of serum were afterwards classified in the literature as Factor VII deficiency. As mentioned previously, Hougie and Graham (Hougie, et al., 1957; Graham, et al., 1957) and Telfer, et al. (1956) found that plasma from some patients with prolonged one-stage prothrombin time could normalise the one-stage prothrombin time in other patients. It was found that a prolonged one-stage prothrombin time which was normalised by serum could also be due to Factor X deficiency (=Stuart factor).

Girolami, et al. (1970b) described a family with Factor X deficiency where the evidence obtained suggested that the defect was due to an abnormal Factor X. Denson, et al. (1970) have found at least five different types of Factor X defect. They also believe that it is a question of an abnormal protein and that the different types are due to different genetic mutations. Denson, Conard and Samama (1972) also recently suggested that the Factor VII defect is not due to lack of synthesis of Factor VII and that several genetic variants may occur.

Patients with Factor VII deficiency and Factor X deficiency have exactly the same clinical symptoms. The defects are equally common among males and females. The bleeding symptoms usually appear early in childhood and consist of an increased tendency to haematoma and nose-bleeding, menorrhagia, gastro-intestinal bleeding and copious bleeding after trauma, surgical operations and tooth extractions. A few single cases have been described with haemarthrosis. But the bleeding

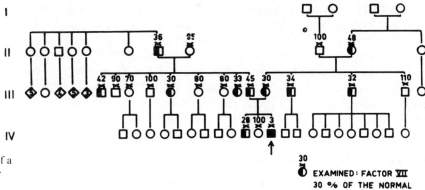

Fig 31. Pedigree of a family with Factor VII deficiency. Symbols as in Fig 26, page 66.

symptoms are relatively mild and resemble most closely those seen in mild haemophilia. The differential diagnosis between Factor VII deficiency and Factor X deficiency is based on laboratory findings.

In Factor VII deficiency the coagulation time is normal or slightly prolonged, the one-stage prothrombin time is prolonged, and the P&P value is low. The Stypven time is normal. The thromboplastin generation test is normal. Exact determination of Factor VII content is possible if plasma is available from a patient with congenital deficiency of Factor VII activity (for references on congenital Factor VII deficiency see Owen, et al., 1964; Marder and Shulman, 1964; Mandelli, et al., 1969).

Factor X deficiency is characterised by a mildly prolonged coagulation time, prolonged one-stage prothrombin time and decreased P&P value. The Stypven time is prolonged. The thromboplastin generation test is said to give abnormal values if the test is performed with the patient's serum. The exact amount of Factor X can be determined if the examiner has access to plasma from a patient with congenital Factor X deficiency (for references on congenital Factor X deficiency see Graham, et al., 1957; Lechler, et al., 1965; Kurz, et al., 1969).

Most authors are of the opinion that the diseases are inherited as autosomal recessive characters.

In Sweden we know of four families with Factor VII deficiency in which the disease is transmitted by an autosomal recessive gene. Fig. 31 shows the pedigree for a Factor VII deficiency family. The proband in this family was a 4-year old boy with nose-bleeding, haematoma and bleeding after tooth extraction. He was the only member of the family with manifest bleeding symptoms, but we have found several members of his family with decreased Factor VII values between 25–50 per cent of the normal. Thus, the mother and the father and the paternal grandfather and maternal grandmother had Factor VII deficiency. It is thus only homozygotes who have bleeding symptoms. In some of the cases with Factor VII deficiency immunologic prothrombin determination was done according to Ganrot and Niléhn. Normal values were found. In Sweden we know of only one family with congenital Factor X deficiency.

Factor VII deficiency and Factor X deficiency are treated in the same way. In bleedings and surgical operations plasma may be given as substitution therapy, but it need not be fresh plasma. Even concentrates of prothrombin factors of such types as PPSB, Konyne, and Oxford 'routine', all of which have a high activity of Factor VII and Factor X may be used to advantage. The half-life of Factor VII has been reported as 4 hours initially and then 20 hours (Bowie, et al., 1967). The half-life of Factor X has been given as 35–50 hours (Bowie, et al., 1967).

3. Congenital Factor V deficiency

Congenital Factor V deficiency was first described by Owren (1947) in Oslo. He called the disease parahaemophilia. It is an extremely rare disease. So far, only about 30 families with the condition have been recorded. The bleeding symptoms may resemble those of haemophilia, but no associated joint bleedings have been reported. The disease is characterised by a prolonged one-stage prothrombin time, which is corrected by addition of adsorbed prothrombin-free plasma, but not by addition of stored plasma (for references see Ratnoff, 1960a; Lopez, et al., 1969). Factor V is a labile substance and for treatment of the condition fresh plasma must be used. The half-life of Factor V has been described as 16 hours (Bowie, et al., 1967). The exact mode of inheritance is not known. According to some authors, it is transmitted by an autosomal recessive gene (Kingsley, 1954), while other authors believe that it is transmitted by a dominant gene (López, et al., 1969).

C. *Defects in phase III—conversion of fibrinogen to fibrin*

Coagulation defects in this phase comprise conditions associated with a fibrinogen deficiency or with a fibrinogen defect and conditions with lack of fibrin stabilising factor (Factor XIII). A decreased content of fibrinogen due to fibrinolysis or intravascular coagulation is discussed in a separate chapter (page 111).

1. Congenital afibrinogenaemia and hypofibrinogenaemia

Congenital absence of fibrinogen is rare and, so far, only 60 cases are on record (Rabe and Salomon, 1920; Prichard and Vann, 1954; Soulier, et al., 1955; Bommer, et al., 1963, and others). The mode of inheritance is not known with certainty, but cumulative evidence suggests that its transmission is recessive and not sex-linked. Thus, in at least 7 of the reported families the patients were children of cousins, and in at least 4 of the cases low fibrinogen values have been demonstrated in both parents. It is thus believed that patients with afibrinogenaemia are homozygotes and that the heterozygotes, at least in some cases, have hypofibrinogenaemia. It appears that patients with congenital deficiency of fibrinogen cannot synthesize fibrinogen. Infused fibrinogen has a normal survival. Patients with complete afibrinogenaemia have bleeding symptoms of the type seen in haemophilia, but much less severe than those in the severe form of haemophilia. Joint bleedings may occur, but not permanent joint deformities. Cases have been published in which the patients have died from umbilical cord bleeding, and in one case from a cut in the finger. Women with afibrinogenaemia have been described as having normal menstruations.

Patients with afibrinogenaemia have incoagulable blood, but the coagulation process is otherwise normal. Addition of thrombin does not result in clotting of the blood. Heating of plasma to 56°C for 10 minutes does not result in the formation of any precipitate. Immunochemical methods have, however, often revealed traces of fibrinogen (for references see Jackson, et al., 1965). The coagulation time, recalcification time and one-stage prothrombin time are infinite. The bleeding time is usually normal. Values found for the other coagulation factors are normal. Patients with protracted bleeding or undergoing surgery should be treated with fibrinogen.

Patients with *congenital hypofibrinogenaemia* have fibrinogen values between 0·01 and 0·10 g/100 ml plasma. Only 20 cases of congenital hypofibrinogenaemia have been reported in the literature (see Hasselback, et al., 1963; Phillips, et al., 1963; Ménaché, 1964b; Caen, Castaldi and Inceman, 1965; Nilsson, Niléhn, Cronberg and Nordén, 1966). These patients have only mild bleeding symptoms or none at all. If the fibrinogen content is < 0·05 g/100 ml only small insignificant clots will form, which are difficult to read. Therefore, coagulation analysis often gives prolonged times for coagulation and for the one-stage prothrombin time. Only during operations do these patients require treatment with fibrinogen.

We have had the opportunity of seeing only one patient with congenital hypofibrinogenaemia (Nilsson, Niléhn, Cronberg and Nordén, 1966). The fibrinogen level was 0·02 g/100 ml. He had no bleeding symptoms. But multiple thrombi developed and the patient died after the major part of the small intestine had been resected after having become gangrenous owing to multiple microthrombi. Autopsy revealed multiple thrombi, probably platelet thrombi, and infarcts in all the visceral organs. The liver was necrotic. A similar case has been described by Caen, et al. (1965).

2. Abnormal fibrinogens

Imperato and Dettori (1958), Ménaché (1964b) and Beck, et al. (1965) were the first to draw attention to abnormal fibrinogens. They described, in all, three patients in whom an abnormal structure of the fibrinogen was thought to be the cause of the fibrin abnormality found in these patients.

Clotting of the plasma from these patients required an abnormally large amount of thrombin. The patients had a normal fibrinogen content, as measured by immunological methods. Addition of Reptilase did not result in any clotting, and plasma from the patients inhibited clotting

*Table 8. Character-
istics of congenital
dysfibrinogenemias.*

Name	Thrombin time	Effect on normal clotting	Major defect*	Reference number
Asymptomatic				
Amsterdam	Prolonged	Inhibitory	A	5
Bethesda II	Prolonged	Inhibitory	A	6
Cleveland	Prolonged	Inhibitory	A	7
Los Angeles	Prolonged	Inhibitory	A	8
Nancy	Prolonged	Slight	A	9
Paris I	Infinite	Inhibitory	U	10
Paris II	Prolonged	Inhibitory	U	11
St. Louis	Prolonged	Inhibitory	A	12
Troyes	Prolonged	Unreported	U	13
Zurich I	Prolonged	Inhibitory	A	14
Zurich II	Prolonged	Inhibitory	A	15
Abnormal bleeding				
Bethesda I	Prolonged	Inhibitory	FP	16
Detroit	Prolonged	Inhibitory	FP	17
Leuven	Prolonged	Slight	A?	18
Metz	Infinite	Unreported	U	13
Oklahoma	Normal	None	U	19
Parma	Infinite	None	U	20
Vancouver	Prolonged	None	U	21
Abnormal thrombosis				
Oslo	Shortened	Unreported	U	22
Bleeding and thrombosis				
Baltimore	Prolonged	None	FP	23
Wiesbaden	Prolonged	Inhibitory	A	24

*A = Aggregation of fibrin monomers; FP = fibrinopeptide release;
U = unreported or uncertain.

From Ann. intern. Med. 77:471, 1972 Gralnick & Finlayson

of normal plasma by thrombin, Reptilase and thromboplastin. The defect was congenital and the patients had only mild bleeding symptoms or none at all. Infused fibrinogen had a normal survival time. It was therefore assumed that in these cases it was a question of an inherited functional disorder of the fibrinogen.

Since then all together 21 families with abnormal fibrinogens have been reported (see Gralnick and Finlayson, 1972) (Table 8). Beck (1971) established the convention of naming the new fibrinogens after the town of discovery, e.g. fibrinogen Baltimore, Paris, Detroit, etc. Jackson, et al. (1965) believe that most of the previously reported cases of afibrinogenaemia and hypofibrinogenaemia are not deficiencies, but conditions due to abnormal fibrinogen. These congenital variants of fibrinogen have usually first been noticed in coagulation tests in which plasma fibrinogen is converted to fibrin, namely thrombin time, Reptilase time and the one-stage prothrombin time. These clotting times are generally prolonged and in some cases no clot forms. A characteristic finding in these cases is also that a low fibrinogen level is obtained in assays based on coagulation methods, but a normal fibrinogen level by immunochemical methods. The fibrinogen variants thus react with antisera to normal fibrinogen, but immunoelectrophoretic and other differences have shown that they have distinctive characteristics. Other coagulation factors are normal and there is no increased fibrinolysis. Some patients were investigated because of a tendency to bleed, while in others the defect was an incidental finding. Some of the patients had both a bleeding tendency and thrombosis. In patients with excessive bleeding, treatment with normal fibrinogen has proved effective. The fibrinogen defects appear to be inherited as an autosomal dominant trait and two forms of fibrinogen have been found in heterozygotes.

Attempts have been made to reveal the defect of the fibrinogens. In most of the cases studied the defects seem to delay aggregation of fibrin monomers, while in only a few cases has a decrease been demonstrated in the rate of release of fibrinopeptides A and B. Only in fibrinogen Detroit has a specific amino acid replacement been shown. Blombäck, M., Blombäck, B., Mammen and Prasad (1968) thus discovered an abnormal fibrinogen in a Negro in Detroit in which homozygotes regarding the abnormal allele had a severe haemorrhagic diathesis. In fibrinogen 'Detroit' they could show substitution of an amino acid in the N-terminal disulphide knot of the Aα-chain. An arginine residue had been replaced by a serine fragment, and this prevented effective activation of the fibrinogen molecule. The fibrinogen peptides were split off in a normal way but the reactive centre was not opened after the separation (Blombäck, B., 1969) (see Fig. 22 page 43).

In recent years also abnormal fibrinogens with defective power of polymerisation have been observed in patients with severe liver diseases (Soria, et al., 1970) and in patients with primary hepatoma (von Felten, et al., 1969; Verhaeghe, et al., 1972).

3. Deficiency of fibrin stabilising factor (Factor XIII)

Congenital deficiency of fibrin stabilising factor (FSF) or Factor XIII is the latest hereditary coagulation defect discovered. Altogether some 50 cases from 30 families are known (see Duckert, et al., 1960; Ikkala and Nevanlinna, 1962; Alami, et al., 1968; Lorand, et al., 1970; Aziz and Siddiqui, 1972; Stefanini, et al., 1972). This defect differs from all other known defects. The coagulation mechanism, including the first stage in the formation of fibrin, the aggregation of fibrin monomers, is normal. The fibrinolytic system and platelet function are also normal. But unlike normal platelets, the platelets do not contain Factor XIII. The only abnormal findings are an abnormal thromboelastographic picture and the solubility of the fibrin clot in 30 per cent urea solution or 1 per cent monochloracetic acid. The patients have oozing protracted bleeding from wounds for 24 to 36 hours after injury. Bleedings from mucosa have not been reported. Haematoma, ecchymoses and bleeding after skin incisions are common. The fibrin formed by these patients is not mechanically strong enough, and its structure makes it very sensitive to proteolytic enzymes and less able to serve its physiological purpose. Characteristic of the disease is also poor wound healing. Beck, et al. (1961) have shown that Factor XIII is necessary for the normal growth of fibroblasts.

Most methods for assaying Factor XIII have been based on the ability of the activated factor to convert simple fibrin gels into the acid- or urea-insoluble form. The amount of insoluble clot formed has been taken as an index of cross-linking. Dilution of the factor to a threshold level of activity has provided the basis for quantitative analysis. According to Lorand, et al. (1969), the assays based on clot solubility are particularly difficult to interpret quantitatively when direct testing of the Factor XIII content of plasma is required. With these methods, which have been used in most published cases of Factor XIII deficiency, it has probably been possible to demonstrate only cases with severe Factor XIII deficiency. On addition of only 1 per cent of normal plasma the clots of the patients became insoluble in 5 M urea solution. A new sensitive method based on amine incorporation has been worked out by Lorand, et al. (1969) for measuring the activity of Factor XIII in plasma. This has opened up new possibilities for diagnostic and genetic studies of Factor XIII.

The exact plasma level of Factor XIII necessary to prevent bleeding is not known, but it has been suggested that a level as low as 2–3 per cent is sufficient. Since the half-life of this factor is of the order of 3–6 days, it is easy to maintain a haemostatic level by means of plasma or blood transfusions once every 7–10 days (Ikkala, et al., 1964). The mode of inheritance of the disease is not known with certainty. Recent family studies by Lorand, et al. (1970), however, have shown that the Factor XIII levels, as assayed by the amine incorporation assay, are equally decreased in both fathers and mothers in families with only affected males and in families with affected females, supporting the concept that congenital Factor XIII deficiency is transmitted as an autosomal recessive trait.

Acquired Factor XIII deficiency has been described in patients with myeloma, lead poisoning, pernicious anaemia, agammaglobulinaemia, liver diseases and renal diseases (Lorand and Jacobsen, 1958; Nussbaum and Morse, 1964; Losowsky and Walls, 1969). In patients with acquired Factor XIII deficiency in the plasma, the Factor XIII content of the platelets is normal. Patients with congenital afibrinogenaemia have a normal Factor XIII content (Kiesselbach and Wagner, 1966). In addition, inhibitors may appear in the circulation and interfere either with the activation of Factor XIII or with the action of the formed Factor XIII (Lorand, et al., 1969, 1972). Several of the patients with inhibitors had been treated with isoniazid, which is a substrate for transamidating enzymes. These patients had severe bleeding symptoms.

Fibrinolysis, thrombolysis and defibrination

I. Fibrinolysis and thrombolysis

Fibrinolysis is the process which in health and in disease causes an enzymatic dissolution of fibrinogen and fibrin clots. It is now generally accepted that thrombi formed in the blood stream can be dissolved enzymatically and that the circulation through the vessels can be restored by activation of the fibrinolytic system in the body. It is evident that a defective or deficient function of the fibrinolytic mechanism can favour the growth, and impair the dissolution, of thrombi.

A distinction is generally made between fibrinolysis and thrombolysis. Fibrinolysis is the proteolytic activity arising in the circulating blood on activation of the fibrinolytic system and formation of plasmin. Thrombolysis is the corresponding sequence of events in formed thrombi, and their subsequent dissolution.

A. *The fibrinolytic system*

Plasma normally contains a protein substance, plasminogen, which under the influence of various activators is converted to plasmin, which is a proteolytic enzyme, whose activity resembles that of trypsin (Fig. 32). Plasmin attacks, above all, fibrinogen and fibrin molecules, but can also digest other plasma proteins, such as Factor V and Factor VIII (AHF). Plasmin breaks down fibrinogen and fibrin to fibrin/fibrinogen degradation products, which inhibit the conversion of fibrinogen to fibrin (fibrin/fibrinogen degradation products are discussed separately, see page 127). The activation of plasminogen can be inhibited by inhibitors in the blood or by synthetic substances, such as epsilon-aminocaproic acid (EACA) and its homologues. The action of plasmin can be inhibited by α_2-macroglobulin (immediate reacting antiplasmin) as well as by α_1-antitrypsin (slow reacting antiplasmin).

The presence of free plasmin in the blood results in the creation of multiple defects in the process of haemostasis. The fibrinolytic bleeding defect thus includes 1) dissolution of formed thrombi, 2) breakdown of fibrinogen, Factor V and AHF, 3) inhibition of polymerisation of fibrin by fibrin/fibrinogen degradation products with a defective clot as a result.

A survey of the various components of the fibrinolytic system is given as follows.

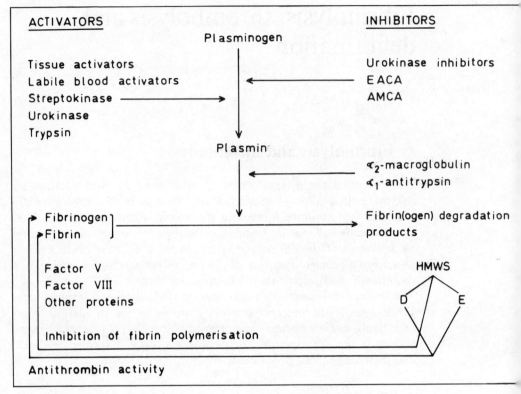

Fig 32. The fibrinolytic system.

1. Plasminogen

Plasminogen (profibrinolysin), the inactive precursor of plasmin, is a β-globulin. Plasminogen can be precipitated from plasma and serum at pH 5·3 and at low ionic strength. It was Milstone (1941) who first observed that the plasminogen resides in the euglobulin fraction from plasma and serum. Remmert and Cohen (1949) concentrated plasminogen 135–165 times by repeated euglobulin precipitation from $(NH_4)_2SO_4$ or ethanol precipitate from human serum and by the use of kaolin as an adsorbent. The method is difficult to reproduce and has not been widely used. Christensen and Smith (1950) showed that plasminogen can be extracted from Cohn's fraction III by diluted mineral acids at pH 2. On the basis of this observation Kline (1953) devised a method for purifying plasminogen. The method includes two extraction procedures with acid. Kline reported a 400-fold higher specific activity of this preparation compared with that of the total plasma protein. But the strong acid environment in the production of preparations by Kline's method gives them undesirable physico-chemical characteristics. These plasminogen preparations are not soluble at neutral pH, but they are soluble at pH below 4 and above 8. The discovery that small amounts of certain amino acids such as lysine, arginine and EACA, markedly increase the solubility of these plasminogen preparations in neutral buffers, was a considerable advance (Alkjaersig, et al., 1959b). Wallén and Bergström (1960) have produced a highly purified plasminogen preparation by adsorbing Cohn's fraction II + III with DEAE-cellulose from a solution in 0·04 M $(NH_4)_2SO_4$ buffer at pH 9 and eluting it with the same buffer containing 0·01 M lysine or 0·01 M EACA. The preparation was purified 500 times, compared with plasma. This plasminogen preparation is stable and soluble at neutral pH. This principle with avoidance of acid extraction has since been utilised in several methods for purifiying plasminogen (Mosesson, 1962; Alkjaersig, 1964; Robbins, et al., 1965).

Estimates of its molecular weight vary because of the difficulty in obtaining plasminogen in pure form (Barlow, et al., 1969; Robbins and Summaria, 1971). During preparation, proteolytic degradation may occur by autocatalytic activation (Wallén and Wiman, 1972). Wallén and Wiman (1970) have produced evidence of the existence of different native components of plasminogen, which can be separated by starch gel-electrophoresis. Other components may appear owing to proteolytic degradation during isolation procedures. These workers give molecular weights ranging from 90.000 to 115.000 in the presence of EACA, whereas Robbins and Summaria (1971) give 81.000. Robbins, et al. (1967) described the plasminogen molecule as a single polypeptide chain with 22 disulphide bonds. The molecule contains an arginyl-valine bond, which can be cleaved by an activator converting the plasminogen to a plasmin molecule.

Bovine plasminogen cannot be activated directly by streptokinase, but only after addition of human globulin. Astrup (1956) and Müllertz and Lassen (1953) therefore assumed that streptokinase was active only in the presence of a factor occurring especially in human plasma. They called this factor proactivator. It has, however, not been possible to separate plasminogen and proactivator. It is now widely believed that the properties of plasminogen differ with species and that plasminogen and proactivator activity are linked to different active centres of the plasminogen molecule (Kline and Fishman, 1961; de Renzo, et al., 1965). Plasminogen as well as plasmin has a high affinity for fibrinogen and fibrin. Preparations of fibrinogen are therefore contaminated with plasminogen. Several methods have been devised for eliminating such contamination, e.g. precipitation with ethanol in the presence of lysine or EACA, chromatography, gel-filtration, adsorption to charcoal and bentonite (see page 39).

Plasminogen contaminating fibrin can be destroyed by heating (Lassen, 1952), but the fibrin is thereby partly denatured and less sensitive to plasmin.

The fibrin plate method (Astrup and Müllertz, 1952; Lassen, 1952) is based on the fact that ordinary preparations of human and bovine fibrinogen are contaminated with plasminogen, which makes it possible to measure not only plasmin activity, but also the plasminogen activator activity of plasma. By denaturing the plasminogen by heating the fibrin plates, it is possible to measure plasmin activity separately.

The site of production of plasminogen is still debatable. According to Barnhart and Riddle (1963), it is synthesized in eosinophilic leukocytes, but is is more probably produced in the liver cells (Johnson, Skoza and Tse, 1969).

The concentration of plasminogen is most often given relative to that in a normal standard pool. Absolute values have been given by Sherry (1968a), Schwick and Heimburger (1969), Rabiner, et al. (1969) and Collen, et al, (1972b). Its concentration in healthy adults is about 200 μg/ml plasma. Collen, et al. also studied the metabolism of human plasminogen labelled with radioactive iodine. They found the half-life of the plasma radioactivity in healthy adults to be $2 \cdot 21 \pm 0 \cdot 29$ days. The plasminogen turnover rate was studied in one healthy adult who was given heparin, and in one patient with low circulating plasminogen activator activity. Plasminogen metabolism was found to be normal in both, and it was therefore concluded that the bulk of plasminogen is not catabolised by primary fibrinolytic activation or by consumption secondary to intravascular coagulation. The synthesis of plasminogen is rapid, as is apparent from its quick recovery after treatment with streptokinase; it rises from practically nil to normal within 12–24 hours (Fletcher, et al., 1959; Robertson, et al., 1970).

Jacobsen (1968) described six families in which several of the members had a low plasminogen level. The clot lysis times were prolonged, even after addition of urokinase, and several other tests also showed these persons to have an abnormally low fibrinolytic activity. No symptoms of disease were observed. This is the first time that congenital deficiency of the fibrinolytic system has ever been reported.

2. Plasmin

Plasmin (fibrinolysin) is the active proteolytic enzyme formed by activation of plasminogen. According to Robbins, et al. (1967) and Robbins and Summaria (1971), the underlying chemical change is the cleavage of a single arginyl-valine bond in the plasminogen molecule resulting in a two-chain molecule held together by a single disulphide bond. There is one heavy chain and one light chain. When the disulphide bond is cleaved, plasmin loses its enzymatic activity (Robbins, et al., 1967). The molecular weight of plasmin is now thought to be somewhat lower than that of plasminogen, 75.000, and this has raised the question whether a peptide is split off from the plasminogen molecule during activation. Human plasmin contains a single proteolytic active centre (Robbins and Summaria, 1971).

Plasmin catalyses the hydrolysis of α-amino substituted lysine and arginine esters (Sherry, et al., 1966). It thus attacks the lysyl-lysine or lysyl-arginine bonds of the fibrinogen and fibrin molecules and breaks them down into fibrin/fibrinogen degradation products.

Plasmin can, as already pointed out, attack not only fibrinogen and fibrin, but also other coagulation factors such as Factor V and Factor VIII and even other proteins such as gelatin and casein.

3. Activators

The conversion of plasminogen to plasmin is brought about by various activators. As already mentioned, the activation is due to the cleavage of the single arginyl-valine bond in the plasminogen molecule. Plasminogen activators occur naturally in many tissues (tissue activator), in the circulating blood (blood activator), in urine (urokinase) and in some other body fluids. There are also other activators such as streptokinase and trypsin.

Tissue activator. Astrup and coworkers (Astrup and Permin, 1947; Albrechtsen, 1957; Astrup, 1966) have published extensive studies on the tissue activators. They have demonstrated, first, the presence of a potent acid stable activator of plasminogen in KSCN extracts of many tissues; second, a selective localisation of this agent to the intima of large veins; and third, a direct correlation between the fibrinolytic activity of a tissue and its content of vascularised connective tissue. The tissue activator was barely soluble in physiological saline.

The location of fibrinolytic activity in the tissues has been facilitated since the introduction of Todd's histochemical method (Todd, 1959). It is now known (Astrup, 1966; Pandolfi, et al., 1969) that the tissue activator is related chiefly to structures of the endothelial cells of the capillaries. Plasminogen activators have, however, recently been found in certain epithelial, synovial and mesothelial cells. The exact chemical nature of the tissue activator is not yet known. Kok and Astrup (1969) isolated and purified it and estimated the molecular weight at about 60.000. It is probably different from urokinase (Kok and Astrup, 1969, 1972).

Blood activator. Much suggests that the fibrinolytic activity in the blood is derived from activators produced in the endothelium of small vessels and that the activators are continuously presented to the blood stream (see Fearnley, 1965; Nilsson and Pandolfi, 1970). This was first suggested by Mole (1948), who thought the fluidity of cadaveric blood to be due to liberation of fibrinolytic agents from the vessel walls. Pandolfi (1970), Åstedt, et al. (1971a) and Åstedt and Pandolfi (1972) have produced evidence, also in tissue culture, that these activators are synthesized by vascular epithelium and are continuously released from the cells into the culture medium. It has been shown that different stimuli causing quick changes in the calibre of the blood vessels, such as injections of vasoactive drugs, enhance the release of these activators into the blood stream. The blood activator is labile (Müllertz, 1956). Müllertz found a similarity between plasminogen activator obtained from post mortem globulin preparations and activator obtained by the action of streptokinase on human globulins. Recently a labile plasminogen activator has been obtained by post mortem perfusion of vessels with saline; it is probably identical with the blood activator (Aoki and von Kaulla, 1971a). The molecular weight of this vascular activator, as estimated by gel filtration, was about 65.000 (Aoki and von Kaulla, 1971b).

The spontaneous fibrinolytic activity in the blood is normally low, due partly to the influence of inhibitors. The effect of inhibitors can be diminished by dilution of the plasma, or by separation of activators from the inhibitors by euglobulin precipitation. The fibrinolytic activity of the blood can be enhanced by a variety of stimuli, such as physical exercise, emotion, surgical operations, electric shock, pneumoencephalography and ventriculography, pyrogens, and venous occlusion. Many compounds, such as epinephrine, nicotinic acid, histamine, acetylcholine, carbacholine and several other vasoactive drugs, enhance the blood fibrinolytic activity of the blood *in vivo* (for references, see Nilsson and Pandolfi, 1970).

The vasoactive drugs have no such effect on blood *in vitro*. Unlike the spontaneous fibrinolytic activity, the activity demonstrable after these stimuli is so elevated as to permit measurement of intra- and inter-individual differences. It is above all, nicotinic acid, epinephrine, exercise, and venous occlusion of the limbs that have been used for estimating the fibrinolytic capacity of a given person.

The relationship between the stable tissue activator and the labile blood activator is unknown. In some tissues Albrechtsen (1958) observed two types of plasminogen activator, an acid stable one resembling that assayed with KSCN extraction and a labile one obtained by saline extraction. He thought that the latter might be identical with the labile blood activator. Nilsson, et al. (1970) feel that the endothelium of small vessels contains an activator of plasminogen, which is bound to other proteins or lipids and which has different properties when bound than when it is free (stable tissue activator extractable with KSCN). The activator is released in a labile form into the blood stream and maintains the spontaneous fibrinolytic activity of the blood. They think that the release of labile plasminogen activator into intracellular spaces may account for the quota of labile activator demonstrated by Albrechtsen (1958) in saline extracts of some tissues. Kucinski, et al. (1968) have also suggested the possibility that 'plasma activator is probably derived from tissue activator, especially that found in relation to blood vessels'.

Urokinase. Macfarlane and Pilling (1947) reported that human urine possesses fibrinolytic (and tryptic) activity. Somewhat later three research groups (Williams, 1951; Astrup and Sterndorff, 1952; and Sobel, et al., 1952) demonstrated that this activity was due to an activator in the urine which could convert plasminogen to plasmin. Urokinase is now the most thoroughly investigated human plasminogen activator. It is a protein with a β-globulin mobility and the molecule is built up of a single polypeptide chain. It has been prepared in a highly purified and crystalline form (Lesuk, et al., 1965; White, et al., 1966). Its molecular weight has been given as 53.000 (Lesuk, et al., 1967), whereas White, et al. described two main components, one with a molecular weight of

32.500, the other with a molecular weight of 54.700. The enzyme is very stable and tolerates temperatures up to 50°C within a wide pH range. It has not been found in the blood, not even in renal venous blood (Kucinski, et al., 1968).

Urokinase activates plasminogen by an enzymatic mechanism. In addition, it has esterase activity and hydrolyses arginine and lysine esters. These esters act at the same time as competitive inhibitors of the plasminogen activation by urokinase.

In a recent review, Astrup and Thorsen (1972) stated that the origin of urokinase is debatable. It is probably not extracted from the blood, but several studies indicate that the kidney and possibly the glomeruli may be the source (for references, see Astrup and Thorsen, 1972; Åstedt, 1972).

Streptokinase. Streptokinase is a well defined protein obtained from β-haemolytic streptococci; it has an electrophoretic mobility corresponding to that of the serum α_2-globulins and a molecular weight of 47.000 (Heimburger, 1971). As pointed out already, streptokinase can activate human, but not bovine, plasminogen to plasmin. It was therefore assumed that human blood contains a special component, proactivator, that forms a complex with streptokinase, which in turn enzymatically converts plasminogen to plasmin. But it is now well established that this component is an equimolar complex of streptokinase with plasminogen or plasmin (de Renzo, et al., 1965; Tomar and Taylor, 1971). The activation of human plasminogen is at present the subject of much debate. It is assumed that streptokinase might activate plasminogen directly or by reacting with a specific 'proactivator' (Takada, et al., 1971, 1972) different from plasminogen. Reddy and Markus (1972), however, claim that all proactivator activity can be explained by plasmin or plasminogen. Since streptokinase can form stable complexes with plasminogen and plasmin, they also feel that it is not necessary to assume that streptokinase plays an independent enzymatic role. In their tentative description of the mechanism of the streptokinase activation of human plasminogen the first step is the formation of a streptokinase-plasminogen complex that possesses the active centre. In the second step this complex converts plasminogen to plasmin, and in the third, it may itself be converted to the complex streptokinase-plasmin.

4. Inhibitors of fibrinolysis

Inhibitors of fibrinolysis inhibit the activation of plasminogen to plasmin or act upon the plasmin already formed. Synthetic inhibitors are also available.

The inhibitory effect of the blood on plasminogen activation can be measured from its capacity to inhibit urokinase-induced fibrinolysis (urokinase inhibitors). This inhibitory capacity has been utilised in the elaboration of several methods of determination (Paraskevas, et al., 1962; Lauritzen, 1968). Nilsson and Hedner (1972) who used ion-exchange chromatography and gel filtration, recently purified an inhibitor of urokinase-induced plasminogen activation with α_2-globulin mobility. They also prepared a rabbit antiserum against this inhibitor fraction. Aoki and von Kaulla (1971c) separated an inhibitor (molecular weight about 80.000) acting mainly on plasminogen activation. This anti-activator was found to have an inhibitory effect on plasminogen activation induced by saline extracts from the human vessel wall.

The significance of inhibitors of plasminogen activation has been demonstrated in some patients with severe thrombotic disease (Nilsson, et al., 1961; Brakman, et al., 1966; Pandolfi, et al., 1970). Hedner, et al. (1970) reported a low content of fibrinolytic inhibitors in four patients with high fibrinolytic capacity.

There are mainly two *circulating inhibitors* (*antiplasmins*) of already formed plasmin. They react with plasmin to form a fibrinolytically inactive complex. One of them, α_2-*macroglobulin* (α_2M) (molecular weight 845.000) is thermostable and reacts instantaneously and reversibly with plasmin. The other α_1-*antitrypsin* (molecular weight 47.000) is thermolabile and reacts slowly and irreversibly with plasmin (Rimon, et al., 1966; Ganrot and Niléhn, 1967). During infusion of streptokinase, the concentration of α_2M, which is presumably the most important plasmin inhibitor, after complexing with formed plasmin, rapidly decreases, while α_1-antitrypsin is essentially unaffected (Niléhn and Ganrot, 1967).

Some *synthetic amino acids* have a strong inhibiting effect on fibrinolysis. The most important of these substances are epsilon aminocaproic acid (EACA, Epsikapron®), 4-aminomethyl-cyclohexane-carbonic acid (tranexamic acid, AMCA, Cyclokapron®) and p-amino-methyl benzoic acid (PAMBA), all of which exert their effect by competitively inhibiting the activation of plasminogen. They have therefore been utilised clinically as antifibrinolytics (see page 140).

A distinction is made between *general fibrinolysis* and *local fibrinolysis*. In general fibrinolysis the fibrinolytic activity resides in the circulating blood and is due to release of usually labile activators from tissue to the blood stream, which results in an activation of the fibrinolytic system. In local fibrinolysis no abnormal fibrinolytic activity is demonstrable in the circulating blood. The process is localised to the tissue that is damaged and where the activators of the cells come into contact with locally formed fibrin clots and dissolve them.

B. *Mechanism of thrombolysis*

Opinions differ on the mechanism of thrombolysis. Since it has not been possible to study the mechanism of thrombolysis in the human body, our understanding of the mechanism is based on studies of clots and experimental thrombi. It is generally accepted that a thrombus can be dissolved enzymatically in two ways, namely 1) the fibrin in the thrombus may be attacked from the outside by plasmin ('external lysis'), and 2) activators may diffuse into the thrombus and activate the plasminogen present in the thrombus to plasmin, which afterwards dissolves the fibrin in the thrombus ('internal lysis'). It was Sherry and coworkers who launched the intrinsic clot lysis theory (Alkjaersig, Fletcher and Sherry, 1959a; Sawyer, Alkjaersig, Fletcher and Sherry, 1961; Sherry, 1968a). This theory has attracted much attention and is now accepted by most workers in this field. They based their theory on the observation that on clot formation about 30 per cent of the total amount of plasminogen in the plasma is adsorbed to the fibrin, and on the observation that thrombolysis may occur even in the absence of demonstrable amounts of plasmin in the blood. According to this group, then, the ability of plasma to lyse thrombi is dependent directly on its activator content and is relatively independent of its proteolytic activity. Adherents of this school do not think that plasmin preparations should be used in thrombolytic treatment because the plasmin has only little thrombolytic effect and, second, because the high proteolytic activity in the blood during treatment with plasmin results in severe coagulation defects and the risk of a haemorrhagic diathesis difficult to control. They believe, instead, that activators, as a rule streptokinase or urokinase, should be given in excess, with the result that practically all plasminogen will be bound to streptokinase with the formation of an activator complex, which can diffuse directly into the thrombus. In this way only small amounts of plasmin would form in the blood and interfere with haemostasis. The extrinsic clot lysis theory put forward by Ambrus and Markus (1960), has hitherto had only few adherents. These authors believe that a plasmin-antiplasmin complex plays an important role in thrombolysis. They have found that active plasmin is bound to antiplasmin in the circulation but is dissociated from it when the complex comes into contact with fibrin, because plasmin has a greater affinity to fibrin than antiplasmin. Therefore, according to them, plasmin digests the thrombi from the surface inwards.

In recent years, however, Sherry's intrinsic clot lysis theory has been criticised. It has been shown by various groups (Fantl, 1962; Hedner and Nilsson, 1965; Ogston, et al., 1966) that the plasminogen content of the plasma and that of serum are the same and that plasminogen is thus not consumed in the coagulation of the blood. Only traces of plasminogen have been demonstrated in clots and thrombi (Hedner, et al., 1966). These findings thus argue against the assumption that large amounts of plasminogen are incorporated in the fibrin during clot formation. In a series of experiments concerning the dissolution of experimental thrombi in rotating glass tubes (Chandler's tubes), it has also been shown that dissolution of thrombi always starts from the outside and proceeds inwards. Incubation of thrombi in a plasmin solution resulted in marked thrombolysis, while activator solutions such as streptokinase and urokinase had only an insignificant effect (Jacobsen and Chandler, 1965).

The above observations make it difficult to accept intrinsic clot lysis as the most important mechanism of dissolution of thrombi *in vivo*. On the other hand, they lend support to the extrinsic clot lysis theory, accord-

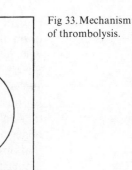

Fig 33. Mechanism of thrombolysis.

ing to which, fibrin thrombi and fibrin clots are digested mainly from the outside by plasmin. In fresh and unretracted clots and thrombi whose loose fibrin network contains plasma or serum components, it is only natural that activators can diffuse into, and activate the serum plasminogen in the clot or thrombus, and thereby bring about intrinsic dissolution. In model experiments it has also been shown that streptokinase and urokinase can dissolve such fresh, unretracted clots. In our opinion, then, retracted thrombi and clots are digested mainly from the surface by plasmin, while fresh unretracted clots and thrombi can be digested by intrinsic activation of the plasminogen in the clot or thrombus (Fig. 33).

The nature of the mechanism of thrombolysis is of considerable importance in the planning of thrombolytic therapy. If the mechanism of thrombolysis is mainly extrinsic, plasmin should be indicated; if it is intrinsic, activators such as streptokinase and urokinase are indicated. It is difficult to produce pure plasmin free from activators, and only few clinical trials have been performed with pure glycerol activated plasmin. Storm, et al. (1971) used porcine plasmin, obtained by trypsin activation and reported a good clinical effect. Most authors have, as mentioned, used activators, such as streptokinase and urokinase. Since the production of urokinase is very complicated and expensive, streptokinase has been most widely used. I believe that streptokinase can have both an extrinsic and intrinsic effect in the dissolution of thrombi. Most authors have used large doses of streptokinase to lower the plasminogen content to very low levels and thereby prevent plasmin formation. Plasminogen is synthesized very rapidly, and even if the plasminogen content is lowered to practically nil, plasminogen will be produced continuously and some will in practice always be present during treatment with streptokinase. The most important antiplasmin, $\alpha_2 M$, falls rapidly as soon as treatment with streptokinase has been started. In contrast with most other proteins, $\alpha_2 M$ is synthesized slowly in the course of 3–4 weeks. This means that even if the plasminogen content is low during treatment, the plasmin formed will not be inactivated by $\alpha_2 M$, but will be adsorbed to the fibrin in the thrombus, where it can cause thrombolysis.

g 34. Haemostatic
echanism in DIC.

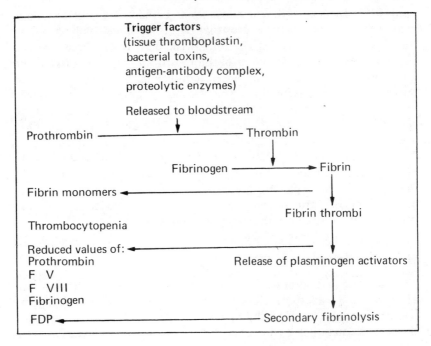

Trigger factors
(tissue thromboplastin,
bacterial toxins,
antigen-antibody complex,
proteolytic enzymes)

Released to bloodstream

Prothrombin ———————————— Thrombin

Fibrinogen ——————→ Fibrin

Fibrin monomers ◄————————————————

Fibrin thrombi

Thrombocytopenia

Reduced values of: ◄————————————
Prothrombin
F V   Release of plasminogen activators
F VIII
Fibrinogen

FDP ◄————————————————— Secondary fibrinolysis

II. Defibrination or disseminated intravascular coagulation (DIC)—pathogenesis

In the literature defibrination or disseminated intravascular coagulation (DIC) has most often been defined as a pathological process, which leads to activation of coagulation with the formation of thrombin in the circulating blood and of thrombi situated in small vessels and consisting of platelets and fibrin. According to the most modern concepts, defibrination is better defined as pathological formation of fibrinogen derivatives, usually due to excessive enzyme-induced proteolysis.

Defibrination has been studied in greatest detail in animals, where it has been induced by injection of thrombin, tissue thromboplastin or blood or bacterial endotoxins in prepared animals (Shwartzman reaction).

A. *Mechanism of haemostasis in DIC*

Activation of the coagulation process in the circulating blood may produce a 'consumption syndrome' with reduced content of those factors normally consumed in the coagulation of blood, i.e. reduced content of prothrombin, Factor V, Factor VIII, fibrinogen and platelets (Fig. 34). But since activation may occur in any one or more stages of the coagulation process, these factors need not all be decreased at the same time. It is regarded as characteristic of these conditions that fibrinogen derivatives and fibrin monomers can be demonstrated in the blood (Godal and Abildgard, 1966; Lipinski and Worowski, 1968; Latallo, et al., 1971; Godal, et al., 1971). It is generally believed that DIC is associated with secondary fibrinolysis (McKay, 1965). The fibrinolytic activity has been ascribed partly to release of activators of fibrinolysis from the injured tissue and partly to activators from the vessel endothelium as a consequence of the intravascular coagulation. The secondary fibrinolysis can partly or completely dissolve any fibrin thrombi present. Such dissolution results in the formation of fibrin/fibrinogen degradation products. They are regarded as characteristic of conditions with associated DIC.

The bleeding defect that develops in DIC may thus comprise a variety of abnormalities, namely 1) thrombocytopenia, 2) secondary fibrinolysis, 3) reduced content of prothrombin, Factor V, Factor VIII and fibrinogen, 4) inhibition of fibrin polymerisation by fibrin/fibrinogen degradation products with a defective fibrin clot as a result.

B. *Microthrombi and DIC*

The haemorrhagic diathesis is only one aspect of DIC. The most important disorder is the widespread formation of microthrombi obstructing the microcirculation and contributing to the development of hypovolaemic shock. Such obstruction can impair the supply of blood and cause tissue necrosis of various organs. Those organs which, according to McKay (1969a, b), are usually first involved are the lungs, kidneys, gastro-intestinal tract, adrenals, brain, liver, pancreas and skin. According to McKay, the localisation of the microthrombi varies considerably not only from one disease to another, but also in one and the same disease.

The most reliable evidence of DIC ought to be histopathological demonstration of widespread thrombi in the microcirculation. McKay (1965, 1969a, b) stated that the histopathological findings in the organs involved may vary from negligible or uncertain changes, to capillary platelet and fibrin thrombi, focal haemorrhage and necroses. Schneider (1951) and Hardaway (1966) like McKay, demonstrated fibrin deposits in capillaries and other small vessels in organs with focal necrosis in patients with DIC. But some authors regard these thrombi and fibrin deposits as secondary to necrosis (Ober, et al., 1956).

In most clinical syndromes believed to be caused by intravascular coagulation, it has, however, not proved possible to demonstrate thrombi in the circulation (Robboy, et al., 1972). Even in dogs given sublethal doses of various substances inducing coagulation, only few or even no thrombi have been demonstrable microscopically (Ratnoff, 1969). Various explanations have been offered for this lack of thrombi. It has been assumed that in several cases the thrombi formed have been dissolved by secondary fibrinolysis. This assumption is supported by the demonstration of fibrin/fibrinogen degradation products in the blood (Steichele, 1969). According to Lee, Prose and Cohen (1966) and Walsh and Barnhardt (1969), a major part of the fibrin aggregates formed in intravascular coagulation, is phagocytosed by the RES. McKay (1969a, b, c) stressed

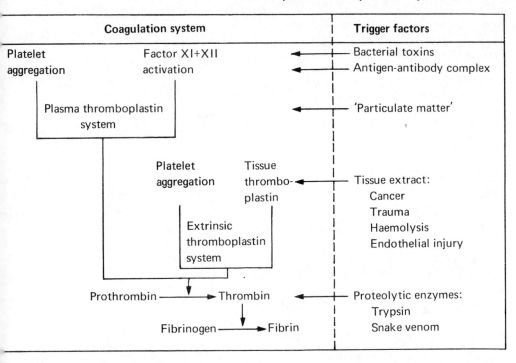

| Coagulation system | Trigger factors |

Fig 35. Trigger mechanisms in DIC.

that the thrombi may be submicroscopic and demonstrable only with the electron microscope.

In an electron microscopic investigation Margaretten, Csavossy and McKay (1967) found thrombi consisting of fibrin, platelets and granulocytes in the small vessels in the renal cortex in thrombin-induced DIC in rabbits. These authors as well as Skjörten (1966) have electron-microscopically demonstrated such thrombi also in the adrenals, heart and brain in persons with the Shwartzman reaction.

C. *Trigger mechanism of DIC*

What is the cause of DIC? Various trigger mechanisms have been assumed. They fall into two groups, *viz.*, direct and indirect (Müller-Berghaus, 1969; Rodriguez-Erdmann, 1969; Evensen and Jeremic, 1970; and Evensen and Hjort, 1970) (Fig. 35). Müller-Berghaus and Evensen and co-workers divided the trigger substances into two groups, namely direct and indirect. Direct triggers are such agents that can initiate or accelerate coagulation when added to blood *in vitro*. Indirect triggers are agents that have no effect on the coagulation process *in vitro*, but only if they are given *in vivo*. These indirect triggers are believed to act by the release, into the blood, of a mediator which can in turn act as a direct trigger.

1. Direct triggers

The most important direct trigger is thromboplastin (Fig. 35, Table 9).

Direct	Indirect
Thromboplastin:	Bacterial toxins
Cancer	Antigen-antibody complex
Trauma	'Particulate matter':
Haemolysis	Amniotic fluid
Endothelial injury	Liquid
Proteolytic enzymes:	
Trypsin	
Snake venom	

Table 9. Trigger factors.

Tissue thromboplastin can be released into the blood stream on disintegration of cells by e.g. trauma, operations, burns, necrosis and anoxia. Leukocytes in patients with leukaemia, and cancer cells, possess high thromboplastic activity, and on disintegration of these cells, thromboplastin may be released into the blood stream. Normal leukocytes have little or no thromboplastic activity (Rapaport and Hjort, 1967). Endothelial cells contain thromboplastic activity, and in endothelial injury the coagulation process may be activated.

Haemolysate of red blood cells possesses coagulation activity, and its effect resembles that of platelet factors 3 and 4. In haemolysis, then, activation of the coagulation process may be expected. This is probably not a very potent trigger mechanism, because most patients with haemolysis show no signs of DIC. In this connection it might not be out of place to mention that it has been shown that intravascular coagulation *per se* causes structural changes in the red blood cells ('burr cells') and haemolysis (Brain and Hourihane, 1967).

Various proteolytic enzymes, such as trypsin and those contained in certain snake poisons, can activate the conversion of prothrombin to thrombin. Certain snake poisons, such as that of *Bothrops jararaca*, contain an enzyme with a thrombin-like effect.

2. Indirect triggers

The coagulation process can probably be activated by a variety of indirect trigger mechanisms. Our knowledge of such mechanism is still very limited. The indirect triggers that have received most attention are bacterial toxins, antigen-antibody complexes, and 'particulate matter'. 'Particulate matter' is here to be understood as including substances such as amniotic fluid and synthetic polymers e.g. Liquoid.

Bacterial toxins. Of bacterial toxins, Gram-negative endotoxins have been studied most. The experimental model used in experiments is the Shwartzman reaction. A sublethal dose of endotoxin is injected into rabbits, for example, and after an interval of 24 hours, a second similar injection is given. The first injection, the so-called preparative dose, produces only a mild reaction. The second, however, causes platelet aggregation and activation of the coagulation process, which results in generalised deposition of fibrin in several organs and often necrosis of the renal cortex. Endotoxin is believed to activate the coagulation process by several mechanisms, *viz.*, platelet aggregation with release of platelet factors 3 and 4, activation of Factor XII and release of thromboplastin from endothelial cells injured by the toxins. The last component is probably the most important one.

Injection of disintegrated platelets alone does not cause DIC. Neither is it possible to prevent a Shwartzman reaction in rabbits rendered thrombocytopenic (see Evensen and Hjort, 1970). Intravenous injection of substances that activate Factor XII *in vitro* does not produce a Shwartzman reaction.

Granulocytes are necessary for induction of the Shwartzman reaction, but it is not known whether they release any mediator necessary for the coagulation process. In the Shwartzman reaction there is haemolysis, which is secondary to the initiated intravascular coagulation. Distintegrated blood cells can, as mentioned, have some accelerating effect on coagulation.

It is important for the clinician to bear in mind that DIC can be elicited not only by endotoxin, but also by other bacterial toxins. Pneumococcal and streptococcal sepsis may thus result in intravascular coagulation.

Antigen-antibody complex. Intravenous injection of antigen-antibody complex into experimental animals produces thrombocytopenia, reduction of coagulation factors and renal injury resembling that seen in the Shwartzman reaction. It is believed that the antigen-antibody complex can induce activation of the coagulation process in the same way as endotoxin. The coagulation stimulating effect of these complexes is, however, not so pronounced as that of endotoxin. In clinical practice this might perhaps be of importance in certain cases of auto-immune diseases.

'Particulate matter'. It is not known how these substances activate coagulation. Liquoid, a synthetic polymer with anticoagulant properties *in vitro*, can induce DIC and a Shwartzman reaction in rabbits. Müller-Berghaus (1969) assumes that this substance acts via the contact phase in the coagulation process.

Table 10. *Modifying factors in DIC.*	Predisposing and stimulating	Inhibiting
	Activation of coagulation system	Anticoagulating factors
	Reduced fibrinolytic activity in vessel walls	Fibrinolytic activators
	High content of fibrinolytic inhibitors	RES stimulating
	Blocking of RES	Blocking of adrenergic system
	Vasoactive substances, e.g. epinephrine	
	ACTH, cortisone	
	Hyperlipaemia (?)	

D. *Factors deciding the severity of the reaction in DIC—modifying factors*

Another question of importance is which factors determine the severity of the reaction and the spread of DIC. It is known from animal experiments and clinical experience that the severity of DIC varies little with the amount of trigger substance given. The reaction in DIC can be influenced by the coagulation system, the reticulo-endothelial system (RES), the fibrinolytic system, pregnancy, vascular factors and possibly lipids (Table 10).

The coagulation system. Coagulation defects offer protection against intravascular coagulation. It is thus not possible to induce a generalised Shwartzman reaction in warfarin-treated rabbits. The platelets are not of the same importance. DIC can thus be induced in thrombocytopenic rabbits. The clinical conditions, which may be complicated by DIC, e.g. pregnancy, malignant disease, renal disease and infections, are, as a rule, associated with a high content of several coagulation factors. Some workers (Penick, et al., 1966; Lasch, 1969a) believe that high values of prothrombin, Factor VIII, and Factor V predispose to DIC. In conditions with an increased content of coagulation factors it is difficult to judge the coagulation status in acute situations. A normal content of factors in such patients may mean that they have been reduced by DIC.

The reticulo-endothelial system. This system plays an important role in DIC and Shwartzman reaction. RES can absorb endotoxin, intermediary coagulation products, thromboplastin, platelet material, fibrin monomers, fibrin and fibrinogen degradation products from circulating blood (Walsh and Barnhart, 1969). When the first preparative dose of endotoxin is given in the Shwartzman reaction a certain activation of the coagulation process may occur, but both endotoxin and the products of coagulation are removed from the blood by the RES. When the provoking dose of endotoxin is given, the RES is completely or partly blocked and the classical picture of Shwartzman reaction can develop. The first preparative dose of endotoxin may be replaced by substances that block RES. Thorotrast, trypan blue, carbon and cortisone, for instance, have been described as capable of causing such blocking. The RES thus normally offers good protection against intravascular coagulation by removing coagulation components and fibrin activated by trigger substances. It is not known how much fibrin is necessary to block the RES or how long such blocking lasts. Further, hardly any information is available about the functional capacity of RES in different diseases.

The fibrinolytic system. This system is important for the regulation, formation and localisation of fibrin thrombi. All organs of the body except the liver, placenta and renal cortex contain potent activators of fibrinolysis. These occur in the endothelium in small vessels and in the vasa vasorum of larger vessels. These activators may be released by certain stimuli and then cause dissolution of local fibrin deposits (Nilsson and Pandolfi, 1970). In some conditions the content of inhibitors of fibrinolysis in the blood is increased and thereby impairs or prevents fibrinolysis.

Isacson and Nilsson (1972b) found that 73 per cent of patients with idiopathic venous thrombosis had a low fibrinolytic activity in the vessel walls. It is noteworthy that prednisone lowers the fibrinolytic activity of the vessel walls (Isacson, 1970). In uraemia and renal diseases as well as during rejection of renal grafts the fibrinolytic activity in the vessel walls is normal, but inhibitors of fibrinolysis in the blood are markedly increased (Isacson and Nilsson, 1969; Larsson, et al., 1971a, b; Ljung-qvist, et al., 1969). In reactive processes, e.g. malignant tumours and infections, the content of inhibitors of fibrinolysis is, as a rule, also markedly increased (Olow, 1963; Hedner and Nilsson, 1971a).

In all conditions with decreased fibrinolytic activity in the vessel walls or markedly increased content of inhibitors of fibrinolysis in the blood there is thus a risk of fibrin thrombi not being dissolved. In rabbits pre-treated with EACA a single preparative dose of endotoxin may thus be sufficient to induce the Shwartzman reaction and DIC. Margaretten, et al. (1965) also induced DIC in cortisone treated rabbits after admini-stration of only the preparative dose of endotoxin. Administration of streptokinase, on the other hand, can prevent the development of DIC in rabbits. In human beings with an intact fibrinolytic system the risk of development of persistent fibrin thrombi on activation of the coagulation process is negligible. Patients treated with snake venom with a thrombin effect (Arvin) as a prophylactic measure against thrombosis have thus not developed DIC (Bell, et al., 1968a, b).

Pregnancy. It is known that pregnancy predisposes to DIC. In preg-nant animals the preparative dose of endotoxin may be sufficient to provoke the Shwartzman reaction. The fibrinolytic activity in the vessel walls is markedly reduced in pregnancy (Åstedt, et al., 1970).

On the other hand, the capacity of the RES is normal during pregnancy.

Vascular factors. Much suggests that the adrenergic system is of importance in the development of fibrin deposits in DIC, especially in the localisation of such deposits. McKay (1969a, b) has shown that DIC can be produced in rabbits by a single preparative dose of endotoxin if noradrenalin is given at the same time. On the other hand, it has proved possible to prevent the development of DIC by administration of substances that block the adrenergic system.

Lipids. It has been assumed that lipids may increase the susceptibility to DIC, but the effect of lipids has not been studied in detail.

III. Fibrin/fibrinogen degradation products (FDP)

The breakdown of fibrinogen by the proteolytic enzyme, plasmin, results in the formation of high molecular weight products, which Marder, et al. (1967) called X (molecular weight 240.000) and Y fragments (mole-cular weight 155.000). X fragments are still coagulable with thrombin,

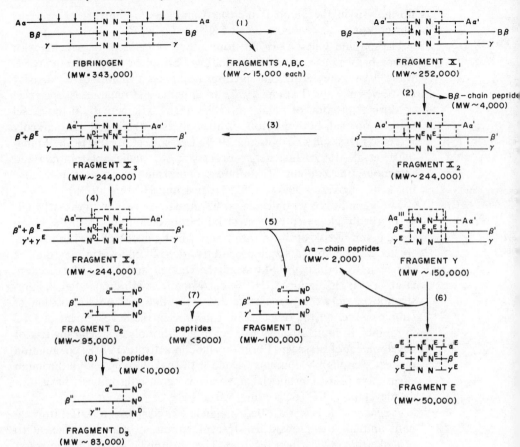

Fig 36a. Digestion of fibrinogen by plasmin. The vertical arrows indicate approximate sites of cleavage by plasmin. The 'N' represents the amino terminus of each chain. The vertical dashed lines indicate the approximate site of the minimal number of disulfide bonds required to fulfil the analyses of the sub-unit structures of the digestion products. The superscript above the 'N's, i.e., 'N^D' or 'N^E' represents the new amino termini which appear in fragments D and E, respectively.

This scheme was kindly given by Dr. P. A. McKee, Durham, North Carolina (*J. Biol. Chem.* 1973).

though slower than undigested fibrinogen, while Y fragments are uncoagulable. Recently Pizzo, et al. (1972) have shown that at least four different X fragments may exist. The molecular weight of the X product has been described as varying between 240.000 and 260.000 (Marder, 1971). According to Pizzo, et al. (1972), the α-chain of the fibrinogen is most susceptible to digestion by plasmin. On degradation of the α-chain the peptides A, B and C (Marder, 1971) each with a molecular weight of 15.000, are split off. The X products may thus consist of fragments from which the A, B and C peptides of the two α-chains in the fibrinogen molecule have been split off (fragment X$_1$ according to Pizzo, et al., with a molecular weight of 252.000), but X fragments with a varying degree of breakdown of the α-chain also occur (Mosesson, et al., 1972a).

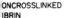
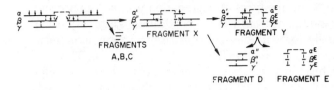

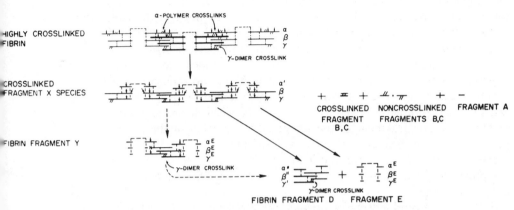

Fig 36b. Digestion of non-crosslinked and highly crosslinked fibrin by plasmin. The symbols are the same as for Fig 36a. The crosslinks are indicated by parallel, slightly angled lines between fibrin monomers.

This scheme was kindly given by Dr. P. A. McKee, Durham, North Carolina (*J. Biol. Chem.* 1973).

The next step in the breakdown process is degradation of the β-chain in the fibrinogen molecule (fragments X_2 and X_3 according to Pizzo, et al., 1972, are of molecular weight 244.000). Fragment X may also contain different varients of X_1 and X_2 and possibly also fragments with a partially digested γ-chain called X_4 (Fig. 36a).

When fragment Y (molecular weight 150.000) is formed, a D fragment is split off simultaneously (Marder, et al., 1967; Pizzo, et al., 1972; Furlan and Beck, 1972). Complete degradation of the fibrinogen molecule gives rise to D and E fragments, both of which have antigenic determinants in common with fibrinogen (Nussenzweig, et al., 1961; Marder, et al., 1967). The molecular weight of fragment D varies between 83.000 and 100.000 (Pizzo, et al., 1972) depending on the degree of degradation of the γ-chain. The same research group also showed that the D product obtained on degradation of fibrin by plasmin differs from that obtained on the breakdown of fibrinogen in that it contains a dimer of the digested γ-chain containing the cross-linking site of the γ-chain (Fig. 36b). Fragment E has been shown to be made up of the disulphide link of the fibrinogen molecule (Pizzo, et al., 1972; Furlan and Beck, 1972) and to have a molecular weight of 50.000. Taylor, et al. (1972) have shown that the E product obtained on degradation of fibrin is identical with that obtained on digestion of fibrinogen by plasmin. The X and Y products are generally called high molecular weight degradation products and the D and E fragments 'end products' (Marder, et al., 1967).

Fragments X and Y are the types of degradation products that occur most often in the blood in various clinical conditions. They may occur separately, but usually form a complex with soluble fibrin monomers and fibrinogen (Lipinski, et al., 1967).

According to Niléhn (1967a, b), about 50 per cent of the high molecular weight products are retained in the clot on coagulation of the blood, but only about 10 per cent of the D and E products. Larrieu (1971) has found that 70 per cent or more of fragment X is retained in the clot. On the other hand, addition of fragment Y to blood is followed by a larger increase in the amount of degradation products in serum than that corresponding to the amount of fragment Y added, and thereby suggests complex formation between fragment Y and fibrinogen.

Serum may thus contain small amounts of fragment X, fragment Y, and D and E products as well as a complex between fibrin monomers or fibrinogen and fragment Y and fragment X. Since all of these components have antigenic determinants in common with fibrinogen, Merskey, et al. (1971) believe that it would be more correct to call such components 'fibrinogen-fibrin-related antigen' or abbreviated, FR-antigen in serum.

FDP have several effects on coagulation (Niléhn, 1967c; Marder, 1971; Larrieu, et al., 1972) and vasomotor function of the blood vessels (Malofiejew, 1971). The prolongation of thrombin and Reptilase times depends on two effects, namely inhibition of the proteolytic activity of thrombin on fibrinogen and inhibition of the polymerisation of fibrin. The former effect has been ascribed to the D and E fragments which also have an antithromboplastin effect. However, Larrieu, et al. (1972) have produced evidence that fragments D and E differ distinctly in anticoagulant action, fragment D being an inhibitor of fibrin polymerisation, fragment E acting like an antithrombin. The inhibition of fibrin polymerisation is exerted mainly by fragment Y, which is the most potent anticoagulant degradation product. Since fragment Y probably consists of a single fragment D and a single fragment E, Larrieu, et al. (1972) thought that it might possess the anticoagulant properties of both fragments D and E. As to the effect of FDP on platelets, Niléhn (1967c) was not able to demonstrate any decrease in platelet adhesiveness by FDP, whereas Kowalski (1968) found that both early and late FDP had such an effect. Larrieu (1971) demonstrated that low molecular weight fragments inhibit platelet aggregation.

Malofiejew (1971) has reported on the pharmacological properties of FDP. These effects are diverse, including vasoconstriction by stimulation of vasoactive peptides, influence on blood pressure and capillary permeability.

A. *Methods for determining FDP*

Serum is used for determining FDP. Since some degradation products can be retained in the clot on coagulation of the blood, it would have been more correct to determine FDP in plasma. But this is not possible because FDP and fibrinogen have the same antigenic determinants. It might, however, be mentioned that Fletcher, et al. (1970) divised a method utilising Bio Gel-chromatography for demonstration of early fibrinogen degradation products in plasma.

Most authors recommend *addition of thrombin to the blood in the determination of FDP*. This eliminates the risk of incomplete coagulation and of persistent fibrinogen in the serum.

It is also important that the blood samples be collected in tubes containing *an inhibitor of fibrinolysis such as EACA*. Otherwise plasminogen in the samples may be activated with too high a value as a result.

The four methods described below are those most widely used today.

1. Tanned red cell hemagglutination inhibition immunoassay (TRCHII)

This method, which is based on the Boyden-technique, was introduced in 1966 by Merskey, (Merskey, et al., 1966). In this method the serum to be tested is incubated with a highly diluted antifibrinogen serum. Afterwards fibrinogen-coated red blood cells are added. The consequent degree of inhibition of aggregation is a measure of the amount of FDP or FR-antigen in the sample. Normal citrated plasma with a known fibrinogen content is used as a standard. Merskey (Merskey, et al., 1969; Merskey, et al., 1971) recently modified the method. He now uses human O-blood cells instead of sheep cells. The method has also been automatized. The method can measure concentrations down to about 0·5 μg/ml.

Merskey's method is probably the one that is most widely used. The advantages of the method are that it is sensitive and fairly quick (2–6 hours). The method does not measure E products and is not very sensitive to D products, especially if the D product is the only antigen (Rayner, et al., 1969; Bouma. 1971).

2. Staphylococcal clumping test

In this method fibrinogen, fibrin monomers and fragments X and Y can be aggregated by certain strains of *Staphylococcus aureus* (Hawiger, et al., 1970). The highest dilution of serum that produces aggregation is determined. A solution of fibrinogen is used as a standard. The method is quick (30–45 minutes). It is said to be able to measure concentrations down to 0·5–1 μg fibrinogen/ml. No reaction is obtained with D or E products. The method is difficult to standardize because the results may vary with the batch of *Staphylococcus aureus*. In clinical trials it has proved to give positive results in some cases where other methods have given negative results and to give negative results in cases where Merskey's method has given positive values (Thomas, et al., 1970; Donati, et al., 1971).

SERUM OR URINE SAMPLE
+ ANTIFIBRINOGEN
INCUBATION > 3 MIN.

0.1 ML SERUM- ANTI-
FIBRINOGEN MIXTURE
+ 0.1 ML "FIBRINOGEN-COATED"
LATEX

SAMPLE ROCKED FOR 2 MIN.

Fig 37.   Agglutination inhibition test for FDP.

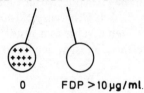

0   FDP >10 µg/ml.

3. Latex agglutination methods

Allington (1971) and Svanberg, et al. (1973) have devised quick latex agglutination inhibition methods using latex particles coated with human fibrinogen (Fig. 37). The serum to be tested is first incubated with highly diluted antifibrinogen serum. The fibrinogen-coated latex particles are afterwards added. The inhibition of the aggregation thereby produced is a measure of the FDP in the sample. A solution of human fibrinogen is used as standard. The method measures fibrinogen with an accuracy of 10 µg/ml. Results in good agreement with those obtained with Niléhn's immunochemical method have been reported (Svanberg, et al., 1973).

Melliger (1970) has described a direct latex agglutination test using latex particles coated with γ-globulin isolated from antifibrinogen serum. Agglutination occurs in the presence of fibrinogen and its degradation products. According to Melliger the method is quick and its reproducibility is as good as that of the TRCHII method.

A suspension of latex particles coated with a mixture of anti-D and anti-E antibodies is now commercially available (Thrombo-Wellcotest). Quick slide tests for detecting FDP with these antibody-coated latex particles have been described (Garvey and Black, 1972; Arocha-Pinango, 1972; Hulme and Pitcher, 1973). The sensitivity of the methods has been given as 2–5 µg fibrinogen/ml. The results have been described as agreeing well with those obtained with the TRCHII method.

These latex agglutination methods should be useful for screening in acute cases.

4. Niléhn's immunochemical method

Niléhn's method (Niléhn, 1967b) is based on Laurell's technique, according to which a glass plate is covered with agarose gel containing specific antibodies (anti-D). Serum from the patients to be tested is placed in a hole punched in the gel (Fig. 38). With the aid of an electric current the

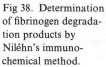

Fig 38. Determination of fibrinogen degradation products by Niléhn's immunochemical method.

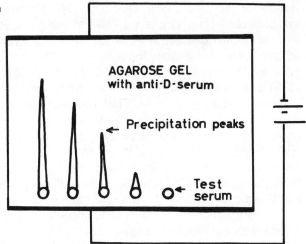

test serum is forced into the gel. If the sample contains degradation products, they will form peaks resembling rockets in the electrophoretic pattern. The height of these peaks varies with the concentration of the antigen. High molecular weight degradation products are used as a standard since they occur mainly in the serum in various diseases. The occurrence of degradation products in urine may be determined in the same way. With this method FDP can be measured down to a concentration of 5 μg/ml. In normal persons no degradation products can be demonstrated in serum or urine with this method. The method determines high molecular weight FDP as well as D products.

Bouma, Hedner and Nilsson (1971) have recently modified this method so that FDP in serum and urine can be typed. In the modified method serum and urine are added to agarose plates containing antifibrinogen serum, anti-D serum and anti-E serum, respectively. Fibrinogen is used as standard for all the plates. The appearance of single peaks or double peaks in the various plates reveals the types of degradation products present, and their concentrations can be measured. If the sample contains high molecular weight degradation products plus D, for example, two peaks will appear in the pattern of the plates with antifibrinogen and anti-D because the D product and high molecular weight degradation products differ in molecular weight and diffusibility in the gel. In doubtful cases the answer may be obtained by addition of fibrinogen, high molecular weight degradation products and D and E products, respectively, to the sample. Addition of the substance present in the sample will increase the peak. If the substance added is not identical with that in the sample, the electrophoretic pattern will show a double peak.

B. *Occurrence of FDP*

The concentration of FDP in normals was first given as 0–10 μg/ml serum (Merskey, et al., 1966; Das, et al., 1967; Catt, et al., 1968). Merskey and coworkers (Merskey, et al., 1971; Merskey and Johnson, 1971) now give the normal concentration as less than 5 μg/ml serum. The survival of high molecular weight degradation products in the blood has been given as 24–48 hours, while that for the end products is much shorter (Niléhn and Robertson, 1965; Fisher, et al., 1967).

Urine normally contains no FDP. In conditions with a high concentration of D and E products in the blood, e.g. during treatment with thrombolytics, these products may be excreted in the urine (Bouma, et al., 1971). High molecular weight degradation products cannot be excreted in the urine (Rayner, et al., 1969). When found in the urine they may derive from the breakdown of local deposits of fibrin in the kidneys or from fibrinogen filtered through damaged glomeruli.

In recent years various clinical conditions have been studied for FDP, usually with the TRCHII method.

We have published the results of examination of FDP with Niléhn's method in 3.075 patients with various diseases (Hedner and Nilsson, 1971b). Our results are largely in good agreement with those obtained by other authors. The most important conditions in which we and others have found FDP are summarised below.

1. Malignant diseases

FDP are often demonstrable in patients with malignant diseases (Table 11). They have thus been found in 60 per cent of 346 patients with various sorts of *cancer* in different stages (Hedner and Nilsson, 1971b; Åstedt, et al., 1971b; Carlsson, 1973). Merskey, et al. (1966) and Colman, et al. (1970) have also reported FDP in cancer.

Åstedt, et al. (1971b, 1972) routinely measured FDP in patients with palpable ovarian tumours and found FDP in 82 per cent of those who were afterwards proved to have ovarian carcinoma but no FDP in those who were found to have benign tumours. After successful treatment with surgery and radiotherapy the FDP disappeared, but reappeared in association with recurrences of the tumour. Examination for FDP in patients with suspect malignant tumours may be of diagnostic value and also helpful for assessing recurrences.

It is possible that FDP in patients with cancer originate from extravascular fibrin broken down by malignant cells. Several authors have shown that certain tumours contain fibrinolytic substances (Cliffton and Grossi, 1955; O'Meara, 1958; Rudenstam, 1968; Peterson, 1968).

2. Renal diseases

Several reports of FDP in renal diseases have been published during the last few years (Wardle and Taylor, 1968; Braun and Merrill, 1968; Rayner, et al., 1969; Larsson, et al., 1971c; Clarkson, et al., 1971; Preston, et al., 1971; Hedner and Nilsson, 1971b; Stiehm, et al., 1971; Chirawong, et al., 1971; Ekert, et al., 1972; Vermylen, et al., 1972).

Table 11. *FDP in sera from patients with different diseases.*

	No. of patients	Pos (%)	Range (μg/ml)
Cancer	162	61	10–170
Renal diseases	150	37	10–80
Acute thromboembolic diseases	150	72	10–160
Collagen diseases	30	38	10–50
Sepsis	75	98	10–1000
Miscellaneous infections	140	56	10–40
Postoperative bleedings with shock	50	95	10–500
Liver cirrhosis	183	25	10–30
Complications of pregnancy (toxicosis and hepatosis)	323	75	10–200

The origin of FDP in these conditions, the type of FDP in the urine and the diagnostic and prognostic value of determinations of FDP in the serum and urine in various forms of renal disease have been the subject of much debate.

Intraglomerular fibrin deposits have been demonstrated in glomerulo-nephritis, nephritis in lupus erythematodes and eclampsia (Vassalli, et al., 1963; Koffler and Paronetto, 1966; Humair, et al., 1969; Clarkson, et al., 1971; Chirawong, et al., 1971). Fibrin deposits have also been demonstrated in the haemolytic-uraemic syndrome (Habib, et al., 1969; Liebermann, 1972). It has been assumed that the fibrin deposits are the results of disseminated intravascular coagulation, precipitated by the primary disease. However, most kidney diseases are characterised by a normal platelet count, high levels of AHF and fibrinogen, high or normal levels of Factor V, prothrombin and plasminogen, low fibrinolytic activity and no fibrin monomers in the circulating blood, even if FDP are present in the serum and urine. It has been questioned whether disseminated intravascular coagulation really is necessary for the formation of fibrin deposits in the kidney and whether it might not simply be due to local coagulation. The primary factor may thus be endothelial injury in the glomeruli owing to an antigen-antibody complex, for example. This endothelial injury leads to exposure of the basement membrane. The collagen of the basement membrane is an extremely strong trigger factor for platelet aggregation. Platelets therefore aggregate at the site of the exposed basement membrane, and this in turn leads to deposits of fibrin and formation of thrombi (Gilchrist and Liebermann, 1969; Rodriguez-Erdmann and Guttman, 1969; Nilsson, 1970; Merskey and Johnson, 1971; Franklin, et al., 1972).

A prerequisite for local deposition of fibrin in the kidneys to give rise to FDP is that the fibrin be dissolved.

In the kidney there are two types of fibrinolytic activators, namely tissue fibrinolytic activator and urokinase. With histochemical methods the tissue fibrinolytic activator has been found to be localised mainly in the intrarenal blood vessels between the medulla and cortex, while human glomeruli are inactive (Kwaan and Fischer, 1965; Pandolfi, et al., 1971). In contrast with what is seen in normal kidneys, the renal cortex has been found to acquire fibrinolytic properties in chronic inflammation and during rejection of renal grafts (Pandolfi, et al., 1971). Uro-kinase is probably produced by the glomeruli, as shown in tissue culture, while in renal disease the production of urokinase disappears (Carlsson, et al., 1970; Åstedt, 1972). But because of the persistence of tissue fibrinolytic activator in the diseased kidney, dissolution of fibrin/fibrinogen is possible.

In renal disease the fibrinolytic activity in the circulation is markedly reduced (McNicol, et al., 1965; Larsson, et al., 1971a, b; Ito, et al., 1972). This reduction is due to an increased amount of inhibitors of fibrinolysis (Larsson, et al., 1971a, b, c) and not to deficient synthesis of activators of fibrinolysis (Isacson and Nilsson, 1969).

Another possible reason for the occurrence of FDP in the urine is filtration of fibrinogen through damaged glomeruli and then further degradation of the fibrinogen in the kidneys.

FDP in uraemia. FDP have been demonstrated in the serum, parti-cularly in *acute renal insufficiency* (Wardle and Taylor, 1968; Larsson, et al., 1971c; Hedner and Nilsson, 1971b; Ekert, et al., 1972). For instance, we found FDP in the serum in 78 per cent, and in unconcentrated urine in 57 per cent of patients with acute uraemia (Larsson, et al., 1971c) (Table 12). The concentration of FDP in the urine was usually higher than in the serum. The urinary FDP have been found to be predominantly of high molecular weight type (Bouma, et al., 1971).

Determination of FDP in such patients has proved useful for following the course of the disease and the effect of therapy (Larsson, et al., 1971c; Hedner, et al., 1973a).

In *chronic uraemia* FDP are more often demonstrable in the urine than in the serum (Rayner, et al., 1969; Preston, et al., 1971; Hedner and Nils-son, 1971b). We found FDP in the serum in 37 per cent and in uncon-centrated urine in 39 per cent of patients (Table 12). The amount of FDP has been shown to vary with the activity of the disease (Stiehm, et al., 1971; Hedner and Nilsson, 1971b; Larsson, et al., 1971c; Clarkson, et al., 1971; Preston, et al., 1971). The urinary FDP have been shown to be of the high molecular weight type (Bouma, et al., 1971). Gel filtration on Sephadex G-200, and typing, showed that FDP in the urine in chronic uraemia consist of both X and Y fragments. Low molecular weight products could also be demonstrated but in low concentrations (Hedner, 1973).

Renal disease	Total no. of cases	FDP/s % pos	FDP/s Range µg/ml	FDP/u % pos	FDP/u Range µg/ml	Type
Chronic uraemia	76	37	5–60	39	10–100	X, Y (D, E)
Acute uraemia	18	78	10–80	57	20–350	X, Y (D, E)

Table 12. FDP serum and urine patients with ren[...] diseases (Hedn[...] and Nilsson).

FDP in glomerulonephritis. FDP have also been related to the histological findings in renal disease (Clarkson, et al., 1971; Chirawong, et al., 1971). FDP in the serum as well as in the urine have been found predominantly in the proliferative types of glomerulonephritis and most often in the acute forms of this type of nephritis, but less often in membranous glomerulonephritis and minimal renal lesions (Clarkson, et al., 1971; Stiehm, et al., 1971; Preston, et al., 1971; Ekert, et al., 1972).

To ascertain whether FDP are demonstrable in the urine early in the development of glomerulonephritis we studied 24 patients without signs of renal insufficiency (Hedner, et al., 1973a) (Table 13). We found no FDP in unconcentrated urine from these patients, while all but one (18 of 19) of those with a proliferative glomerulonephritis and 2 out of 5 with membranous forms of glomerulonephritis had demonstrable FDP in concentrated samples of the pooled 24-hour urine. Typing with the method of Bouma showed the FDP in the concentrated urine to be mainly of high molecular weight type. We have never been able to demonstrate FDP in concentrated urine from normals. Recently we also investigated concentrated urine from patients with pyelonephritis but without uraemia. No FDP were found.

FDP in the haemolytic-uraemic syndrome. FDP in the serum are common in the haemolytic-uraemic syndrome (Luke, et al., 1970; Katz, et al., 1971).

FDP in the urine have, however, not been studied so extensively as in other renal diseases. We have followed ten patients with the syndrome and found that such repeated determinations can be of great value for estimating the prognosis and the effect of therapy.

FDP in renal transplantation. FDP in the serum have been demonstrated during the first postoperative week and during episodes of rejection (Braun and Merrill, 1968; Antoine, et al., 1969; Rosenberg, et al., 1969; Carlsson, et al., 1970; Bouma, et al., 1971). The occurrence of FDP in the urine in such patients is now considered much more informative. The occurrence of FDP in the urine later than two weeks after operation has been regarded as a sign of rejection (Braun and Merrill, 1968; Antoine, et al., 1969; Carlsson, et al., 1970; Clarkson, et al., 1970). Immunochemical

Table 13. *FDP and okinase activity in ine in patients with oliferative glomeronephritis and with embranous glomernephritis* (*Hedner d Nilsson*)

Diagnoses	FDP/s µg/ml	FDP/u uncon- centrated µg/ml	FDP/u concen- trated µg/24 hrs	FDP type	Urokinase activity Ploug units/ml
Proliferative glomerulonephrit. (19)	0	0	90–1,650	HMWS (17)	0·9–6
Membranous glomerulonephrit. (5)	0	0	30–70	HMWS (3)	1–3·2
Control (19)	0	0	0		>6

typing has shown the FDP in the urine to be of high molecular weight type (Bouma, et al., 1971; Hedner, 1973).

3. Leukaemia and blood diseases

FDP have often been demonstrated in leukaemia (Merskey, et al., 1966; Colman, et al., 1970). We have found FDP in the serum with a frequency of 42 per cent in acute leukaemia and of 22 per cent in chronic leukaemia (Table 11). Fibrinogen and plasminogen are usually decreased, and the fibrinolytic activity in the blood is periodically increased, i.e. the disease includes a fibrinolytic component—primary or secondary. We have only occasionally found FDP in the serum in thrombocytopenia, thrombocytosis, haemolytic and aplastic anaemia, agranulocytosis and polycytaemia.

4. Thrombo-embolic diseases

Of 75 patients with acute thrombo-embolism, most (72 per cent) were found to have FDP in the serum (Hedner and Nilsson, 1971b) (Table 11). On the other hand, no such products were found in serum in patients with thrombotic disease and examined at least three months after the acute thrombo-embolic episode. Cash, et al. (1971) sometimes found a marked increase in FDP postoperatively. Further investigation showed that these patients had thrombo-embolic complications. FDP in the acute stage of thrombo-embolism can probably be ascribed to spontaneous dissolution of the fresh thrombus.

In myocardial infarction, on the other hand, FDP are not seen initially except in patients who have been resuscitated (Almér, et al., 1972). In the differentiation between myocardial infarction and pulmonary embolism, determination of FDP with a quick method in the acute stage may be of value immediately after the attack.

Later, more than one third of all patients with myocardial infarction have FDP in a concentration of 10–40 μg/ml serum. The infarctions are significantly larger in patients belonging to this group than in those who do not develop FDP (Almér, et al., 1972).

5. Dysproteinaemias

FDP are fairly common in collagenosis (Merskey, et al., 1966; Fisher, et al., 1967; Colman, et al., 1970). We found FDP in the serum of 38 per cent of a series of patients with collagen diseases (rheumatoid arthritis, SLE, polyarteritis nodosa) (Table 11). In most of the patients with FDP the disease was in the acute stage.

Patients with myeloma, macroglobulinaemia and arteritis (Takayasu's disease) usually have no FDP in the serum.

6. Liver diseases

FDP have often been found in liver cirrhosis and have been regarded as a consequence of either primary or secondary fibrinolysis (Merskey, et al., 1966; Fisher, et al., 1967; Colman, et al., 1970). In an investigation of a large series of liver cirrhosis we found FDP in the serum in only 19 per cent.

7. Sepsis and infections

FDP are a common finding in sepsis with shock (Merskey, et al., 1966; Abildgaard, Ch., 1969; Lasch, 1969a; Cronberg and Nilsson, 1970; Hedner and Nilsson, 1971b). FDP in the cases with sepsis are believed to originate from microthrombi, dissolved by the activators of fibrinolysis in the vessel walls.

We were unable to demonstrate FDP in most patients with broncho-pneumonia. Of patients with other infections (cholecystitis, obscure diseases with fever, urinary tract infections etc.) we found FDP in the serum in 50 per cent. This finding is probably due to secondary dissolution of fibrin deposits.

8. Shock, trauma, postoperative complications

Patients with haemophilia and other haemorrhagic diseases do not usually have FDP in association with bleeding (Hedner and Nilsson, 1971b). FDP have only occasionally been demonstrable in patients with menorrhagia and gastro-intestinal bleeding. But the occurrence of FDP is one of the characteristic coagulation findings in shock due to haemorrhage, trauma and postoperative complications (Lasch, 1970).

In our series of postoperative bleeding all of those patients who showed signs of shock were found to have FDP in the serum. Most of these patients also had thrombocytopenia and decreased Factor V and prothrombin.

According to Lasch (1970) and several other authors, shock is associated with generalised intravascular coagulation with disseminated micro-thrombosis. FDP most probably originate from the dissolution of these fibrin thrombi by secondary fibrinolysis.

After uncomplicated operations only small amounts (5–25 $\mu g/ml$) of FDP are demonstrable, and then only for a short time (Hedner and Nilsson, 1971b; Cash, et al., 1971).

9. Obstetric complications

Several authors have demonstrated FDP in high concentration in serum from patients with obstetric complications such as ablatio placentae and missed abortion (Merskey, et al., 1966; Woodfield, et al., 1968; Bonnar, et al., 1969; Kleiner, et al., 1970). The occurrence of FDP in these cases shows that the conditions are associated with defibrination and/or fibrinolysis.

Hedner and Åstedt (1970) published determinations of FDP with Niléhn's method in the serum and in the urine from 1001 women in the third trimester of pregnancy. None of the patients had FDP in the urine, 99 had FDP in the serum and 85 per cent of them developed conditions such as toxicosis, hepatosis and Rh-immunisation. In a series of toxicosis and hepatosis, Hedner and Nilsson (1971b) found that 68 per cent of those with toxicosis and 81 per cent of those with hepatosis had FDP (Table 11). In these cases the concentration of FDP varied with the course of the disease. McNicol, et al. (1971) also found that an increasing amount of FDP during pregnancy is a sign of complications. It is also known that fibrin deposits and microthrombi occur in the kidneys and liver in toxicosis. The FDP probably originate from dissolution of such fibrin deposits.

10. Comments

The occurrence of FDP indicates intravascular or extravascular dissolution of fibrinogen or fibrin. Repeated demonstration of FDP is a sign of a disease requiring further investigation. It is probable that in certain cases routine determinations of FDP may be of value as a diagnostic screening method. It has already proved informative in the investigation of suspect malignant disease, renal disease, postoperative complications and sepsis and pregnancy.

IV. Synthetic antifibrinolytics
HANS KJELLMAN

In the beginning of the 1950s it was found that some amino acids such as ornithine and lysine, inhibit the activation of plasminogen *in vitro*. But the effect of these amino acids proved too weak to be utilised in the treatment of fibrinolytic haemorrhagic conditions. In systematic investigation in 1953 by a group in Japan under the direction of S. Okamoto it was shown that several mercapto- and aminocarbonic acids have an antifibrinolytic effect. Of these substances, epsilon aminocaproic acid (EACA) had the strongest effect (Fig. 39). This acid has since been widely used clinically. But as the treatment of fibrinolytic haemorrhagic conditions requires large doses of preparations, 8–30 g a day, a search has been made for other substances with a stronger antifibrinolytic effect (Markwardt, et al., 1967; Okomoto, et al., 1962, 1968). Two such substances have been found and used clinically, AMCA and PAMBA.

The antifibrinolytic activity of 4-amino-methyl-cyclohexane-carbonic acid (AMCHA) was reported in 1962. This compound contains two stereoisomers. Independently of each other, Kabi's research department (Melander, et al., 1965) and Okamoto, et al. (1964) found that only the *trans*-form was antifibrinolytically active. The antifibrinolytically active form was called tranexamic acid (AMCA or trans-AMCHA).

The antifibrinolytic activity of p-amino-methyl bensoic acid (PAMBA)

Fig 39.

$$H_2N-CH_2-CH_2-CH_2-CH_2-CH_2-COOH$$

epsilon aminocaproic acid, EACA, Epsikapron®

$$H_2N-CH_2-\langle\!\langle\bigcirc\rangle\!\rangle-COOH$$

p—aminomethyl benzoic
acid, PAMBA

trans-aminomethyl cyclohexane
carbonic acid, tranexamic acid,
AMCA, Cyclokapron®

has been studied by the Markwardt group (Markwardt, et al., 1967). Their preparation has been used particularly in Eastern Europe.

AMCA, EACA and PAMBA are said to exert their antifibrinolytic effect by competitively inhibiting the activation of plasminogen (Alkjaersig, et al., 1959b; Andersson, et al., 1965). According to Abiko, et al. (1969), AMCA inhibits the activation of plasminogen by forming a plasminogen inhibitor complex, which presumably causes conformational changes in the plasminogen molecule. Collen, et al. (1972b) found that 3 g AMCA taken each day by mouth increased the turnover of labelled plasminogen in one of three volunteers. When 6 g AMCA was given, it accelerated the turnover of plasminogen in both of two persons studied.

EACA and AMCA are weak, non-competitive inhibitors of plasmin (Alkjaersig, et al., 1959b; Andersson, et al., 1965). According to some investigators (Okamoto and Okamoto, 1962, and others), EACA and AMCA primarily inhibit plasmin. The difference, according to them, depends on the choice of substrate, enzyme and activator used in the test system. It is, however, generally claimed that the concentrations of EACA and the cyclic inhibitors of fibrinolysis necessary to inhibit plasmin are 10–100 times higher than those necessary for inhibition of activation of plasminogen (Markwardt, et al., 1967). The inhibiting effect of AMCA and EACA on trypsin and pepsin is weak or very weak (Alkjaersig, et al., 1959b; Markwardt, et al., 1967).

Comparative investigations *in vitro* of the inhibiting effect of AMCA, EACA and PAMBA on plasminogen activation induced by streptokinase or physiological activators, such as urokinase or tissue activators, have given different results, presumably because of differences in the test methods used. The effect of AMCA on streptokinase-induced plasminogen activation has been described as 6–40 times stronger than that of EACA and the effect of AMCA on urokinase-induced plasminogen activation as 6–100 times stronger than that of EACA (Andersson, et al., 1965; Okamoto, et al., 1968). Opinions differ on the antifibrinolytic activity of PAMBA compared with that of AMCA or EACA. As a rule, however, AMCA is claimed to be twice as strong as PAMBA *in vitro* (Maki and Beller, 1966).

In the appraisal of the antifibrinolytic effect of AMCA and EACA on fibrin plates, where the plasminogen is activated by activators from human tissues, AMCA has been found to be 10 times stronger than EACA (Andersson, et al., 1968).

Investigations of the variation of the antifibrinolytic effect of synthetic inhibitors of fibrinolysis with their molecular structures have shown that the antifibrinolytic effect is due to the presence of free amino and carboxyl groups and that the effect is strongest when the distance between them is about 7 Å, as it is in AMCA, EACA and PAMBA. The stronger antifibrinolytic activity of AMCA and PAMBA can probably be ascribed to the greater rigidity of the molecule (Markwardt, et al., 1967).

A. *Toxicology*

All three antifibrinolytics, AMCA, EACA and PAMBA, are of low acute toxicity (Melander, et al., 1965). In rats and mice the LD_{50} of AMCA by mouth is about 12.500 µg/kg and given intravenously is 800 and 1.300 µg/kg, respectively. The LD_{50} of EACA given orally to rats and mice is 12.000–16.000 µg/kg and intravenously about 3.000 µg/kg. The acute toxicity of PAMBA is of the same magnitude. In toxicity tests of AMCA carried out on dogs and rats and continued for some months, neither macroscopic nor microscopic examination of several organs revealed any toxic injuries. In the female dogs, however, the ovaries were always smaller than in the controls. Daily treatment of dogs with AMCA for 1 year by mouth and for seven days intravenously in amounts correspond- ing to respectively 7 and 18 times the maximal doses per kg body weight recommended for man has been reported to produce retinal changes. Such changes did not occur in dogs or rats that received respectively 3·5 and 7 times the maximal dose by mouth for 1 year and for 22 months, respectively, or in monkeys who were given 18 times the maximal dose intravenously for 7 or 14 days (Kjellman, 1972).

No retinal changes have been reported or seen at examination of patients treated with Cyclokapron® for several weeks to months. Patients who are to be treated continuously for several weeks should preferably be examined ophthalmologically (visual acuity, colour vision, fundus oculi, field of vision, etc.) before, as well as at regular intervals during treatment.

Adenoma and adenocarcinoma of the liver have been reported in rats after 22 months' oral treatment, but not after 12 months, with about 27 times the maximal dose of AMCA per kg body weight recommended for man. No such tumours have been seen in rats given 6 times the maximal daily dose per kg body weight recommended for human beings (Kjellman, 1972).

Light microscopic examination of tissues and organs from dogs that had been given 110 or 220 mg AMCA per kg body weight a day for 14 days, showed no deposits of fibrin. Electron microscopic examination showed little evidence of fibrin deposits in the kidneys. AMCA in a dose of 500 mg/kg a day by mouth caused oedema of the subendothelial layer the aorta and swelling of subendothelial cells, and infiltration of inflammatory cells in rabbits (Kato, et al., 1970). Carroll and Tice (1966) found that doses of 0·33–1·4 g EACA per kg given intravenously to nephrectomised dogs produced hyperpotassaemia. The authors feel that EACA is taken up by muscle cells and thereby increases the escape of intracellular K^+. Garrett, et al. (1968) found administration of 50–200 mg EACA per kg body weight to have a diuretic effect on dogs with an increased excretion of Na^+, Cl^- and, to some extent, also of K^+. Muscle pain with increases in the serum enzymes, creatinine phosphokinase and aldolase have sometimes been reported in clinical investigations with EACA in patients with hereditary angioneurotic oedema (Frank, et al., 1972). In one case Korsan-Bengtsen, et al. (1969) demonstrated Zenker's hyaline degeneration in muscle cells in a muscle biopsy specimen.

Experiments on rats, mice and rabbits for any teratogenic effect of the preparations in doses of up to 500 mg AMCA/kg a day revealed no foetal abnormalities. Neither has EACA been found to have any teratologic effect. EACA given to dogs and female rats in large doses has resulted in a reduction of fertility by 50 per cent, but the reduction was reversible (Eneroth and Grant, 1966).

In the rat, mouse and dog EACA releases noradrenalin from the heart (Lippman and Wishnick, 1965), but not from the brain. Subendothelial haemorrhages, particularly on continuous intravenous infusion in the dog, have been ascribed to this release of catecholamines. It has also been shown that EACA, like guanethidine, blocks not only the depots of amines, but also the transport of catecholamines through the cell membranes. Comparative investigations of the effect of AMCA and EACA on the release of noradrenalin from the heart and brain in the rat have shown that AMCA in doses up to 1.000 mg/kg does not reduce the noradrenalin content of such tissues. On the other hand, EACA lowers the noradrenalin content of the heart (Granstrand, et al., 1966).

In the rat, administration of EACA in a dose of 2 g/kg intravenously is followed first by a sympathomimetic phase and later, within six hours, by a 20 per cent reduction of the blood pressure (Andén, et al., 1968). Hedwall, et al. (1968), however, have not been able to demonstrate an increase in blood pressure and a later decrease. AMCA given intravenously to the cat and rat in a dose of 30 mg/kg has a certain pressure effect if the injection is given relatively quickly. Cummings and Welter (1966) showed that the blood pressure in the dog is not affected by intravenous or repeated oral administration of EACA. On the other hand continuous intravenous infusion raises the blood pressure in the cat and the dog. Gabryelewicz, et al. (1967) found that the arterial blood pressure increased in patients with a low blood pressure treated with 100 mg EACA per kg body weight a day for four days.

B. *Pharmacokinetics*

The absorption, distribution and excretion of EACA given intravenously and by mouth have been studied in man by McNicol, et al. (1962) and

Nilsson, et al. (1960). Intravenous administration of 10 g EACA or 100 mg/kg produces an initial serum concentration of about 15.000 μg/ml serum and after 3–4 hours, about 35 μg/ml (McNicol, et al., 1962; Andersson, et al., 1968). About 80–100 per cent of the dose of EACA given is excreted unchanged in the urine within 3·5–6 hours, respectively, after intravenous injection (McNicol, et al., 1962). Andersson, et al. (1968), however, found that only 71 per cent of the dose given was excreted in the urine within 24 hours of an intravenous injection. The biological half-life and volumetric distribution volume have been found to be about 77 minutes and 0·28 1./kg, respectively. When given by mouth EACA is rapidly absorbed, and almost entirely from the gastro-intestinal tract. A maximum serum concentration of about 200 μg/ml is reached 1–2 hours after a therapeutic dose (McNicol, et al., 1962). The concentration of EACA in the urine is about 100 times higher than that in plasma. 80 per cent of the dose given is excreted within the first four hours of administration (McNicol, et al., 1962). According to Andersson, et al. (1968), only about 60 per cent of the dose given is excreted during the first 24 hours after administration.

On intravenous administration of 10 mg AMCA/kg, the serum concentration was 18, 10 and 5 μg/ml 1, 3 and 5 hours, respectively, after the injection. About 55 per cent was excreted unchanged during the first three hours after the injection and about 90 per cent within 24 hours. In a cross over examination of twelve volunteers that had received a single dose of two tablets of Cyclokapron® (total dose 1.000 mg AMCA) and 1.000 mg AMCA in the form of a water solution in the fasting state the maximal plasma concentrations noted were respectively 8·4 and 8·2 μg/ml. Both preparations reached their maximal plasma concentration within about 3 hours. About 40 per cent of a given dose is excreted in the urine (Andersson, et al., 1968). As mentioned, AMCA has been reported to be about 10 times more active than EACA, both *in vitro* and *in vivo*. Since AMCA is not so readily absorbed as EACA, when given by mouth, AMCA is only 3 times as active as EACA. The biological half-life is given as 1–2 hours in patients with normal renal function (Andersson, et al., 1968). If renal function is impaired, the half-life is longer, and the interval between the doses should therefore be prolonged (Andersson, et al., 1971).

In the treatment of local fibrinolysis due to an abnormal release of tissue activators, it is important to know how long the fibrinolytic inhibitor persists in different tissues. The concentrations of AMCA and EACA in serum and in pieces of human tissue, e.g. large intestine, kidneys and prostate obtained at operation, have been determined by Andersson, et al. (1968) with high-voltage electrophoresis. AMCA was given 36–48 hours before the operation in four doses of about 10–20 mg AMCA/kg body weight. The corresponding dose of EACA was 100 mg/kg body weight. The last dose was given at a varying interval before the operation. The results showed that the antifibrinolytically active concentration of AMCA (10 μg/ml) persisted longer in the tissues examined than did the corresponding concentration of EACA (100 μg/ml). AMCA has thus not only a higher antifibrinolytic activity than EACA but it also persists longer in the different tissues.

AMCA passes transplacentally to the foetus (Kullander and Nilsson, 1970). After intravenous injection of 10 mg/kg body weight the concentration in the foetal serum may be anything between 4 and 31 μg/ml. Tovi, et al. (1972a, b) have shown that if AMCA is given intravenously in a dose of 1 g six times a day to patients with subarachnoid haemorrhage, it enters the cerebrospinal fluid. After treatment for some days the concentration in the cerebrospinal fluid is 2–5 μg/ml.

PAMBA, in contrast with AMCA and EACA, is excreted partly in acetylated form (Andersson, et al., 1971). After oral administration of 20 mg PAMBA/kg body weight 53 per cent was excreted within 24 hours and 17 per cent of it as antifibrinolytically inactive acetyl-PAMBA. These values agree with those given by Markwardt, et al. (1967). On oral administration of 20 mg PAMBA/kg body weight the maximal serum concentration, 5–10 μg/ml, was noted after 2 hours (Andersson, et al., 1971). 50–70 per cent of an intravenous dose of PAMBA is excreted within 24 hours and 30–50 per cent as metabolites, mainly acetyl-PAMBA.

V. Fibrinolysis and defibrination from a clinical standpoint

Though the fibrinolytic and coagulation systems consist of different plasma proteins, much suggests that both systems can be activated by similar mechanisms. When tissues are injured by trauma, for example, the fibrinolytic system may be activated by release of tissue activators of fibrinolysis, and the coagulation system can be activated by release of tissue thromboplastin. Clinically, it is therefore difficult to decide whether fibrinolysis and defibrination occur together or one after the other.

Several clinical syndromes are probably associated with some degree of both fibrinolysis and defibrination.

Conditions with associated fibrinolysis and defibrination can be roughly classified as follows:

1. *Fibrinolysis.* Bleeding conditions in which systemic fibrinolysis is the primary and main cause of the bleeding. The fibrinolysis may be classified as acute or chronic according to the duration of the condition.

2. *Local fibrinolysis.* The bleeding is confined to a single organ and is due to local release of activators of fibrinolysis. The fibrinolytic activity in the blood is not increased.

3. *Defibrination with or without secondary fibrinolysis.* Conditions in which an abnormal activation of the coagulation process is regarded as the primary haemostatic disorder. Systemic or local fibrinolysis may develop secondarily to this process. The defibrination syndrome may also be classified as acute or chronic according to the duration of the condition.

4. *Local deposition of fibrin.* Conditions with signs of fibrin deposition only in a *single organ* without concomitant signs of systemic intravascular coagulation.

A. *Fibrinolytic bleeding conditions—systemic fibrinolysis*

In *acute* fibrinolysis the plasminogen is rapidly and markedly activated to plasmin, which results in pronounced hypofibrinogenaemia and even afibrinogenaemia. The activation of the fibrinolytic system has been ascribed to a sudden release of labile activators of plasminogen into the circulation. The haemorrhages are severe and may often be fatal. As a rule, there is generalised bleeding—blood oozes from all mucosae—and there is diffuse bleeding from wounds and the operative field. Severe acute fibrinolysis has been observed in profound shock, obstetric complications and in association with operations, particularly of the chest, pancreas, prostate and thyroid (for references, see Pechet, 1965; Fearnley, 1965; Fletcher, 1966; Nilsson, Andersson and Björkman, 1966; Fisher, et al., 1967; Johnson and Merskey, 1970).

Fibrinolysis of *chronic* type, often with remissions and exacerbations, has been reported in several conditions such as liver diseases, malignant tumours, especially of the prostate and the pancreas, leukaemia, Boeck's sarcoid, lymphogranulomatosis and polycythaemia (for references, see Fearnley, 1965; Pechet, 1965; Nilsson, Andersson and Björkman, 1966; Ogston, et al., 1968; Mathur, et al., 1968; Brakman, et al., 1970). In these conditions, the fibrinolytic activity in the blood is, as a rule, lower than in acute fibrinolysis and in the mild cases the fibrinogen content need not be reduced. Large haematomas and oozing haemorrhages from mucosal and local lesions are common.

Characteristic laboratory findings in systemic fibrinolysis are as follows:
1. Fibrinolytic activity in the blood, both activator and plasmin activity.
2. Decreased content of plasminogen.
3. Decreased content of the factors which can be broken down by plasmin, i.e. fibrinogen, AHF and Factor V.
4. High content of fibrin/fibrinogen degradation products (FDP).
5. Prolonged thrombin time and Reptilase time.
6. Decreased content of α_2-macroglobulin.
7. Normal platelet count, unless reduced by basic disease.
8. Normal prothrombin, Factor VII and Factor X, unless suppressed by basic disease.

In acute fibrinolysis it is, as a rule, only during a short attack that the activators of fibrinolysis are released. These activators are also quickly cleared from the blood, their half-life being only 13 minutes (Fletcher, et al., 1964). Since blood samples cannot always be obtained at the beginning of the acute bleeding, it is sometimes not possible to demonstrate any increased fibrinolytic activator activity in the blood sample (Fletcher and Alkjaersig, 1966). But even in these cases it is possible to ascertain retrospectively whether fibrinolysis has occurred by determining the plasminogen content and the occurrence of FDP. A reduced plasminogen value is an important diagnostic sign of fibrinolysis. As previously mentioned, plasminogen is not consumed during coagulation of the blood. It is possible that several of the cases classified as primary fibrinolysis included intravascular coagulation. A specific indicator of *in vivo* fibrinolysis might be obtained in the future by determining fibrinogen-D products and fibrin-D products, respectively.

The differentiation between systemic fibrinolysis and defibrination and the treatment of conditions with systemic fibrinolysis are discussed together with defibrination, since these conditions are related to one another in several respects.

B. *Local fibrinolysis*—See page 155

C. *Defibrination with or without secondary fibrinolysis*

In recent years conditions with intravascular coagulation or defibrination have attracted extensive attention. Various clinical reviews of defibrination have been published in the last few years (Hjort and Rapaport, 1965; Verstraete, et al., 1965; Merskey, 1968; Verstraete and Vermylen, 1968; Steichele, 1969; Ratnoff, 1969; Abildgaard, Ch., 1969; McKay, 1969a, b; Owen, et al., 1969; Didisheim, et al., 1969; Lasch, 1970; Colman, et al., 1972). Several authors feel that primary fibrinolysis is extremely rare and even question whether haemorrhage is ever due to primary fibrinolysis alone (Verstraete, et al., 1965; Merskey and Johnson, 1966; Verstraete and Vermylen, 1968; McKay, 1969a, b; Abildgaard, Ch., 1969; Lasch, 1969a, b, 1970). They thus ascribe most of the acute bleeding conditions with low fibrinogen, to intravascular coagulation.

The defibrination syndrome was first described from a clinical point of view by Schneider (1951) in a woman with abruptio placentae and amniotic fluid embolism. As pointed out in the previous section on the defibrination process, there are several different mechanisms which may lead to activation of the coagulation process *in vivo*. Considering this, the spectrum of diseases in which defibrination or intravascular coagulation has been found is extremely wide. McKay (1965, 1969a, b), Hardaway (1966) and Ch. Abildgaard (1969) believe that intravascular coagulation plays an important role in most clinical syndromes, namely, shock of varying etiology, burns, trauma, fat embolism, postoperative complications, haemorrhages, extracorporeal circulation, renal diseases, pulmonary insufficiency, heart diseases, hypertension, liver diseases, pancreatic diseases, acute adrenal insufficiency, thrombo-embolism, haemorrhagic gastritis, enterocolitis, haemolytic syndrome, obstetric complications, toxicosis, malignant diseases, leukaemia, large haemangiomas, *purpura fulminans*, various types of infections, e.g. malaria, mycoses, rickettsia, viral and bacterial infections, amyloidosis, snake bite, hyaline membranes (in newborns), heat stroke, and rejection of transplants. Merskey, who is one of the pioneers in the field of defibrination, definitely refrains from classifying most of the known diseases with associated intravascular coagulation. He claims that in most of these conditions the blood shows no changes suggesting intravascular consumption of coagulation factors and that there is no certain evidence of disseminated thrombosis.

We, like several other researchers, now feel that the primary cause is the basic disease. In some cases this may lead to release of thromboplastin into the blood stream (cancer, trauma, amniotic emboli) and in other cases the basic disease results in vascular injury, which initiates thrombus formation. It is extremely important for the clinician to be aware of the fact that *defibrination should not be regarded as a separate disease or diagnosis, but only as a complication or as part of the clinical picture of a particular disease*.

Judging from our clinical experience, *systemic defibrination may above all be induced by the following clinical conditions*:

Acute systemic defibrination
1. Sepsis of varying origin.
2. Haemorrhagic shock, trauma and postoperative complications, following incompatible blood transfusions, and anaphylactic shock.
3. Widespread tissue damage, e.g. burns and multiple fractures.
4. Obstetric complications, particularly ablatio placentae, aminotic fluid embolism, missed abortion, eclampsia and toxicosis.
5. Purpura fulminans.
6. Following extracorporeal circulation.
7. Snake bite.

Subacute or chronic systemic defibrination
1. Malignant diseases, especially disseminated cancer.
2. Acute promyelocytic leukaemia.
3. Thrombotic thrombocytopenic purpura.
4. Missed abortion.
5. Giant haemangioma.

In this connection it should be stressed that pregnancy, blocking of the RES, cortisone and catecholamines increase susceptibility to defibrination.

It is still an open question whether the intravascular coagulation in the Shwartzman reaction is the cause of shock. McKay and Hardaway believe it is, while others (Lerner, et al., 1968) have shown that intravascular coagulation and endotoxin shock are independent manifestations of endotoxinaemia. According to them, the precipitation of fibrin is not the cause of death in endotoxin shock. Salzman (1968) has studied haemorrhagic shock in man and he, too, arrived at the conclusion that the eventual intravascular coagulation has nothing to do with the shock and fatal issue. Attar, et al. (1970), who studied the coagulation and fibrinolytic systems in 294 patients with shock of various origins, concluded that DIC does not play any notable role in the irreversible stages of shock in man. According to Lasch (1969b), no unequivocal evidence has been produced to show that changes in the haemostatic mechanism are of significance in the pathogenesis of shock. He says: 'Anticoagulants, like heparin, which are only administered after the onset of shock may interrupt consumption coagulopathy, but do not have any effect whatsoever on the onset of shock'.

Clinical findings in defibrination. The symptoms are normally those characteristic of the primary disease together with symptoms compatible with widespread microthrombosis and necrosis in various organs. Such symptoms may be shock, peripheral circulatory disorders, oliguria and anuria, cerebral affection, liver insufficiency, abdominal symptoms and adrenal insufficiency (McKay, 1969c). According to Lasch (1969a, b), anuria is the most serious complication. In several of the acute types of defibrination the symptoms of the underlying disease are so pronounced that the defibrination is unsuspected, since it adds little or nothing to the clinical picture. Haemorrhagic diathesis may occur, but severe bleeding tends to occur only in cases with a considerable fibrinolytic component and in those patients who have primarily had a bleeding defect, such as thrombocytopenia in leukaemia.

Also in the subacute and chronic cases with defibrination bleeding is generally not the predominant symptom. If bleeding occurs, it is usually from some local injury such as ulcerating cancer in the gastro-intestinal canal. But the patients often have multiple thrombi involving both veins and arteries with local symptoms as a result. The defibrination fairly often causes no additional symptoms, and the syndrome is suspected only because of the associated disease or from the coagulation analysis. Intravascular coagulation can cause haemolysis (McKay, 1969a) and the occurrence of burr cells is said to be characteristic of defibrination.

Characteristic laboratory findings in systemic defibrination are as follows:

1. Thrombocytopenia.
2. Decreased fibrinogen.
3. Decreased Factor V and prothrombin.
4. Usually increased AHF related antigen.
5. No increase in the fibrinolytic activity in the blood.
6. Normal or moderately decreased plasminogen.
7. Fibrin monomers in the plasma.
8. Fibrin/fibrinogen degradation products (FDP) in serum.
9. Prolonged thrombin time and Reptilase time.
10. Decreased content of α_2-macroglobulin.

Not all of these findings are necessary since the activation of the coagulation may start at different stages. Thus, the platelet count may be normal if the activation begins in one of the later stages of coagulation. But the diagnosis can be established only if it can be shown that *degradation of fibrinogen* has occurred. This may be done by demonstration of fibrin monomers in the protamine sulphate precipitation test (Latallo, et al., 1971) or ethanol gelation test (Godal, et al., 1971), low fibrinogen levels and fibrin/fibrinogen degradation products, for example. Furthermore in mild defibrination and in brief attacks of defibrination, fibrinogen and other coagulation factors need not be decreased because the synthesis of such factors may exceed their consumption. The fibrinogen level may also be normal in acute episodes in patients with initially markedly increased values, e.g. in pregnancy and in reactive processes. In such

Table 14.

	Systemic fibrinolysis	Defibrination syndrome	Local fibrin deposition (f ex renal diseases)
Platelet count	normal unless reduced by the basic disease or following massive transfusions	reduced (normal)	normal as a rule
Prothrombin group (Factors II, VII, X)	normal unless reduced by the basic disease	reduced (normal)	normal or increased
Factor V	reduced	reduced (normal)	normal or increased
Fibrinogen	reduced (normal)	reduced (normal)	increased
Fibrinolysis	**increased**	not increased	not increased
Plasminogen	**reduced**	moderately reduced	normal
FDP in serum	**increased**	**increased**	**increased**
Ethanol gelation test	usually neg	pos	neg—pos
Thrombin time	prolonged (normal)	prolonged	ev slightly prolonged
Reptilase time	prolonged (normal)	prolonged	ev slightly prolonged

cases an increased consumption of the factors is demonstrable only by administration of radioactively labelled factors. In the evaluation of decreased platelet counts and various coagulation factors it must be checked whether the patient already had low values because of his basic disease, e.g. hepatocellular damage. The prolonged thrombin and Reptilase times have been ascribed to FDP. α_2-macroglobulin can bind both plasmin and thrombin and may thus be reduced in fibrinolysis as well as in defibrination (Ganrot and Niléhn, 1967).

In most clinical conditions with associated systemic defibrination, fibrinolysis (primary or secondary) is apt to appear. This component can be assessed from the plasminogen content and the amount of FDP. A low plasminogen value and high content of FDP show that the fibrinolytic component of the syndrome is considerable.

Table 14 gives a survey of the most important criteria for differentiation between systemic fibrinolysis and generalised and local defibrination. *Most cases include both components,* but knowledge of the ratio between them is desirable. In doubtful cases the analysis should be repeated to find out which course the condition is pursuing.

Complete investigation of the coagulation and fibrinolytic status is not possible in situations with severe acute bleeding. In most cases, however, certain screening tests will furnish sufficient information for deciding further treatment. The screening analyses we use are: platelet count, Owren's P&P test or thrombotest or normotest, fibrinolysis test (preferably euglobulin clot lysis time, which gives a relatively quick answer), determination of the fibrinogen (rapid method, e.g. Schneider), thrombin time, Reptilase time, a quick method for FDP and test for fibrin monomers (Godal's ethanol gelation test). Further methods are given on page 216.

The results of these analyses can be obtained within 20–30 minutes.

If the tests show a normal platelet count, normal P&P or thrombotest or normotest, fibrinolysis, decreased fibrinogen, prolonged thrombin and Reptilase times (caused by FDP if the fibrinogen is not markedly decreased) and the presence of FDP, the bleeding is probably due mainly to fibrinolysis.

If the tests show a decreased platelet count ($< 100.000/mm^3$) and the reduction cannot be explained by the basic disease or by repeated blood transfusions, decreased values for P&P or thrombotest or normotest, no increase in the fibrinolytic activity, decreased fibrinogen, prolonged thrombin and Reptilase times, a positive quick test for FDP and a positive ethanol gelation test, there is reason to assume that the syndrome includes defibrination. It is often useful to repeat the analysis to assess the further course of the condition.

D. *Local deposition of fibrin*

Several conditions are associated with signs of fibrin deposition only in a *single* organ without concomitant evidence of intravascular coagulation. The following *clinical conditions may include local deposition of fibrin*:
1. Renal disease. Deposits of fibrin have been demonstrated in renal biopsy specimens of patients with acute glomerulonephritis and tubulo-nephritis (McCluskey, et al., 1966).
2. Haemolytic-uraemic syndrome (Gilchrist and Liebermann, 1969).
3. Rejection of renal grafts. It has been clearly shown that rejection of renal grafts is accompanied by the appearance of thrombi of platelets and fibrin in the vessels and in the graft (see Kincaid-Smith, 1969a, b).
4. Toxicosis and hepatosis of pregnancy. These complications are attended by deposition of fibrin in the liver and kidneys (McKay, 1965).

These patients, except those with a low platelet count, show no evidence of an increased bleeding tendency. Most of these patients have markedly increased values for fibrinogen, AHF and prothrombin, e.g. in renal diseases. FDP are, as a rule, demonstrable in the circulating blood. In local defibrination in the kidney FDP can be demonstrated in the urine (see also page 134).

E. *Considerations on the treatment of conditions with associated defibrination and fibrinolysis*

What is the most adequate treatment for patients with signs of disseminated or local defibrination? It is widely agreed that the most important thing is to *treat the basic disease* in the hope that it will abolish the trigger mechanism. Anticoagulant therapy with heparin has often been recommended to counteract intravascular coagulation. Many reports have been published on the use of heparin in the treatment of patients with obstetric complications, shock and bleeding after operations, burns, sepsis, cancer, liver diseases, renal diseases, etc. (Verstraete, et al., 1965; Johnson and Merskey, 1966; Cohen and Gardner, 1966; McGehee, et al., 1967; Straub and Frick, 1967; Verstraete and Vermylen, 1968; Jimenez and Pritchard, 1968; Doughten and Pearson, 1968; Corrigan, et al., 1968; Brain, et al., 1968; Lechner, et al., 1968; Abildgaard, Ch., 1969; McKay, 1969a, b; Lasch, 1969a, b; Gilchrist, et al., 1969; Katz, et al., 1969; Goldfine, et al., 1969; Rosenmann, et al., 1969; McCracken and Dickerman, 1969; Lo, et al., 1971; Colman, et al., 1972). The results obtained have varied, the mortality of the patients treated has been high, and control series have been lacking or insufficient. The patients treated with heparin have died from haemorrhage, irreversible shock or from their basic disease. In most cases the patients have only a short spell of defibrination and platelets and coagulation factors soon recover normal values after such an attack. In a given case it may therefore be difficult to decide whether recovery of the coagulation status is spontaneous or ascribable to treatment with heparin. This has also been pointed out by McKay (1969a, b).

The effect of heparin is mainly prophylactic. Administration of heparin can prevent continued deposition of fibrin and continued consumption of platelets and coagulation factors. Heparin has no immediate effect on those factors responsible for the bleeding in severe consumption coagulopathy—thrombocytopenia, fibrinolysis, low content of several coagulation factors. If heparin is to have any effect, it must be given early in the disease; if it is given to patients with severe changes in the coagulation system, accentuation of the existing bleeding must be expected.

The use of heparin in the *treatment of acute defibrination,* such as *obstetric bleeding* complications, is now the exception rather than the rule. Schneider (1968) who was the first to describe intravascular coagulation in abruptio placentae now also claims that the most important measure is to remove the foetus as quickly as possible. He thinks that neither heparin nor fibrinogen need be given. Pitney (1971) postulates in a survey that 'Anticoagulant therapy is not indicated in short-lived episodes of acute defibrination such as may occur with premature separation of the placenta. Once the uterus has been emptied, the trigger for vascular clotting no longer exists and continuous haemorrhage is due to depletion of coagulation factors and platelets in the initial defibrination'. In acute defibrination the basic disease (e.g. evacuation of the uterus) and shock must be treated first. The blood loss is first compensated for by transfusions. If the bleeding is heavy, it is important to give fresh blood, possibly platelet-rich suspensions, to control the coagulation defect. Administration of fibrinogen has often been recommended in the treatment of acute obstetric complications. In our opinion, fibrinogen is absolutely forbidden if the clinical picture includes signs of defibrination. Administration of fibrinogen will only result in continued deposition of fibrin. If fibrinogen must be given, the patient should first receive heparin.

Judging from our experience, defibrination as a postoperative complication should not be treated with heparin. In such cases heparin will only lead to uncontrollable bleeding in the area of the wound and intra-abdominally and thereby worsen the patient's condition. Vigorous treatment of the shock and infusion of fresh blood to counteract the coagulation defect must first be tried.

The most positive effect of heparin with normalisation of the coagulation status and clinical improvement has been reported in *septic shock, purpura fulminans, thrombotic thrombocytopenic purpura, thrombotic microangiopathy* and *acute renal diseases* (Hjort, et al., 1964; Allanby, et al., 1966; Abildgaard, Ch., 1969; Lasch, 1969b; Kincaid-Smith, 1969a; Little, 1969; Larsson, et al., 1971d). In these cases it is not the haemorrhagic symptoms that are predominant—many of the patients have no haemorrhage at all—but those of disseminated thrombosis. It should, however, be mentioned that Corrigan and Jordan (1970) have shown that heparin treatment of sepsis with signs of DIC has no effect on the mortality despite normalisation of the coagulation status.

Some authors have reported a good effect of heparin on *chronic defibrination* in patients with *cancer* (Rosner and Ritz, 1966; Miller and Davison, 1967; Mosesson, et al., 1968), while other authors have found heparin to have no therapeutic effect, but often to accentuate the bleeding (Sigstad and Lamvik, 1963; Lechner, et al., 1968; Owen, et al., 1969; Didisheim, et al., 1969). It has been assumed that bleeding in promyelocytic leukaemia is due to defibrination (Didisheim, et al., 1964; Hirsh, et al., 1967; and others). But no dramatic effect of heparin on promyelocytic leukaemia has ever been reported (Straub and Frick, 1967).

Opinions differ on the effect of heparin in *haemolytic-uraemia*. According to some authors (Künzer and Aalam, 1964; Piel and Phibbs, 1966; Gilchrist, et al., 1969; Liebermann, 1972) treatment with heparin can reduce the mortality among children with the haemolytic-uraemic syndrome, while others have found no such effect with heparin (Giromini and Laperrouza, 1969; Katz, et al., 1969; Lo, et al., 1971).

As pointed out earlier, in cases with *severe bleeding* it is important to assess the degree of fibrinolysis in the syndrome. In clinical conditions with severe bleeding and in which the patients have signs of both intravascular coagulation and fibrinolysis (primary or secondary) we, like several other authors (Sherry, et al., 1964; Bonnar and Crawford, 1965; Fletcher and Alkjaersig, 1966; Owen, et al., 1969; Lasch, 1969b; Abildgaard, Ch., 1969), feel that combined treatment with inhibitors of fibrinolysis (EACA or AMCA) and heparin is indicated. Several authors have warned against the use of inhibitors of fibrinolysis in the treatment of the defibrination syndrome, on the ground that it might lead to the development of permanent fibrin deposits. If inhibitors are given to a patient with considerable fibrinolysis (primary or secondary) the risk of existing fibrin deposits is probably small. In such acute cases a single dose of EACA or AMCA is, as a rule, sufficient to control the bleeding. The fibrinolytic activity in the body will be reduced for only about 4 hours if renal function is normal. Further deposition of fibrin can be counteracted by simultaneous administration of heparin. We have not seen any complications of such treatment with EACA or AMCA in patients with signs of defibrination associated with pronounced fibrinolysis and bleeding (Niléhn and Nilsson, 1964; Nilsson, Andersson and Björkman, 1966; Hedner and Nilsson, 1971b).

Summing up, patients with defibrination offer difficult diagnostic and therapeutic problems. Bleeding and thrombosis in such patients are manifestations of underlying disorders and every effort should be made to treat such disorders. Treatment of shock is essential. It must be borne in mind that heparin administration is one aspect of a many-sided therapeutic approach and should not be relied upon as the only specific drug for this complication. There are indications for treatment with heparin in certain patients with defibrination. Heparin should not be given if there is undue risk of haemorrhage from the operative area, ulcerative cancer and dangerous local defects in the vessels. Such treatment is risky and should be given only under supervision of a physician well versed in the management of such cases. It cannot be emphasised enough that the effect of heparin is mainly prophylactic. Heparin has no effect on existing fibrin thrombi or organic changes thereby produced. Heparin should be given in doses sufficient to maintain a coagulation time of 20–30 minutes permanently. The heparin should preferably be given by continuous intravenous infusion. A dose of 10–15 units/kg body weight/hour is usually sufficient. One might give the patient 25–50 units heparin/kg body weight at 4 hour intervals. At signs of bleeding the effect of the heparin should be neutralised by immediate administration of protamine chloride. Treatment with heparin should, when possible, be continued until the coagulation status has become normal. If the patient has severe thrombocytopenia and a coagulation defect, fresh blood, possibly platelet-rich plasma, should be given simultaneously. If there is reason to assume a considerable fibrinolytic component, it might be indicated that heparin combined with EACA or AMCA should be given, because of the high risk of bleeding. But neither EACA nor AMCA should be given in renal insufficiency.

It might be questioned whether heparin is the most suitable, or the only anticoagulant that should be used in the treatment of conditions with defibrination. The initial stage in the formation of all thrombi is adhesion and aggregation of platelets on the vessel wall. Heparin has no effect on this stage. Characteristic of several cases with defibrination, and often also the first sign in the analysis of the coagulation system, is a rapid fall of the platelet count. Dextran with a molecular weight of 70.000 (Macrodex®) inhibits the adhesion and aggregation of the platelets and has been used in the prophylaxis of thrombosis (Ahlberg, et al., 1968). Cronberg and Nilsson (1970) described a case of pneumococcal sepsis and typical signs of a generalised Shwartzman reaction and defibrination. That patient was successfully treated with Macrodex alone and antibiotics. It is possible that treatment with Macrodex or Macrodex + heparin can more effectively prevent the formation of widespread microthrombi. In cases with signs of widespread microthrombi it would, theoretically, be more correct to give agents capable of dissolving thrombi, and Lasch (1969b) suggested treatment with streptokinase. He gave this to some patients with shock of varying origin and reported good results. This form of treatment deserves further trials.

There are also some points on the general treatment of patients with defibrination syndrome. Certain drugs may accentuate the defibrination. Cortisone suppresses the fibrinolytic activity of the vessel walls and should be given only when absolutely necessary for the basic disease (Isacson, 1970). Adrenergic substances stimulate defibrination and are therefore not recommended. Instead, substances should be given that block the adrenergic system (e.g. chlorpromazin).

In patients with evidence of only *primary fibrinolysis* inhibitors of fibrinolysis should be given in adequate doses (0·1 g Epsikapron®/kg body weight intravenously at 4–6 hour intervals or 0·01 g Cyclokapron®/kg body weight intravenously at 4–6 hour intervals in acute situations; otherwise Epsikapron® and Cyclokapron® can be given by mouth (see pages 143–145).

VI. Local fibrinolysis
LENNART ANDERSSON

As mentioned in an earlier section, most human tissues and body fluids contain activators of plasminogen. The highest concentrations occur in the uterus, adrenals, lymph nodes, prostate and thyroid (Albrechtsen, 1957). The urine has a high fibrinolytic activity owing to its content of urokinase (see page 116). Urokinase is excreted by the kidneys. Activators also occur in the watery secretion of the lacrimal glands, cerebrospinal fluid, milk and other body fluids.

The physiological purpose of these activators is apparently to dissolve fibrin precipitates in the tissues and to maintain the patency of the urinary pathways and excretory ducts. But it also maintains and prolongs various forms of haemorrhage. The normal fibrinolytic activity does not, however, cause haemorrhage in intact tissues.

Recent research has shown that a variety of drugs can inhibit both normal and, in certain situations, increased fibrinolytic activity in tissues and body fluids and thereby stop or suppress bleeding.

A. *Substances inhibiting fibrinolysis*

The drugs used today are given in Fig. 40.

Epsilon aminocaproic acid (EACA), *trans*-amino-methyl-cyclohexane-carbonic acid (tranexamic acid, AMCA) and p-amino-methyl bensoic acid (PAMBA) inhibit the activation of plasminogen. Trasylol® and Iniprol® counteract activation of plasmin as well as of formed plasmin (see also page 140).

B. *Effect of inhibitors on tissue activators*

The inhibiting effect of EACA, PAMBA and AMCA on various tissue

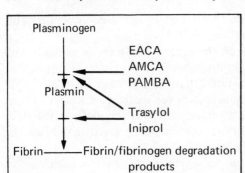

Fig 40. Mode of action of anti-fibrinolytic preparations now used.

activators has been studied by Andersson, et al. (1968, 1971). Standardised drops of a suspension of tissue activators from various human organs were deposited on fibrin plates containing one of the inhibitors in varying concentration. The fibrin plates were incubated at 37°C for 18–20 hours, after which the size of the zones dissolved was measured. Activator from porcine myocardium extracted with potassium rhodanide solution was used as reference. The inhibitory effect of PAMBA was found to be 3–4 times that of EACA and 10 times that of AMCA.

To study the situation *in vivo*, Andersson, et al. (1968, 1971) gave EACA (100 mg/kg body weight). PAMBA (20 mg/kg) or AMCA (10 mg/kg) to a number of patients about to undergo operations. During the operation, biopsy specimens of various tissues were obtained. A sample of venous blood was also obtained. Determinations were made of the concentrations of the respective substances in the tissues and in the serum. Administration of AMCA produced a satisfactory anti-fibrinolytic activity for 7–8 hours in the serum, for up to 17 hours in the tissue and for up to 48 hours in the urine. EACA produced a satisfactory antifibrinolytic level for 3 hours in the serum, for 6 hours in the tissues, and for 24 hours in the urine. Judging from tests on fibrin plates, the concentrations in the tissues after administration of these doses of AMCA and EACA could inhibit the tissue activators by 80–90 per cent. The values found for PAMBA were the same as for EACA (Table 15).

	AMCA	PAMBA	EACA	
				Table 15. *Duration in hours of 80 per cent inhibition of tissue*
Colonic mucosa	>17	~6	~6	*activator in various*
Colonic muscle	>17	~6	~6	*human organs after*
Lung	>14		~6	*preoperative admini-*
Thyroid	~13		~4	*stration of AMCA,*
Urinary bladder	>9	~7	~7	*PAMBA or EACA.*
Prostate	>9	~9	~6	*Concentration of*
Kidney	>7		>6	*inhibitor substance*
Stomach	>4		~3	*determined in tissue*
Abdominal wall muscle	>17	~6	~6	*specimens obtained at operation.*

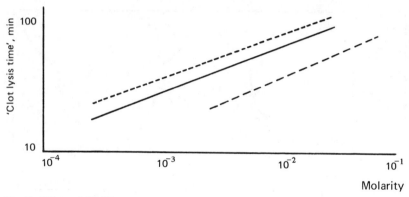

Fig 41. Effect of EACA (— — —), PAMBA (———) and AMCA (- - -) on urokinase, examined with clot lysis method. Increasing concentration of inhibitor substance in clotting system (abscissa) prolongs the clot lysis times (ordinate). AMCA is the strongest inhibitor— longest lysis times at same molar concentration. PAMBA is about 5 times as strong, and AMCA 8–10 times as strong an inhibitor of urokinase as EACA.

C. *Effect of inhibitors on urokinase*

The effect of EACA, PAMBA and AMCA on urokinase *in vitro* was studied by Andersson (1962) and Andersson, et al. (1968, 1971) who used the clot lysis method (Andersson, 1962). The inhibitory effect of AMCA on urokinase was found to be 8–10 times as strong as that of EACA and about twice as strong as that of PAMBA (Fig. 41).

In an attempt to find out whether the fibrinolytic activity of urine can be inhibited we gave EACA, PAMBA, AMCA or Trasylol® to healthy adult volunteers. EACA and AMCA were given by mouth or intravenously, PAMBA only by mouth because it is not readily soluble and can be given intravenously in only small doses. Trasylol® (like Iniprol®) can only be given intravenously. The fibrinolytic activity of the urine was measured with the clot lysis method before, and at various intervals after, the medication. EACA, PAMBA or AMCA markedly suppressed the fibrinolytic activity in the urine for several hours. Trasylol® , on the other hand, had no such effect with certainty.

The low molecular weight substances, EACA and AMCA, are excreted unchanged and PAMBA is largely excreted in unchanged form by the kidneys; they competitively inhibit the activity of the urokinase. Trasylol® and Iniprol® are high molecular weight substances and are not excreted in active form by the kidneys.

D. *Clinical use of inhibitors*

1. Urinary pathways

Blood clots are dissolved by urine because of its urokinase content. As mentioned above, treatment with AMCA, PAMBA and EACA can markedly suppress the fibrinolytic activity in the urinary pathways.

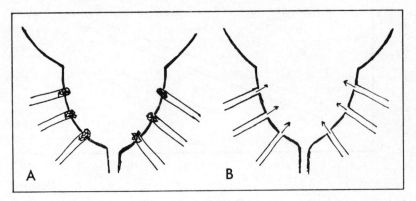

Fig 42. Prostatic cavity after enucleation of prostate (A). Dissolution of haemostatic plug results in continued bleeding (B).

Therapeutically, we have aimed at reducing the fibrinolytic activity by at least 80 per cent.

Lower urinary pathways

Prostatectomy. At enucleation of an adenoma of the prostate, numerous blood vessels in the prostatic bed are opened. As a rule, only the larger vessels require surgical haemostasis, bleeding from the small vessels ceasing spontaneously. When urine flows through the cavity it comes into contact with haemostatic clots and dissolves them (Fig. 42). This maintains the bleeding during the postoperative period. The tissue activators, which are abundant in the walls of the prostatic bed, probably contribute towards the maintained bleeding.

It has been shown in several investigations that medication with EACA

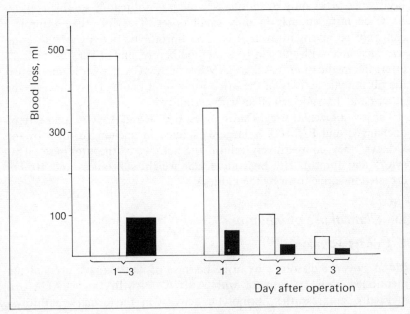

Fig 43. Average bl loss on first day af prostatectomy in t groups of patients. one (■) the patien were treated with EACA in a mean of 20 g a day; in th other (□), no anti fibrinolytic therap was given. The postoperative bloc loss in the treated group was about 2 of that in the cont

or AMCA after prostatectomy reduces postoperative bleeding. Fig. 43 refers to an investigation by Andersson (1964), where the blood loss after prostatectomy was substantially reduced by treatment with EACA. AMCA has a similar effect (Hedlund, 1969). An adequate dose of AMCA in this situation is 1 g, twice a day, by mouth if the patient's condition permits the use of this route, otherwise intravenously.

Investigations with the double blind method have shown that such antifibrinolytic treatment in association with prostatectomy does not raise the frequency of postoperative thrombo-embolism (Vinnicombe and Shuttleworth, 1966).

The value of this treatment is to be seen not only in its effect on post-operative bleeding, but also in its favourable effect on drainage of the urinary bladder and thereby reduction of the risk of infection.

Operations on the urinary bladder. The principles of treatment for reducing postoperative blood loss after prostatectomy holds also for various operations of the bladder, such as extirpation of diverticula, tumours, etc.

Spontaneous bleeding from the prostate or bladder wall. Bleeding, spontaneous or after catheterisation, from a hyperaemic mucosa or varicose vessel in the neck of the bladder is a fairly common complication of prostatic hyperplasia or *prostatic cancer.* Such bleeding usually ceases spontaneously. Occasionally, however, it may be obstinate or abundant. In such situations, treatment with AMCA or EACA may be useful. This also applies to spontaneous bleeding in diseases of the bladder wall. In cancer, however, and particularly in teleangiectasis or necrosis of the bladder wall after radiotherapy of cancer of the bladder or uterus, treatment with such inhibitors has little or no effect.

Bleeding of the upper urinary pathways

Some cases of coagulopathy, such as haemophilia or hypopro-thrombinaemia are on record where inhibitors of urokinase have been given because of haematuria. The bleeding has often ceased or diminished, but in some cases clots have been retained in the kidneys. These clots have, as a rule, been broken down and passed spontaneously within a few days of withdrawal of the drug. The condition is, however, painful and the possibility of irreversible renal injury cannot be excluded. Therefore, *antifibrinolytic therapy should be used with caution in the treatment of profuse renal bleeding.* Such preparations can, however, be used to control bleeding from the upper urinary pathways if the bleeding is scanty, but long or recurrent and therefore producing anaemia. In-hibitors have also had a good effect on patients with prolonged bleeding after renal trauma, with cystic kidneys and with so-called essential haematuria (Andersson, 1962).

The most important indication in urinary tract diseases is, however, bleeding from the lower urinary pathways. If clots should form in the bladder they can be easily removed with the aid of a somewhat rigid catheter or cystoscope.

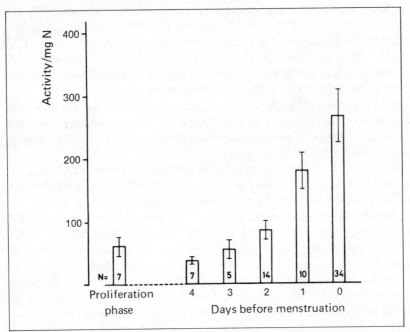

Fig 44. Mean value (with standard deviations) of plasminogen activator activity in endometrium during menstrual cycle. On the days before menstruation the activity increased considerably. The activity increased notably during the days before menstruation (Rybo, 1966).

2. Uterus

The concentration of activators of plasminogen in the endometrium is high. The fibrinolytic activity is lower in the proliferation phase of the endometrium and increases successively in the secretory phase (Fig. 44). It is highest at the beginning of menstruation (Rybo, 1966). This fibrinolytic activity explains why the blood lost at menstruation is normally not clotted.

Profuse menstrual bleeding is a common cause of iron deficiency anaemia in women of fertile age. Hallberg, et al. (1966) found that about two thirds of all women with anaemia lost 80 ml of blood or more at every menstruation. It has also been found that many women with menorrhagia have an abnormally high fibrinolytic activity in the endometrium (Rybo, 1966).

Double blind investigations have shown that treatment of so-called essential menorrhagia with EACA or AMCA, significantly reduces the bleeding at menstruation. Administration of 3–6 g AMCA a day for 4 days diminishes the blood loss by 35–50 per cent (Nilsson, L. and Rybo, 1967). Such treatment should not be started before menstruation is well under way. Treatment should preferably be continued for four days.

Inhibitors of fibrinolysis have also been used successfully in the treatment of uterine bleeding in women with haemorrhagic diathesis (Nilsson and Björkman, 1965) and of haemorrhagic complications after insertion of intrauterine contraceptives.

Some authors have found inhibitors to be useful in the treatment of metrorrhagia in women with myoma or other uterine changes. It should, however, be stressed that, as in all types of palliative treatment, the cause of the bleeding should first be ascertained in order to avoid delay of the diagnosis of a tumour or other serious disease.

3. Digestive tract

Kwaan, Cocco and Mendeloff (1964) in histochemical studies, found that the concentration of activators of plasminogen is abnormally high in the rectal mucosa in patients with active ulcerative colitis. It is not known whether such high fibrinolytic activity is of aetiological significance in the disease or whether it is produced by micro-abscesses in the mucosa.

Bleeding from the mucosa of the colon and impaired absorption of iron are the main causes of the anaemia commonly found in patients ulcerative colitis. Such bleeding often ceases or diminishes if the patients are treated with EACA or AMCA (Nilsson, Andersson and Björkman, 1966). Side effects such as nausea or orthostatic symptoms have been reported relatively often. The haemostatic effect has, however, proved so good that such treatment can be recommended in those cases of ulcerative colitis where rectal bleeding is the main symptom.

Antifibrinolytic therapy has also been used successfully in the treatment of recurrent bleeding of *gastric* or *duodenal ulcers* and of acute erosive gastritis. Cox, Poller and Thomson (1967) studied the fibrinolytic activity in blood obtained from stomach veins at explorative surgery. They found the activity to be higher in patients with ulcers than in those with other abdominal diseases. Judging from their findings, the fibrinolytic activity in the gastric mucosa is abnormally high in patients with gastric ulcers.

4. Intracranial haemorrhage

Lewis and Ferguson (1950) and Moltke (1957) showed that activators of plasminogen occur in the meninges and in the *choriod plexus*. Later Takashima, Koga and Tanaka (1969) and Tovi (1972) histochemically demonstrated that the cerebral tissues also possess fibrinolytic activity. On the other hand, no plasminogen activator activity has been found in normal cerebrospinal fluid (C.S.F.). In intracerebral bleeding, as in subarachnoid bleeding, however, fibrinolytic activity appears in the cerebrospinal fluid (Takashima, et al., 1969).

Tovi and coworkers (Tovi, 1972, Tovi, Nilsson and Thulin, 1972a, b) have recently studied the mechanism of fibrinolysis in subarachnoid haemorrhage. They found little or no increase of the fibrinolytic activity in the circulating blood in patients with subarachnoid bleeding from a ruptured arterial aneurysm, but they did find an increase in the activity in the cerebrospinal fluid as determined by the appearance of FDP in the C.S.F. Patients who survived the acute haemorrhage are initially in a very poor condition, because of, among other things, vascular spasm. They generally improve successively within the following weeks. But bleeding very often recurs within the first three weeks, presumably because the haemostatic clot has not been organised but dissolved. It is believed that the fibrinolytic activity of the cerebrospinal fluid in these situations is a strong contributory cause of the recurrent bleeding.

To reduce the risk of recurrences of subarachnoid bleeding after a ruptured aneurysm, the use of inhibitors of fibrinolysis has been suggested. Since EACA does not normally pass the blood/C.S.F. barrier, but after haemorrhage it passes into the C.S.F., Norlén and Thulin (1969) and others gave EACA for 2–3 weeks after subarachnoid haemorrhage. But a number of recurrent haemorrhages were noted in their group.

In clinical investigations, Tovi and coworkers have shown that AMCA also passes the blood/C.S.F.-barrier in patients with subarachnoid bleeding and then accumulates in the cerebrospinal fluid after repeated injections. Tovi and his coworkers (1971) have shown that complete inhibition of the activity in the C.S.F. requires administration of large doses of AMCA (15 mg/kg body weight 6 times a day intravenously) during the first eight days. Such treatment effectively prevented early recurrent bleeding during the first week after the initial bleeding.

Though antifibrinolytic treatment cannot replace surgery it might facilitate the choice of a less risky time for the operation.

Thrombosis and treatment of thrombosis

I. Mechanism of thrombosis

Platelets are of central significance in the initial stages of haemostasis and thrombosis. When platelets come into contact with an injured vessel wall they adhere to the exposed collagen. This initiates a process, which leads to the formation of a white platelet plug (see page 3). Such a plug invariably constitutes the primary and proximal part of a thrombus. Platelet aggregation is normally followed immediately by coagulation of the blood with the formation of fibrin. This results in the development of a red thrombus consisting of red blood cells and fibrin and built up on the initial white platelet plug. The result is thus a mixed thrombus consisting of a white head and a red body and tail, as described 75–100 years ago by Virchow, Welch, Zahn, and others. This structure of thrombi has been confirmed by electronmicroscopic studies of both true and experimental thrombi.

Though all thrombi form in essentially the same way, arterial and venous thrombi differ from one another in their relative amounts of platelets, leukocytes, red blood cells, and fibrin. Arterial thrombi are built up mainly of platelets and have only an insignificant red part. On the venous side thrombi form in slowly flowing blood. In such a thrombus the head contains only a small amount of platelets and the thrombus consists mainly of a red body and tail, which initially floats in the blood stream.

It should, perhaps, be stressed from the very beginning that a clot formed *in vitro* differs essentially from a thrombus. A clot is of uniform structure and the formed elements of the blood are distributed equally in the fibrin network. A thrombus consists of two parts, the white platelet thrombus and the red thrombus, composed of red blood cells and fibrin.

The mechanisms involved in the development of thrombosis are discussed below. Mainly problems bearing directly on venous thrombosis will be dealt with. The three most important causes are: 1) changes in the blood flow, 2) changes in the circulating blood, and 3) changes in the vessel wall.

A. *Changes in the blood flow*

The significance of venous stasis in the causation of thrombosis is well known. The pathogenesis of thrombosis complicating surgery and cardiac insufficiency always includes some degree of venous stasis. But it is still debatable whether retardation of the blood flow can by itself cause thrombosis. Wessler and Deykin (1958), for example, could not induce thrombosis in dogs by stasis alone but only by stasis combined with injection of a coagulative serum fraction. Neither is it properly understood why immobilisation favours thrombosis in some patients, but not in others.

B. *Changes in the circulating blood*

The most important changes suspected of predisposing to thrombosis are as follows:
1) changes in platelet adhesiveness,
2) increased content of one or more coagulation factors,
3) decreased content of inhibitors in the coagulation system,
4) decreased fibrinolytic activity and increased content of inhibitors of fibrinolysis, and
5) increased content of serum lipids.

1. Changes in platelet adhesiveness

Platelets play an important role in the initial stage of all sorts of thrombosis. There is thus reason to suspect that changes in the adhesiveness of platelets are of significance in thrombogenesis.

In recent years much attention has been given to determination of platelet adhesiveness and aggregation in various diseases. Mainly the methods described by Hellem (1960), Salzman (1963), Moolten, et al., (1949) and Wright (1941) for measuring the adhesion of platelets to glass, and Born's method (Born, 1962) for assessing platelet aggregation, have been used in these investigations. Several authors using different methods have found platelet adhesiveness to be increased in acute thrombosis (Moolten, et al., 1949; Bobek and Cepelak, 1958; Hume and Chan, 1967; Bygdeman and Wells, 1969). Only a few investigations have been carried out on patients with recurrent thrombosis in remission. Bobek and Cepelak (1958) found platelet adhesiveness to be increased in acute thrombosis but not in 'aged, non-active, or healed thrombosis'. Hirsh and McBride (1965) reported increased platelet adhesiveness in nine cases of idiopathic recurrent venous thrombosis. Isacson and Nilsson (1972a) examined platelet adhesiveness with the method of Hellem in 117 patients with idiopathic recurrent venous thrombosis (Table 16). At examination 3 months after the episode of acute thrombosis, platelet adhesiveness was increased in 14 per cent, and after 5 months in 3 per cent.

Several authors have found that increased platelet adhesiveness is relatively common in conditions regarded as thrombogenic, e.g. after operation and post-partum, and in patients with malignant diseases and different arteriosclerotic manifestations (Owren, 1965; Emmons and Mitchell, 1965; Bygdeman, et al., 1966; Nilsson, 1967; Hellem, 1968;

Table 16. *Pathological findings in* 117 *patients with recurrent 'idiopathic' deep venous thrombosis or superficial thrombophlebitis.*

	Number of patients
Platelet adhesiveness $> 52\ \%$	16
Factor VIII $> 160\%$	20
P&P $> 120\%$	5
Fibrinogen $> 0\cdot42$ g/100 ml	14

Nilsson and Isacson (1972a)

McKenzie, et al., 1969; Jacobsson, 1969a, b). Bygdeman, et al. (1966) claimed to have found a correlation between increased platelet adhesiveness and the appearance of clinical signs of thrombosis. Negus, et al. (1969) and Becker (1972), however, were unable to demonstrate any correlation between increased platelet adhesiveness and postoperative venous thrombosis diagnosed with the ^{125}I-labelled fibrinogen uptake method or phlebography. The other investigations did not include analyses of increased platelet adhesiveness and thrombosis for any correlation.

The finding of increased platelet adhesiveness in acute thrombosis and in diseases or conditions believed to predispose to thrombosis has resulted in the assumption that increased platelet adhesiveness is an important predisposing factor in the development of thrombosis. But so far no evidence has been produced that increased adhesiveness alone can cause venous thrombosis. One would therefore expect the adhesiveness to be increased also in patients with idiopathic recurrent thrombosis in remission, and a direct correlation between increased platelet adhesiveness and the incidence of venous thrombosis in other pathological conditions. Most cases probably require not only increased platelet adhesiveness but also some other predisposing factor, such as damage to, or decreased fibrinolytic activity in, the vessel walls. In such predisposed individuals thrombosis can probably be explained by increased platelet adhesiveness in association with a reactive process (e.g. after operation). In arterial thrombotic conditions the adhesiveness and aggregation of platelets very probably play a much greater role.

2. Increased content of one or more coagulation factors

Conditions associated with an increased content of coagulation factors are called hypercoagulable states. Several investigators have tried to find out whether any association exists between an increased content of one or more coagulation factors and an increased tendency to thrombosis. Coagulation has been studied in patients with conditions known to predispose to thrombosis—postoperative, post-partum, fractures, ulcerative colitis, acute pancreatitis and malignant diseases and, second, in patients with verified or assumed acute thrombosis or thrombophlebitis (for references see Nilsson, 1967; Isacson and Nilsson, 1972a). These investigations have shown that an increased content of one or more coagulation factors is common in these conditions. As a rule, increased values have been noted for fibrinogen, Factor V, Factor VII and Factor VIII and in some investigations accelerated thromboplastin generation and increased tolerance to heparin. In addition, families have been described with a predisposition to thrombosis combined with an increased content of Factor V (Gaston, 1966) or Factor VIII (Penick, et al., 1966). These findings have been regarded as evidence of an increase in one or more coagulation factors, contributing to the causation of venous thrombosis. Yet venous thrombosis is not a *sine qua non,* for most of the patients had not had or did not develop thrombosis. But all of them except the aforementioned families, had a reactive process initiated by cancer, inflammation, trauma or tissue destruction. The coagulation pattern in reactive processes is characterised by an increased content of fibrinogen, Factor VIII and, in some cases, by an increased content of Factors V and VII (Egeberg, 1962; Larsson, et al., 1971a; Isacson and Nilsson, 1972c).

Isacson and Nilsson (1972a) recently studied 91 patients with recurrent phlebographically verified idiopathic venous thrombosis and 26 patients with recurrent histologically verified superficial thrombophlebitis. The investigation was carried out about 3 months after the last acute thrombotic episode. Patients with abnormal values were re-examined after a further 2 months. Only in a few cases were abnormally high values demonstrable (Table 16). In other words, a permanent change in the coagulation factors were relatively rare findings in patients with recurrent idiopathic deep venous thrombosis or superficial thrombophlebitis.

Other authors have also failed to find any causal relationship between intravascular thrombosis and changes in any of the known coagulation factors (Erichson, 1965; Owren, 1965; Fletcher, et al., 1970; Wessler and Stehbens, 1971), both normal and increased values of coagulation factors occurring in patients with and without thrombosis.

In this conjunction it might not be out of place to mention that the first step in the formation of all thrombosis is independent of the plasma coagulation and consists in adhesion of platelets to exposed collagen in the vessel wall. In other words, even if coagulation factors are increased, no thrombus will form unless there is a platelet plug on the vessel wall. On the other hand, *hypercoagulability will very likely favour the growth of red thrombi.*

3. Decreased content of inhibitors in the coagulation system

A decreased content of the anticoagulant factors normally occurring in the blood may predispose to thrombosis. Egeberg (1965a) has described a family in which several members had had thrombosis early in life. The antithrombin III content in the affected members was about 50 per cent of normal. v. Kaulla and v. Kaulla (1967) found a reduced antithrombin III activity in 45 patients with acute thrombo-embolism or myocardial infarction. Abildgaard, et al. (1970), on the other hand, could not demonstrate any such reduction in patients with myocardial infarction. Hedner and Nilsson (1972), who used both an immunological method and a biological method, found the antithrombin III activity to be normal in all 100 patients with recurrent venous thrombosis. Thrombosis due to a genetically low content of antithrombin III, as described by Egeberg, is evidently rare. Fagerhol and Abildgaard (1970) have found the antithrombin III content to be reduced in about 15 per cent of the women using oral contraceptives. They conceived this as a sign of predisposition to thrombosis. Olsson (1963) reported a reduced content of heparin cofactor in the postoperative period, which he believed to be of thrombogenic significance. In these investigations, however, the abnormal findings and the thrombosis were not studied for any correlation.

As pointed out earlier, antithrombin III is also an inhibitor of Factor Xa. Since Factor Xa occupies a key position in the activation of the coagulation process it is very probable that a significant decrease in antithrombin III will enhance coagulation and promote the formation of thrombi. Eika and Abildgaard (1970) have shown that a decrease in antithrombin III also will induce aggregation of platelets.

4. Decreased fibrinolytic activity and increased content of inhibitors of fibrinolysis

Cumulative evidence suggests that the spontaneous fibrinolytic activity in the blood derives from activators of fibrinolysis that are produced by the endothelium of small vessels and released by various stimuli to the blood stream (see page 115). The spontaneous fibrinolytic activity in the blood may be decreased in conditions associated with a decreased content of activators of fibrinolysis in the vessel walls or impaired capacity to release such activators from the vessel walls and in conditions with an increased content of inhibitors of fibrinolysis in the blood.

According to Duguid (1955) and Astrup (1958), mural fibrin deposits are converted to arteriosclerotic plaques. Though this theory is not universally accepted, several investigators believe that in patients with degenerative vascular diseases dissolution of thrombi is impaired and that this is an important factor in the development of thrombotic deposits in the vascular system. Several investigators have studied the fibrinolytic system in patients with various manifestations of arteriosclerosis. These investigations have given confusing results due mainly to differences in the test methods used. Some authors have thus found the fibrinolytic activity to be reduced in old arteriosclerotic patients, while others have found it to be normal (for references, see Nilsson, 1964; de Nicola, et al., 1964; Fearnley, 1965; Chakrabarti, et al., 1968; O'Brien, 1969). Robertson, Pandolfi and Nilsson (1972c) have shown that the fibrinolytic activity of blood obtained from the arms after venous occlusion is higher in the aged than in young persons.

Relatively few studies are available on the fibrinolytic activity in the blood in venous thrombosis and/or pulmonary embolism. Ellison and Brown (1965) reported a low spontaneous fibrinolytic activity in 9 out of 11 patients with clinical evidence of pulmonary embolism. Swan, et al. (1970) found the preoperative fibrinolytic activity in the blood to be low in 2 patients who later developed venous thrombosis after operation. Menon, McCollum and Gibson (1971) found the fibrinolytic activity in 20 patients with deep venous thrombosis of the leg to be lower than in age and sex-matched controls. Isacson and Nilsson (1972b) also found that a group of 117 patients with recurrent venous thrombosis had significantly lower spontaneous fibrinolytic activity than a corresponding control group. Mansfield (1972) recently reported that there is a reduced fibrinolytic activity during the postoperative period and that this occurs earlier and is more marked in those patients who develop venous thrombosis, as shown by the 125 I-fibrinogen test. However, the spontaneous fibrinolytic activity in the blood is normally so low that available methods are not sensitive enough to show with certainty whether it is abnormally low in a given individual.

Inhibitors of fibrinolysis. The role played by inhibitors of fibrinolysis in the aetiology of thrombosis has also been discussed. As previously mentioned, human blood contains two antiplasmins, namely slowly acting antiplasmin (α_1-antitrypsin, or α_1 AT) and quick-acting α_2-macroglobulin (α_2M) and inhibitors of activation of plasminogen ($=$urokinase inhibitors). The antiplasmin activity has been described as raised in several conditions, such as pulmonary fibrosis, cancer, infections, thrombo-embolism, myocardial infarction and after operations (for references, see Nilsson, Krook, Sternby, Söderberg and Söderstrom, 1961). Naeye (1961) has described two cases of thrombosis characterised by a high content of antiplasmin and antiplasminogen. In several of these studies it is not clear what was determined in respect of antiplasmin, antitrypsin, antistreptokinase and inhibitors of plasminogen activation.

Ganrot (1967) studied the α_2M content in various conditions. He found it to be markedly increased in nephrosis and slightly increased in diabetes and during pregnancy. The α_2M content was higher in children and young persons than in adults. In recurrent idiopathic venous thrombosis or thrombophlebitis the content of α_2M is normal (Isacson and Nilsson, 1972b). Oral contraceptives produce a slight increase in α_2M. Horne, et al. (1970) have assumed that the increase in α_2M in association with the use of oral contraceptives might be of thrombo-aetiological importance. But convincing evidence is still lacking.

Cumulative evidence, however, suggests that *inhibitors of plasminogen activation* may be of significance in the causation of thrombosis. Nilsson and coworkers (Nilsson, Krook, Sternby, Söderberg and Söderstrom, 1961; Paraskevas, et al., 1962; Nilsson 1967) have described altogether 5 patients, including 2 uniovular twins who had had recurrent severe venous thrombosis since childhood. These patients were found to have no spontaneous fibrinolytic activity in the blood and a high content of inhibitors of plasminogen activation. Brakman, et al. (1966) have also described some cases of severe thrombotic disease in association with an increased content of inhibitors of activators. Pandolfi, et al. (1970) have described a patient with bilateral occlusion of the retinal veins and a very high level of inhibitors of plasminogen activation. Isacson and Nilsson (1972b) investigated 117 patients with recurrent idiopathic thrombosis and found a high level of inhibitors of plasminogen activation in only three. A markedly increased content of inhibitors of plasminogen activation alone is probably a rare cause of thrombosis. It should be mentioned that these patients had only venous thrombosis. The fact that the fibrinolytic system cannot be activated, can presumably affect only the further growth and dissolution of thrombi containing fibrin, e.g. mainly red thrombi.

Inhibitors of plasminogen activation increase after operation, in infections, in renal diseases and in other reactive processes (Olow, 1963; Hedner and Nilsson, 1971a). In these conditions, however, the values do not reach such excessively high values as in severe thrombosis. Reactive processes are thus accompanied by a hypofibrinolytic condition. No association has been found between these changes in the fibrinolytic system and the occurrence of thrombosis. One might nevertheless imagine that hypofibrinolytic conditions favour the development of thrombi containing fibrin.

Recent research has shown that a *reduced content of fibrinolytic activators in the vessel wall is an important factor predisposing to thrombosis* (see page 170).

5. Increased content of serum lipids

Numerous papers have been published on the effect of various fat substances on the coagulation process and the fibrinolytic process *in vivo* and *in vitro*. The results are contradictory. Some investigators claim that lipaemia accelerates coagulation and reduces the spontaneous fibrinolytic activity of the blood. But most authors have found that ingestion of a fatty meal and infusion of lipids have no effect on the coagulation process or the fibrinolytic process (Merskey and Marcus, 1963; Howell, 1964; Cronberg and Nilsson, 1967). Bang and Cliffton (1960) have found that clots formed in lipaemic blood are resistant to 'standardised fibrinolytic therapy'.

It has been shown by many investigators that the spontaneous fibrinolytic activity is often lower in obese persons than in persons of normal body weight (Warlow, et al., 1972), but it is not known why.

C. *Changes in vessel wall*

It is generally accepted that the commonest cause of thrombosis is changes in the vessel walls. The initial stage of all thrombus formation is, as pointed out previously, adhesion of platelets to exposed collagen. Local injury and inflammation of the vessel wall is often associated with thrombosis. Besides mechanical and chemical injury, changes in the vessel wall, such as atherosclerotic plaques, may cause thrombosis. Otherwise the nature of the changes in the vessel wall is largely unknown. Spaet and Erichson (1965) have discussed the role played by the vessel wall in the pathogenesis of thrombosis. They felt that thrombosis may be regarded primarily as due to vessel injury. In some patients thrombosis occurs in association with local vessel injury such as trauma, tumour or infection. In most patients with thrombosis, however, it is not possible to trace or demonstrate any such predisposing factor. Spaet and Erichson postulate that the commonest cause of thrombosis is local manifestations of a disseminated process of unknown nature in the vessel wall, which leads to exposure of the collagen on the endothelial surface. Platelets can then adhere to such exposed collagen and form thrombi. They believe that such a disseminated process in the vessel wall constitutes 'a thrombotic diathesis' and that this is a common cause of thrombosis. Though this hypothesis is only speculative it offers several interesting aspects. In this connection it might not be out of place to mention that Hedner, et al. (1973b) recently found a connective tissue extract from seven patients with thrombotic disease to have a notably increased capacity to aggregate platelets, compared with connective tissue from age and sex-matched controls. None of these patients had any other disorder known to predispose to thrombosis. This suggests the possibility of a defect in the structure of the collagen or the subendothelial substances.

Activators of fibrinolysis in the vessel walls. In recent years much interest has been focused on activators of fibrinolysis in the vessel walls and the role they play in the development of thrombosis. Astrup and coworkers (see page 115), who used an extraction method, have shown that the adventitia of all vessels has high fibrinolytic activator activity. The intima in the arteries showed only low or no activator activity, while the intima of the larger veins had high activator activity. At roughly the same time Todd (1959), who used a histochemical method, showed that the fibrinolytic activity of a tissue is localised to the small vessels. Kwaan and Astrup (1965) and Todd and Nunn (1967) showed in autopsy specimens and in experimental thrombosis, that activators in the vessel walls play an important role in thrombolysis and recanalisation. Pandolfi, et al. (1969) studied especially the superficial limbs veins with a histochemical method in living material (biopsy specimens). They found that the fibrinolytic activators in these veins were confined mainly to the vasa vasorum in the adventitia.

As mentioned above, cumulative evidence strongly suggests that activators of fibrinolysis in the body are formed in the endothelium of small vessels. Certain stimuli can release these activators into the blood stream. These stimuli act by narrowing or widening the vessels (see page 116). It has long been known that venous occlusion of the limbs is followed by a marked increase in the fibrinolytic activity in the occluded vessels (Clarke, et al., 1960). There is evidence that the increased fibrinolytic

Fig 45. Illustration of the mechanism leading to the formation of localised fibrinolysis in the fibrin slide technique. Plasminogen activator at the active sites of the section transforms the plasminogen contained in the overlying fibrin into plasmin with focal fibrinolysis as consequence.

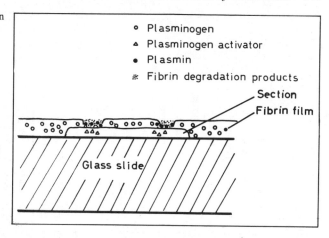

activity in venous occlusion is due to activators of fibrinolysis released from the vessel walls (Fearnley, 1965; Pandolfi, et al., 1967; Nilsson and Pandolfi, 1970).

The importance of activators of fibrinolysis in the vessel walls in the development of venous thrombosis has been studied since 1966 in a series of investigations at the coagulation laboratory in Malmö (Pandolfi, et al., 1967, 1968, 1969; Nilsson and Robertson, 1968; Nilsson and Pandolfi, 1970; Roberston, Pandolfi and Nilsson, 1972a,b,c; Isacson and Nilsson, 1972a,b,c). We have studied the rise in the local fibrinolytic activity on venous occlusion of the arms and legs as well as the content and localisation of plasminogen (fibrinolytic) activators in the vessel walls with Pandolfi's modification (Pandolfi, et al., 1968; Pandolfi, Bjernstad and Nilsson, 1972) of Todd's histochemical method (Todd, 1959) permitting quantitation of the fibrinolytic activity.

Venous occlusion was produced by wrapping a cuff round the thigh or upper arm and inflating it to a pressure midway between systolic and diastolic pressure for 20 minutes. Samples for determining the fibrinolytic activity (resuspended euglobulin precipitate on fibrin plates according to Nilsson and Olow, 1962a) were obtained before application, and immediately before deflation, of the cuff.

The plasminogen activator level in superficial veins of the arms and legs was determined in the following way. A 0·5–1·0 cm long segment of a vein is obtained by biopsy under local anaesthesia and frozen immediately. The specimen is sectioned in a cryostat, after which the sections are incubated in contact with a film of fibrin enriched with plasminogen. The preparations are then incubated for predetermined periods (usually 0, 10, 20 and 30 minutes). If the sections contain plasminogen activators, the plasminogen in the fibrin layer will be converted to plasmin which digests the fibrin (Fig. 45). The preparation is afterwards fixed and stained. The digested areas will appear in the stained fibrin layer as pale zones varying in size with the extent of the activation. The fibrinolytic activity of each slide is evaluated according to the following three grades. Grade I:

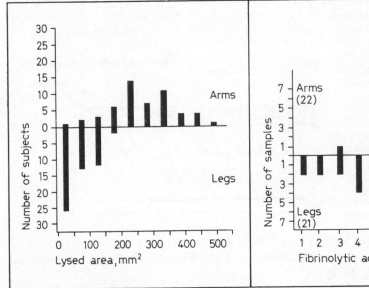

Fig 46. Fibrinolytic activity of resuspended euglobulin precipitate after venous stasis of arms and legs for 20 minutes.

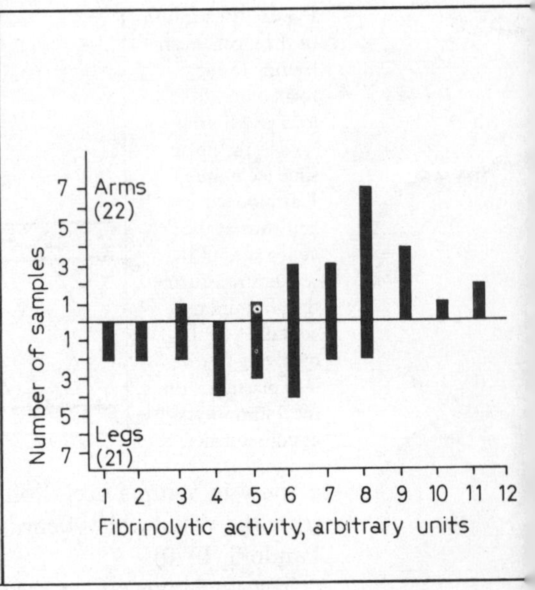

Fig 47. Fibrinolytic activity in arbitrary units superficial arm and leg veins obtained by biops from healthy subjects. The specimens were examine by a modified fibrin slide technique.

microscopic punctate areas of lysis in the majority of the sections (Fig 49); grade II: larger lytic zones or irregular outline, often confluent; grade III: massive digestion of the fibrin over the sections. 1, 2 and 3 points, respectively, are allotted to grades I, II and III. The sum of the points scored by each set of slides (four slides incubated for 0, 10, 20 and 30 minutes, respectively) is taken as a direct measure of the fibrinolytic activity of the specimen. In this way the activity can be expressed in units ranging from 0 to 12. The median value found at our laboratory in 50 biopsy specimens of hand veins from healthy volunteers was 7·5 arbitrary units (range 6–10).

We have so far examined 117 patients with recurrent idiopathic venous thrombosis verified phlebographically and 420 controls. The most important findings were as follows.

The fibrinolytic activity in the arms is 3–4 times as high as that in the legs, as measured with the use of venous occlusion and by direct determination of the activators in biopsy specimens of superficial veins (Figs. 46 and 47). However, in persons who have been confined to bed for more than 14 days with the legs horizontal, the fibrinolytic activity in the legs during venous occlusion is just as high as that in the arms (Karaca and Nilsson, 1971).

In superficial veins of the arms and legs in healthy persons and patients with thrombosis the activity is localised to the vasa vasorum in the adventitia. The media is much less active and the intima only exceptionally

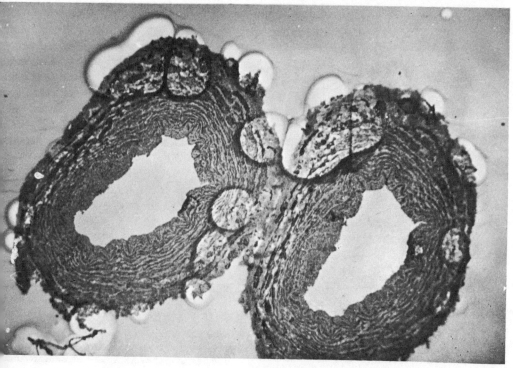

Fig 48. Localisation of fibrinolytic activity (plasminogen activator activity) in superficial veins. Fibrinolysis (white areas) in the adventitia and the media. The intima is inactive. Photo M. Pandolfi.

(Fig. 48). Veins containing fresh obstructing thrombi have little or no activity (Fig. 50). The activity returns on recanalisation of the vessels (Fig. 51).

In the patients with recurrent deep venous thrombosis the fibrinolytic activity in the blood during venous occlusion of the arm was significantly lower (p < 0·005) than that found in a normal series of healthy adult volunteers (Fig. 52). The fibrinolytic activity developed in the arm was thus abnormally low in 38 per cent of the patients. The plasminogen activator content determined histochemically in superficial veins from the arms was significantly decreased (p < 0·005) in 55 per cent of the patients (Fig. 53). In a group of patients in whom the activator content was determined both in arm and leg veins the biopsy specimen was always normal or abnormal in both. A defective fibrinolysis, i.e. a defective release of plasminogen activator from the vein walls during venous occlusion and/or a decreased plasminogen activator content of the vessel vein walls was found in 73 per cent of the patients with thrombosis.

These observations suggest that a decreased content of activators of fibrinolysis in the vessel walls or decreased release of such activators is an important predisposing factor to thrombosis.

The reduced fibrinolytic activity in the veins, which contain fresh

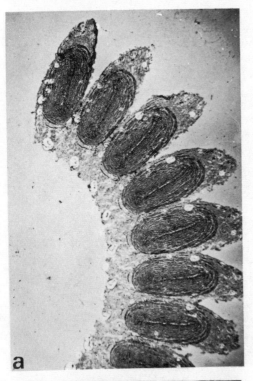

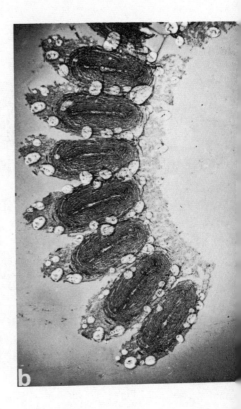

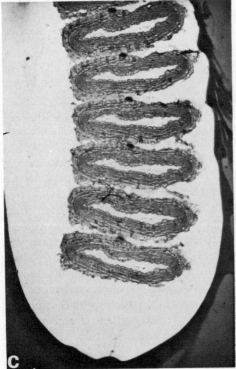

Fig 49. Serial sections of a superficial arm vein dem
strating different degrees of fibrinolysis. In grade 1
small foci of fibrinolysis are visible. Grade 2 (b) is c
racterised by larger lytic areas often confluent. In grade 3
total dissolution of the fibrin film in contact with the secti
is present. × 25. (Photo M. Pandolfi).

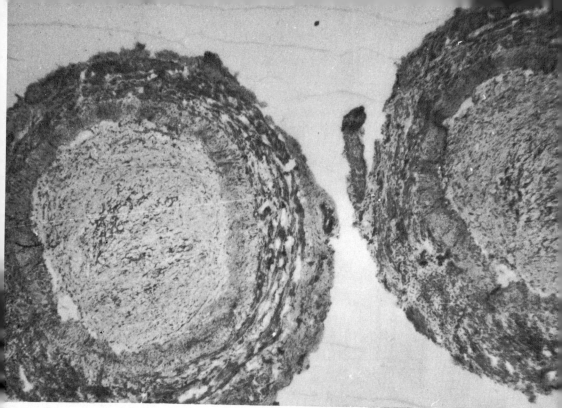

Fig 50. Fresh thrombotised vein. No fibrinolytic activity. Photo M. Pandolfi.

Fig 51. Recanalisation of vein occluded by thrombus. Fibrinolysis adjacent to recanalising vessels. Photo M. Pandolfi.

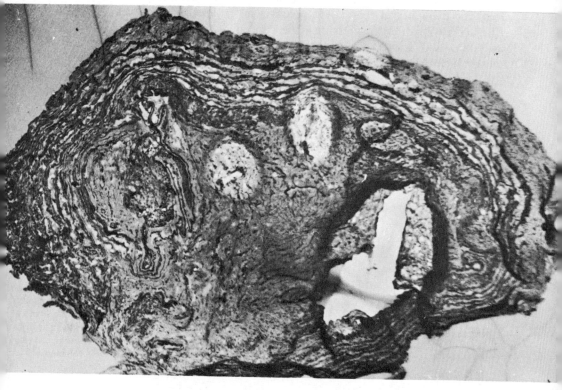

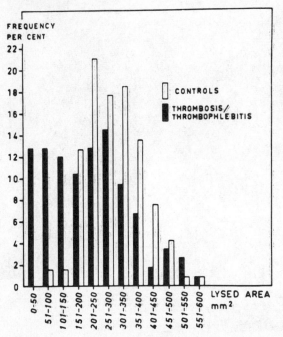

Fig 52. The local fibrinolytic activity in the blood during venous occlusion of the arm, as determined on resuspended euglobulin precipitate on unheated fibrin plates in controls (blank columns) and in patients with venous thrombosis (dark columns).

thrombi, suggests that the vessel walls have consumed their content of plasminogen activators in an attempt to dissolve the thrombus.

Of particular interest is the difference in activity between the arms and legs. The frequency of thrombosis is higher in the less active leg veins. The increased hydrostatic pressure in the legs probably results in a continuous release of activators into the leg veins. This explains the absence of any such difference in patients who have been confined to bed for some time.

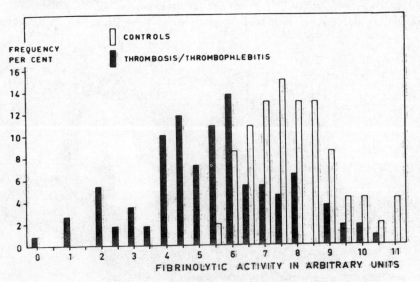

Fig 53. Plasminog activator content, determined histochemically, in bio specimen from the distal part of the cephalic vein in controls (blank columns) and in patients with ven thrombosis (dark columns).

The results obtained may also be of interest in the treatment of thrombosis. It has recently been shown, for instance, that certain oral antidiabetics such as phenformin (Dibein®), combined with anabolic steroids, increases the plasminogen activator content of the vessel walls (Isacson and Nilsson, 1970). Further, in our opinion, demonstration of a low content of fibrinolytic activators in the vessel wall in patients with thrombosis, lends theoretical support to the rationale of treatment of venous thrombosis with thrombolytics. Thrombosis may be regarded as a result of the inability of the vessel to keep itself patent by its own fibrinolytic enzymes.

II. Treatment of thrombosis

To begin with, the diagnosis should be firm. Several investigations have shown that the diagnosis of thrombosis on clinical grounds alone is very uncertain. Phlebography is presumably the most reliable method hitherto available. In recent years much attention has been given to the diagnosis of thrombosis with the use of injection of ^{125}I-labelled fibrinogen, which is enriched in the thrombus, and subsequent scanning of the legs and lungs (Kakkar, et al., 1970). This method cannot, however, be used on patients admitted with symptoms of acute thrombosis, but only for diagnosing, for example, postoperative thrombosis in patients given the ^{125}I at operation.

As a guide in the choice of treatment of a given case of recurrent idiopathic thrombosis, especially in a young person, investigation of the coagulation and fibrinolytic system is indicated.

In the choice of treatment of thrombosis it should be borne in mind that the arterial thrombus is composed mainly of platelets, while the venous thrombus is built up mainly of fibrin. The adhesion of platelets to collagen and the formation of a permeable platelet plug are independent of the coagulation process and cannot be prevented by administration of heparin or dicoumarol preparations. It is thus almost exclusively the last reaction, i.e. coagulation of the blood with the formation of a red thrombus, that is therapeutically blocked by administration of anticoagulants. Prevention of the initial stage of the formation of a thrombus requires administration of substances capable of lowering the adhesiveness of the platelets and their tendency to aggregate.

Anticoagulants and substances lowering platelet adhesiveness can prevent further deposition of platelets, fibrin and erythrocytes on an existing thrombus, and possibly also the development of new thrombi, but they cannot dissolve an existing thrombus. Increased knowledge about fibrinolysis has opened up a new approach to the treatment of thrombosis. By administration of enzymes capable of activating the fibrinolytic system it is possible to dissolve the fibrin in the thrombus, i.e. produce thrombolysis.

In recent years also snake venom with a thrombin-like effect has been tried in the treatment of thrombosis in the hope that the coagulation defect and defibrination thereby produced would have the desired effect.

In the following section a survey is given of the different forms and modes of action of *anticoagulants, agents suppressing platelet adhesiveness, agents stimulating the fibrinolytic activity in the body, agents causing defibrination, and thrombolytic agents,* used in the treatment of thrombosis as well as a brief account of some relevant practical problems.

A. *Anticoagulants*

1. Dicoumarol and indanedione preparations

Dicoumarol consists of a derivative of 4-hydroxycoumarin; indanedion preparations of derivatives of indian-1:3-dione.

Dicoumarol has been used as an anticoagulant for more than 25 years. Given by mouth dicoumarol will suppress the prothrombin activity in blood within 36–48 hours. Addition of dicoumarol to blood *in vitro* will not depress prothrombin. The discoverer of dicoumarol (Link, 1944) therefore thought that dicoumarol inhibits the synthesis of prothrombin. Since vitamin K is necessary, probably as a coenzyme, for the synthesis of prothrombin in the liver, it was assumed that dicoumarol acts as a competitive inhibitor, which prevents one of the enzymes involved in this synthesis from utilising the vitamin.

Later research has, however, shown that dicoumarol does not inhibit synthesis but interferes with it with the formation of an abnormal prothrombin (Niléhn and Ganrot, 1968; Ganrot and Niléhn, 1968b, 1969; Stenflo, 1972a,b) (see also page 38). According to Loeliger and Hemker (1968), treatment with dicoumarol is accompanied by formation of an inactive precursor of prothrombin. It has been shown that dicoumarol inhibits not only prothrombin, but also Factor IX, Factor VII and Factor X. The coagulation time is generally not prolonged before the prothrombin level has fallen to 5 per cent or still lower. Dicoumarol has only a weak anticoagulative effect, but it can inhibit the growth of a red thrombus if the prothrombin values are kept sufficiently low.

Laboratory control. The prothrombin should always be carefully and regularly controlled during dicoumarol therapy.

Prothrombin may be determined by a one-stage or a two-stage method. Two-stage methods are not used routinely for control of anticoagulant therapy.

Quick's classical one-stage method or one-stage prothrombin time measures not only prothrombin specifically, but also Factors V, VII and X and fibrinogen. This method is widely used in the control of dicoumarol therapy. According to this method, optimal amounts of thromboplastin and calcium are added to citrated plasma obtained from venous blood.

P & P-test. A one-stage method, which is more specific and also much more sensitive than Quick's method, is the P&P-test (prothrombin-proconvertin test) devised by Owren and Aas (1951) (see page 215).

		Ordinary dose during first 36–38 hours	Ordinary maintenance dose	Time of maximum
Type	Name	mg/day	mg/day	effect
Dicoumarol	AP	400–500	75 (25–150)	2–3
Acenocoumarol	Sintroma	20–32	4 (2–10)	1·5–2
Phenprocoumon	Marcoumar	27–39	3 (0·75–6)	1·5–2
Warfarin sodium	Waran	25–30	9 (3–21)	1·5–2

Table 17. *Some coumarin derivatives.*

This method measures the sum of prothrombin, Factor VII and Factor X.

The *TT-method* (thrombotest), worked out by Owren, resembles the P&P-test. The reagents are commercially available (Nyegaard & Co., Oslo).

The *Simplastin A-test* (Warner-Chilcott, U.S.A.) is a newcomer which has proved to be a sensitive one-stage method for determining prothrombin (see Korsan-Bengtsen, 1970). Diluted citrated plasma is added to a ready-made, commercially available reagent solution containing fibrinogen, Factor V and thromboplastin.

Owing to differences between the test methods and standards, it has proved extremely difficult to compare the therapeutic concentrations of the factors in patients treated with dicoumarol in different hospitals. The International Haemostasis and Thrombosis Committee has appointed a subcommittee to devise standards for treatment with dicoumarol. Special importance has been attached to the production of a stable brain thromboplastin and reliable, stable standard plasmas. Five thromboplastin preparations for standardisation of laboratory procedures are now available from The Division of Biological Standards, National Institute for Medical Research, Mill Hill, London, N.W.7.

If dicoumarol therapy is to be effective, the P&P and TT-values should lie between 7–15 per cent. The therapeutic range of Simplastin A is somewhat higher, namely 14–35 per cent. The susceptibility to dicoumarol varies from patient to patient. The dose must therefore be adjusted for each patient separately. During the regulation period (1–2 weeks) prothrombin should be determined every third day. Afterwards it is sufficient to check the value once a week for a few weeks and later every 2–3 weeks.

Dicoumarol and indanedione preparations. Table 17 gives the properties of some of the most common oral anticoagulant preparations. Of the aforementioned preparations, only warfarin sodium can be given also intravenously. When given by mouth the preparations are absorbed almost completely and mainly in the duodenum and the oral part of the jejunum, though dicoumarol has been described as somewhat less readily absorbed than the other preparations. All the substances are firmly bound to the plasma proteins, especially dicoumarol and phenprocoumon.

Every physician should preferably use only one of these anticoagulants in order to gain as much personal experience with it as possible.

Releases coumarin derivatives from serum protein bonds:	Inhibits microsomal enzymes of liver:
Salicylates (complex also with vitamin K)	Phenylamidole (Vilexin®)
Phenylbutazone (Butazolidin® , Mobutazon®)	Phenylbutazone
Oxiphenbutazone (Tanderil®)	Oxiphenbutazone

Unknown mechanism:
Kinin, kinidin, corticosteroids, D-thyroxine, clofibrate (Atromidin®)

Table 18.   *Drugs interacting with coumarol derivatives. Increased anticoagulant effect.*

Factors influencing susceptibility to dicoumarol. It is known that the susceptibility of a given patient may vary from one occasion to another. This may be explained by various circumstances.

1. *Effect of concomitant medication.* Various drugs may interact with dicoumarol preparations (see Starr and Petrie, 1972). Simultaneous use of other drugs rarely, if ever, inhibits resorption of dicoumarol. Several drugs, including dicoumarol preparations, utilise serum proteins as depots or carriers (Table 18). Competition between different drugs may break down this linkage to serum proteins with increased release of dicoumarol in active form and increased anticoagulant effect as a result.

Salicylates may compete with vitamin K in the liver. The *increased anticoagulant effect* of dicoumarol preparations in patients using salicylates may thus be explained by vitamin K deficiency in association with release of dicoumarol attached to serum proteins. It is, however, generally accepted that the doses of salicylates must be large if they are to produce this effect. Preparations such as *Butazolidin®* and *Tanderil®* *increase the anticoagulant effect* of dicoumarol, presumably by releasing dicoumarol preparations from serum protein bonds and by inhibiting microsomal enzymes of the liver. *An increased anticoagulant effect* has been observed also after administration of *quinine, quinidine, corticosteroids, D-tyroxin and clofibrate (Atromidin®).* The mechanism of the synergistic effect of these preparations is not known.

Certain drugs such as *barbiturates and chloral hydrate* stimulate microsomal enzymes in the liver with an increase in their capacity to break down a large number of drugs, including dicoumarol (Table 19). This results in a decreased anticoagulant effect of dicoumarol.

2. *Variation of supply of vitamin K and disturbed absorption of vitamin K.* Vitamin K is an antidote for dicoumarol. It is probable that the seasonal

Stimulate microsomal enzymes of liver:	
Barbiturates	(Phenobarbital and others)
Chloral hydrate	(Ansopal® , Mecoral®)

Table 19.   *Drugs reducing anticoagulant effect of coumarine derivatives.*

variation of the supply of vitamin K and variation of diet can explain changes in sensitivity to dicoumarol preparations. Dicoumarol is absorbed almost completely in the intestine, while the absorption of vitamin K varies. The use of a high fat diet increases the absorption of vitamin K with consequent reduction of susceptibility to dicoumarol; on subsequent use of a low fat diet the absorption of vitamin K decreases, and the patient becomes more sensitive to dicoumarol. Certain products such as spinach, are rich in vitamin K and if consumed in large amounts they can depress the patient's susceptibility to dicoumarol.

Vitamin K is synthetised by certain intestinal bacteria. A change in the intestinal flora, such as during antibiotic therapy, may therefore increase sensitivity to dicoumarol.

If adsorption is disturbed, such as during diarrhoea, the sensitivity to dicoumarol may also be increased.

3. *Impaired liver function.* Impairment of liver function and abuse of alcohol increase sensitivity to dicoumarol.

4. *Genetic resistance.* Some families have been described which are resistant to dicoumarol preparations (O'Reilly, 1970).

Indications for dicoumarol therapy

A great deal of literature is available on dicoumarol therapy. Therefore, suffice it here to make a few comments. Readers interested in an excellent survey are referred to 'Current Status of Anticoagulant Treatment' by A. S. Douglas (In Recent Advances in Blood Coagulation. Edited by L. Poller, A. Churchill LTD, London, 1969). The long-term prophylactic use of dicoumarol in patients who have had myocardial infarction and angina pectoris has been thoroughly reviewed by Douglas and will not be treated here.

It should be observed that dicoumarol cannot prevent the development of a thrombus, and that its use is mainly to prevent growth of the red thrombus. The purpose of dicoumarol is thus chiefly to prevent the occurrence of large, red thrombi in veins. The value of dicoumarol in the treatment of arterial thrombosis is debatable.

The most important indications for dicoumarol are as follows:

1. *Acute venous thrombosis and lung embolism.* In the acute stage treatment must be combined with heparin because of the latency of the effect of dicoumarol (2–3 days). Dicoumarol therapy and treatment with heparin are usually started at the same time. Once the prothrombin level has fallen to a satisfactory therapeutic level, heparin is withdrawn and treatment continued with only dicoumarol. In some hospitals dicoumarol is withdrawn as soon as the patient is fully mobilised, while in others dicoumarol treatment is continued for a further 1–3 months. Treatment with thrombolytics has, however, proved therapeutically more effective than heparin combined with dicoumarol.

2. *Recurrent venous thrombosis.* In patients with repeated venous thrombosis, and particularly in those in whom a thorough investigation of the coagulation and fibrinolytic status has revealed changes predis-

posing to thrombosis, continued dicoumarol treatment is indicated unless some other prophylactic treatment is more suitable (see page 188).

3. *Acquired heart disease with risk of embolism, e.g. mitral stenosis.* In this disease continual treatment with dicoumarol is indicated.

4. *Prosthetic heart valves.* Long-term prophylaxis is also indicated in patients with such prosthesis.

5. *Acute myocardial infarction.* In patients with myocardial infarction dicoumarol is indicated chiefly to prevent venous thrombosis of the leg.

6. *Long immobilisation.* This applies mainly to patients immobilised by leg injuries, e.g. fracture of the neck of the femur and unless otherwise indicated, also to patients with hemiplegia or paraplegia. Dicoumarol is used for the prevention of peripheral venous thrombosis.

Inappropriate use of dicoumarol therapy
The most important cases when dicoumarol therapy should not be used are listed below:

1. *Severe arterial hypertension*
2. *Liver diseases*
3. *Haemorrhagic diathesis.* To this group belong patients with thrombocytopenia or other disorders of coagulation.
4. *Peptic ulcer*
5. *Alcoholism*
6. *Poor cooperability*
7. *Pregnancy.* Dicoumarol passes through the placenta with consequent risk of haemorrhage in the foetus. *Dicoumarol* is *not recommended during pregnancy.* Heparin does not pass through the placenta and may be used when anticoagulant therapy is indicated.
8. *Surgical operations.* Surgery should not be performed while the patient is receiving full dicoumarol therapy. In candidates for surgery the prothrombin content should be allowed to rise to about 30 per cent of normal. In the postoperative course the prothrombin level should be about 20 per cent to avoid an otherwise serious risk of bleeding.

Withdrawal of anticoagulant
It has been claimed that abrupt withdrawal of dicoumarol is followed by a rebound phenomenon with increase in the prothrombin level to over 100 per cent and consequent increase in the risk of thrombosis. But convincing evidence of such a rebound phenomenon is still lacking. After abrupt withdrawal of dicoumarol the prothrombin level gradually rises, and does not become normal until some days later. There is thus no reason why dicoumarol should be withdrawn slowly.

Side-effects
Treatment with any kind of anticoagulant involves a risk of bleeding complications. Most authors give a frequency of about 20 per cent. The commonest bleeding complications of treatment with dicoumarol are haematuria, nose-bleeding and haematoma. If the P&P or TT level at

the onset of bleeding is less than 5 per cent, treatment may be withdrawn for 1–2 days and then resumed with a possibly smaller maintenance dose. If the P&P and TT levels lie within the therapeutic range, no special measures are, as a rule, indicated. One should try to avoid unnecessary fluctuation of the activity level. Only if bleeding is severe, should vitamin K be given (Konakion® 10–20 mg intravenously).

It should be pointed out that bleeding in association with dicoumarol treatment may be a sign of a tumour. Repeated bleeding therefore heeds investigating, e.g. urologic examination in the event of haematuria.

All patients should be blood-grouped before treatment with dicoumarol.

Of other side-effects, mention might be made of injury to the haemopoietic organs in patients treated with phenylindanedione preparations.

Information to patients
It is extremely important that patients prescribed continual treatment with dicoumarol be properly informed of the purpose of such treatment. They should know that it is extremely important for them to take the tablets regularly. There are now special dose cards, which make it easier for the patients to know what doses should be taken. The patients must be informed about the risk of bleeding and instructed to contact their physician immediately in the event of bleeding. They should also be informed that they should not have a tooth extracted or undergo any other operation without first informing the dentist or the doctor that they are using dicoumarol. It is also important for them to know that certain other drugs can enhance or depress their susceptibility to the anticoagulant.

2. Heparin

Readers interested in the chemistry of heparin are referred to the excellent survey by Jorpes (1962). Heparin exerts its anticoagulant effect in various ways (see page 47). Heparin thus interferes with the formation of intrinsic thromboplastin and with the conversion of prothrombin. Heparin also acts like an antithrombin, but exertion of its antithrombin effect requires the presence of a cofactor, which occurs in plasma.

Methods of administration of heparin
Continuous intravenous infusion. In principle it is best to give heparin as a continuous infusion. It is advisable to give a primary dose of 5.000 units (50 mg) in order to secure an immediate anticoagulant effect. The infusion is afterwards continued at a rate of 1.500 units (15 mg) per hour. It is advantageous to use a mechanical syringe driver which can be accurately adjusted to deliver small volumes of concentrated solution over a long period. According to this schedule of treatment coagulation times of more than 30 minutes are usually obtained.

Intermittent intravenous injection. Intermittent intravenous treatment with heparin is still the method most widely used. Heparin is then usually given in a dose of 15.000 units (150 mg) every 6th–8th hour intravenously. Heparin begins to act immediately. The effect of a dose of 150 mg lasts for about 6 hours.

Subcutaneous injection in large doses. Heparin may also be given subcutaneously, especially in long-term treatment, and if intravenous administration is for some reason impracticable. According to Engelberg (1963), the coagulation time should be at least twice the original time. A satisfactory prolongation of the coagulation time can, as a rule, be obtained with the following doses: 25.000 units heparin (a heparin solution containing 25.000 units/ml is available for subcutaneous use) on the 1st and on the 2nd day subcutaneously twice a day; 12.500 units heparin (0·5 ml) subcutaneously twice a day on the following 3 days; and 12.500 units heparin once a day on the following days.

The coagulation time should be checked at various intervals after the injection of heparin. If the coagulation time is not twice as long as that found before treatment, the dose must be increased. Overweight persons usually require larger doses.

In a small percentage of patients it is not possible to prolong the coagulation time satisfactorily, presumably because of the presence of some heparin-inactivating enzyme in the subcutaneous tissue. During shock the absorption by the subcutaneous tissue is disturbed and then heparin should be given intravenously.

Subcutaneous injection in low doses. In recent years small doses of heparin have been used in the prophylaxis of postoperative venous thrombosis (see below). A dose of 5000 units subcutaneously at 12 hour intervals is recommended for 1 week starting 1–2 hours before the operation.

Heparin should not be given intramuscularly because it might then cause local haematomas.

The commonest *determinations* used for *controlling the effect of heparin therapy* are coagulation time, thrombin time and activated partial thromboplastin time (see Godal, 1961; Hirsh, et al., 1970a).

Indications for treatment with heparin

1. *Acute venous thrombosis and pulmonary embolism.* The most important indications for heparin are acute venous thrombosis and pulmonary embolism, in which an immediate anticoagulant effect is desired. Heparin has a much stronger anticoagulative effect than dicoumarol and can effectively prevent growth of the red thrombus. In these situations continuous intravenous infusion or intermittent intravenous injection is generally used. In certain cases one may, as mentioned above, also give heparin subcutaneously in large doses. For further information on the clinical effect of heparin reference is made to Bauer (1964).

2. *Introductory to oral treatment with anticoagulants* and *after treatment with thrombolytics* (see page 200).

3. *Haemodialysis* and in cardiac surgery with *extracorporeal circulation*.

4. *Prophylaxis of thrombosis with heparin given subcutaneously in*

low doses. The magnitude of the problem of postoperative deep venous thrombosis has been realised with the advent of the ^{125}I-fibrinogen test. The frequency of postoperative deep venous thrombosis in patients undergoing major surgery has been given as about 30–35 per cent. The low dose subcutaneous treatment with heparin introduced by Kakkar and coworkers for preventing postoperative deep venous thrombosis has attracted much attention. Several trials have shown that the low dose subcutaneous heparin (usually 5000 units subcutaneously 2 hours before operation and then once every 12 hours for 7 days) significantly reduces the incidence of postoperative venous thrombosis as detected by the ^{125}I-fibrinogen test (Kakkar, et al., 1971, 1972; Gordon-Smith, et al., 1972; Nicolaides, et al., 1972). Kakkar, et al. (1972), for example, reported the frequency of deep venous thrombosis as 42 per cent in their control group (patients above 40 years and undergoing major surgery) and as 8 per cent of the patients receiving heparin. It is not yet known with certainty whether low dose heparin can reduce the frequency of fatal pulmonary embolism. Low dose heparin has not been found to have any prophylactic effect in patients with collum fractures or myocardial infarction. It is obvious that if heparin is to have the desired effect, it must be given before the trauma.

Some authors have questioned the value of low dose heparin and claimed that these low doses prevent postoperative changes in radio-activity of the legs but do not confirm the clinical effect. A large scale investigation at various centres has been started to find out whether it has any effect on fatalities due to postoperative pulmonary embolism.

Heparin in such low doses does not prolong the coagulation time, the thrombin time or the kaolin-cephalin clotting time. It has been supposed that Factor X is activated in connection with tissue trauma and that small amounts of heparin are sufficient to prevent the activation of Factor X if they are given before the trauma. This small dose treatment is not accompanied by an increased risk of bleeding.

5. *Prevention of obstruction of catheters and shunts* by thrombi.

6. In *some patients with signs of defibrination* (see page 151).

Large doses of heparin are inadvisable in mainly the same instances as dicoumarol. If such treatment is started on one of the first few days after an operation, it involves a risk of severe bleeding complications.

The side-effects consist of haemorrhages, which are generally more severe than after dicoumarol treatment. Treatment with heparin can be rapidly stopped by injection of *protamine chloride,* which must always be at hand. Patients should always be blood-grouped before treatment with heparin. Heparin should not be given intramuscularly.

Treatment with heparin may, though rarely, cause anaphylactic shock.

B. *Agents reducing platelet adhesiveness*

1. Dextran

It has often been claimed that dextran has a prophylactic effect on thrombosis (Borgström, et al., 1959; Koekkenberg, 1962). It has also been shown that Macrodex® (dextran with a molecular weight of 70.000) reduces platelet adhesiveness *in vivo* (Cronberg, et al., 1966; Bygdeman, et al., 1966; Jacobsson, 1969b) and thereby inhibits the first stage of thrombus formation. Dextran is the most effective agent known for reducing platelet adhesiveness. Dextran also has a well documented effect on the flow, which is produced partly by increase in volume and partly by reduction of viscosity. It is for these two reasons that dextran owes its prophylactic effect on thrombosis.

The greatest disadvantage of treatment with dextran is that the substance must be given intravenously in large quantities every day or every other day and therefore makes long-term treatment impossible or difficult. In addition, a large increase in the blood volume involves risks for patients with heart disease.

The use of dextran in the treatment of thrombosis is theoretically not to be recommended for patients who already have overt venous thrombosis, because dextran exerts its effect on the initial stage of thrombus formation. In thrombosis occurring in the early postoperative stage, when heparin and dicoumarol cannot be used because of the risk of bleeding, dextran may be tried to prevent further deposition of platelets on the thrombus. Villasanta (1965) recommended the use of dextran in the treatment of thrombosis during pregnancy because it does not pass through the placenta.

The most important use of dextran is as a prophylactic against thrombosis. Several workers (Ahlberg, et al., 1968; Johnsson, Bygdeman and Eliasson, 1968) have shown the value of dextran as a prophylactic against postoperative thrombosis in a series of fractures of the femoral neck. Jansen (1968) found in a general surgical series that both Rheomacrodex and Macrodex can reduce the frequency of complicating postoperative thrombo-embolism. Jacobsson (1969b) also showed that Macrodex eliminates the risk of thrombosis following catheterisation for coronary angiography.

In some cases of thrombosis it may be indicated to give combined treatment with dextran and heparin or dextran and dicoumarol.

The dose used for preventing postoperative thrombo-embolism is generally 500–1000 ml of 10 per cent Macrodex® during, or immediately after, the operation and then 500 ml on the first day and on the second postoperative day and, if necessary, a further two doses of 500 ml in the further course of the postoperative period.

2. Acetyl-salicylic acid

In recent years it has been shown that acetyl-salicylic acid affects platelet function by inhibiting the normal release function. Thus, in the presence of acetyl-salicylic acid in Born's aggregometer, no second wave is obtained on addition of ADP and adrenalin to platelet-rich plasma. Platelet aggregation by collagen is also counteracted by acetyl-salicylic acid

(O'Brien, 1968). Even small doses of acetyl-salicylic acid are sufficient to produce this effect both *in vitro* and *in vivo*. Acetyl-salicylic acid can also sometimes prolong the bleeding time.

The possibility of using acetyl-salicylic acid in the prophylaxis of thrombosis has also been envisaged and is now receiving wide spread attention, but so far convincing evidence of any effect of the acid on thrombosis is still lacking.

3. Clofibrate (Atromidin-S®)

According to some authors, clofibrate can reduce the aggregability and adhesiveness of platelet *in vivo*. The changes observed have been insignificant and some investigators have not been able to demonstrate any such effect at all (for references, see Cronberg, 1968; Hellem, 1968). Clinical material to elucidate the effect on the frequency of thrombosis is lacking.

4. Dipyramidole (Persantin®)

Some investigators have found dipyramidole to reduce platelet adhesiveness, while others have not (for references, see Cronberg, 1968; Hellem, 1968). No clinical documentation for either view is available.

C. *Agents stimulating endogenous activators of fibrinolysis*

Various researchers have tried to find drugs capable of stimulating the spontaneous fibrinolytic activity and suitable for use in the prophylaxis of thrombosis. Since impaired fibrinolytic activity in the vessel walls probably predisposes to thrombosis, the search for such drugs has become intense.

It is well known that injection of certain substances such as pyrogens, adrenalin, insulin and nicotinic acid enhances the fibrinolytic activity in the blood (see Weiner, et al., 1958; Sherry, et al., 1959; Fearnley, 1965; Cash and Allan, 1967; Robertson, 1971a), but only for a short time, *viz.*, 2–15 minutes. Plasmin activity can only rarely be demonstrated. The fibrinolytic effect of these substances varies widely from one individual to another. For example, Robertson (1971a) found that 50 mg nicotinic acid intravenously did not produce any such effect in as many as 40 per cent of a group of apparently healthy persons. Repeated injection of nicotinic acid within a period of 14 days had no fibrinolytic effect, not even in those who had responded positively to the first injection. The use of nicotinic acid or pyrogens to induce thrombolysis has been considered. It is probably futile. For, as mentioned, its fibrinolytic effect is very brief. Moreover, when given by mouth nicotinic acid has no such stimulating effect on the fibrinolytic activity except in patients with liver cirrhosis, in whom a slight increase in fibrinolytic activity might be demonstrated.

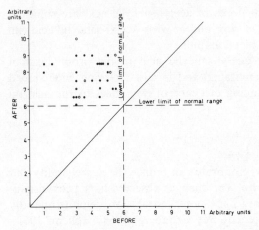

Fig 54. Plasminogen activator content determined histochemically in biopsy specimen from hand veins in 32 patients before and after treatment with phenformin and ethyloestrenol for 12 months (●) and 24 months (○)

Of workers who have devoted much time to the study of fibrinolysis from a pharmacological point of view, mention might be made of Fearnley and coworkers (Fearnley, 1965; Fearnley, et al., 1969; Chakrabarti, et al., 1968, 1970). Fearnley found that 100 mg phenformin plus 8 mg ethyloestrenol a day increases the fibrinolytic activity in the blood. Isacson and Nilsson (1970) studied the effect of this combination more closely. Ten healthy volunteers were given the above combination in the dose mentioned for 30 days. It resulted in an increase of the fibrinolytic activity in the blood, a reduction of the fibrinogen content and *an increased content of plasminogen activators* in the walls of the superficial veins. It also produced a slight reduction of platelet adhesiveness. In both the coagulation and the fibrinolytic system, the combination thus produced changes which should apparently contribute to the prevention of thrombosis. Its prophylactic effect on thrombosis, particularly in patients with thrombosis with a constitutionally low content of fibrinolytic activators, is now being tried out. So far, 32 patients have been treated for 12–24 months and in all the content of fibrinolytic activators in the vessel walls has become normal. No recurrences of thrombosis have occurred (Isacson and Nilsson, 1972) (Fig. 54).

Davidson, et al. (1972) have found treatment with stanozolol alone to enhance the spontaneous fibrinolytic activity of the blood in men with chronic ischaemic heart disease.

D. *Defibrinating agents (snake venom)*

The poisonous secretion of the Malaysian snake (*Ancistrodon rhodostoma*) has a thrombin-like effect and coagulates fibrinogen. It splits off only fibrinopeptide A. This poison has been purified and is commercially available under the name of Arvin® (Reid, et al., 1963; Esnouf and Tunnah, 1967). Injection of Arvin markedly reduces the fibrinogen content of the blood but has no effect on the platelet count or other coagulation factors. Fibrin deposited in the blood stream is believed to be removed partly by secondary fibrinolysis and partly by phagocytes in the reticulo-endothelial system. Fibrin degradation products in high concentration in the serum and reduced plasminogen values have been demonstrated after injection of Arvin (Pitney, et al., 1969a).

In recent years several authors have reported animal experiments and clinical experience with the treatment of thrombosis with Arvin (Bell, et al., 1968; Kakkar, et al., 1969a; Pitney, et al., 1969a; Reid, 1969; Prentice, et al., 1969). There appears to be general agreement that Arvin offers protection against further growth of the thrombi and that the effect is comparable to that of heparin. Arvin has no thrombolytic effect. Kakkar, et al. (1969a) compared the therapeutic effects of heparin, Arvin and streptokinase. They found streptokinase to have the best effect, while heparin and Arvin were roughly equal in effect. It has been pointed out that one of the advantages of Arvin is that it is easier to administer (two doses a day) and it does not cause complicating haemorrhages so often as heparin. Patients may, however, become resistant to Arvin (Pitney, et al., 1969b). It must also be pointed out that Arvin causes disseminated deposits of fibrin in the circulation and must be regarded as a potentially dangerous agent. If Arvin is given to individuals with low fibrinolytic capacity, there may be a considerable risk of the development of permanent fibrin thrombi and organic injury.

Another snake venom with a thrombin-like effect is Reptilase® from *Bothrops jararaca*. Reptilase causes defibrination and has been used in the same way as Arvin in the treatment of thrombosis. Blombäck, M., et al. (1971) has found this poison to have a good clinical effect.

It has recently been claimed that Arvin and Reptilase may be used in preparation for streptokinase therapy and thereby notably reduce the need of streptokinase.

E. *Treatment with thrombolytics*

BERTIL R. ROBERTSON AND INGA MARIE NILSSON

It is only during the last ten years or so that thrombolytic agents have been used in the treatment of thrombosis. This is astonishing since as early as 1933 Tillett and Garner observed that culture filtrates of β-haemolytic streptococci rapidly dissolved the plasma fibrin clot. But there are several reasons why the clinical introduction of thrombolytic agents was so late. First, unlike platelets and the coagulation system, the fibrinolytic system had previously received little attention in thrombosis research. Second, the use of such agents that theoretically appeared to be ideal, created some therapeutic problems because of their antigenicity and side effects, including haemorrhage and fever, problems which have not yet been completely solved.

Owing to stasis or a direct effect on the vessel wall the formation of a thrombus is believed to result in a local release of activators of fibrinolysis from the vasa vasorum in arteries and veins. This fibrinolytic activity may lead to a spontaneous dissolution of a newly-formed thrombus.

Hiemeyer (1967), for example, has shown by angiography that 18 per cent of small arterial emboli and 1 per cent of peripheral arterial thrombi are dissolved spontaneously. Such spontaneous dissolution of thrombi occurs also in veins. Thus, Becker, Borgström and Salzman (1970) found that 16 of 40 postoperative thrombi verified phlebographically had spontaneously disappeared by control phlebography, on the average, 33 weeks later. Kakkar, Howe, Flanc and Clarke (1969b) found that 14 of the 40 cases of deep venous thrombosis diagnosed by phlebography and the isotope technique were dissolved within 72 hours.

Administration of thrombolytic agents aims at dissolving an obstructive thrombus and not, like anticoagulant therapy, at arresting the further growth of a thrombus or preventing embolisation or the development of new thrombi. In the treatment of venous thrombosis such fibrinolytic treatment aims also at preserving the venous valves which are packed in thrombic masses, and thereby at preventing the post-thrombotic syndrome.

Plasmin. It is difficult to prepare human plasmin free from activators. Only a few attempts have been described, and no certain clinical effect has been demonstrated. Some authors have used plasmin preparations obtained by activation of plasminogen with streptokinase or urokinase (Actase, Thrombolysine), but such preparations must be regarded as mixtures of plasmin, plasminogen, streptokinase-activator complex and free streptokinase. According to Deutsch (1967), the thrombolytic effect of such plasmin preparations depends on their content of streptokinase.

Storm, et al. (1971), on the other hand, have described preliminary trials with a highly purified activator-free plasmin of porcine origin and reported promising results.

Urokinase. Pure urokinase preparations have no antigenicity and they are not pyrogenic. The individual differences in anti-urokinase titre (inhibitors of urokinase) are, as a rule, relatively small, for which reason thrombolytic treatment with urokinase is easier to standardise than such treatment with streptokinase.

Urokinase has been used successfully in the treatment of patients with thrombosis of the legs (see Sherry, 1968b) and pulmonary embolism (see Sherry, 1970). Since urokinase is not antigenic it can be used with advantage in the treatment of recurrent thrombosis after thrombolytic treatment with streptokinase (Hess, et al., 1966).

The greatest disadvantage of urokinase preparations is not of medical but of technical nature. The production of urokinase is very complicated and expensive and its supply is limited. This explains why streptokinase (SK), though it is antigenic and though it is not the ideal agent, is the preparation most widely used.

Streptokinase. In 1933 Tillett and Garner observed that filtrates of β-haemolytic streptococci quickly dissolved human fibrin clots. The activator, which is a protein, was called streptokinase (Christensen, 1945). But the streptokinase available at that time was not pure enough for intravenous use. Ten years later Tillett, Johnson, McCarthy and Fletcher succeeded in purifying the preparation further and then streptokinase could be used in clinical trials. In the 1960s highly purified streptokinase preparations became available (Kabikinas®, A.B. Kabi; Streptase®, Behringwerke A.G.; Streptokinase®, Merck, Sharpe and Dome).

Streptokinase is a water-soluble protein, which has proved to be neither toxic nor pyrogenic in animal experiments. Streptokinase is not physico-chemically homogeneous. Its molecular weight is about 47.000. Its activity is measured in international units and determined relative to an international standard, distributed by WHO. One I.U. Kabikinas® corresponds to roughly 0·01 μg protein.

As previously mentioned, streptokinase is antigenic, and in human beings it gives rise to the development of a specific immune antibody (anti-streptokinase) (see Schmutzler, 1969). The content of anti-streptokinase is also increased in streptococcal infections. The anti-streptokinase titre rises rapidly on the 8th–9th day after the beginning of treatment with streptokinase and reaches its maximum within 4–8 weeks, after which it gradually falls to recover its original value after 3–6 months (Schmutzler, 1969).

Infused streptokinase is neutralised by streptococcal antibodies in the blood, and since these occur in most patients, the antibodies must be neutralised before the thrombus can be lysed (Fletcher, Alkjaersig and Sherry, 1959). The titre of the anti-streptokinase varies widely from patient to patient and from one occasion to another in one and the same patient. To neutralise the streptokinase antibodies one must either determine the necessary initial dose of streptokinase by calculating the anti-streptokinase titre in the individual patient (Schmutzler, 1969), or use such a large standardised initial dose of streptokinase as to neutralise an anti-streptokinase titre well above that normally present in most patients (Hirsh, O'Sullivan and Martin, 1970b; Robertson, Nilsson and Nylander, 1970; Olow, et al., 1970). In this connection it should be borne in mind that no generally accepted standardised method is available for determining the initial dose of streptokinase. The methods used vary from one laboratory to another. The tests are based on the same principle, i.e. determination of the smallest dose of streptokinase that will within a certain period (e.g. 10 minutes according to Deutsch and Fischer, 1960; Nilsson and Olow 1962a; or 20 minutes according to Amery, et al., 1963) dissolve a clot formed from the patient's blood.

The various titrated initial doses, hereinafter called TID ('titrated initial dose') are roughly comparable. But when comparing the results and methods of thrombolytic treatment by different research groups the differences in the principles of determination should be borne in mind.

Part of the streptokinase is eliminated quickly from the plasma with a biological half-life of 18 minutes (streptokinase bound to antibodies); the rest slowly, with a half-life of, on the average, 83 minutes. Streptokinase is excreted in the urine and is eliminated rapidly from the liver and

the blood to the extravascular space within 20 minutes of administration
(Pfeifer, Doerr and Brod, 1969).

In an attempt to find out whether streptokinase can pass through the
placenta, Pfeifer (1965) gave 14 pregnant women the titrated dose intravenously in 5 minutes. While the maternal blood showed the expected
reaction, no signs of fibrinolysis were demonstrable in the venous blood
in the umbilical cord. Neither has any notable passage been observed
in animal experiments. Ludwig (1966) reported a passage of 0·01 and
1 per cent of the initial dose.

1. Earlier experience with thrombolytic treatment and diagnosis of throm-
bosis

During the first half of the 1960s many clinical trials to assess the value
of streptokinase in the treatment of both venous and arterial thrombosis
and embolism have been performed, and many good results of treatment
have been reported. But several objections may be raised against the
reported good results of treatment of venous thrombosis. In most
investigations the diagnosis was based only on clinical findings and the
results of treatment were not checked objectively, e.g. by phlebography.
A diagnosis of acute venous thrombosis based only on clinical findings
is very unreliable (see Gormsen and Laursen, 1967; Robertson, Nilsson,
Nylander and Olow, 1967; Robertson, Nilsson and Nylander, 1968,
1970; Kakkar, et al., 1969a). In several investigations reported after
1965 the diagnosis of deep venous thrombosis as well as the results of
treatment with thrombolytic agents was verified phlebographically
(Gormsen and Laursen, 1967; Robertson, et al., 1967, 1968, 1970;
Browse, et al., 1968; Schmutzler, 1969; Olow, et al., 1970).

An objective diagnosis of venous thrombosis can be made not only
with phlebography but also with the ^{125}I-fibrinogen method (Flanc,
Kakkar and Clarke, 1968; Negus, et al., 1968; Browse, 1969; Kakkar,
et al., 1970), plethysmography (Boijsen and Eiriksson, 1968) and ultrasonic method (Browse, 1969). But the isotope method cannot be used
for diagnosing spontaneous thrombosis because the isotope must be
given before the thrombus has developed. Neither the isotope technique,
plethysmography nor the ultrasonic method can be used for diagnosing
high thrombosis in e.g. pelvic veins. It must also be difficult for ultrasonics
and the isotope method to distinguish between a haematoma and acute
thrombosis in association with a fracture of the lower leg or of the femoral
neck. Neither can these methods or plethysmography confirm complete
dissolution of a thrombus after treatment with a thrombolytic agent.
Such verification requires phlebography before and after thrombolytic
treatment. In thrombosis of the lower leg it is, however, often difficult
even for phlebography to demonstrate the thrombus *per primam* because,
as a rule, thrombosis of the lower leg is complicated by such severe
subfascial oedema that the contrast medium fills only the extrafascial
veins. Even if control phlebography after thrombolytic treatment does

show the free deep veins to be intact, it is not possible to conclude that thrombolysis has occurred unless a thrombus had been demonstrated *per primam*. On the other hand, it is usually possible for phlebography to demonstrate thrombosis of the thigh and pelvic veins and to verify the dissolution of such a thrombus after thrombolytic treatment (Robertson, et al., 1970).

2. Indications for thrombolytic treatment

The most widely accepted indications for thrombolytic treatment are:
1. Acute arterial occlusion in the limbs (embolism or thrombosis).
2. Acute venous thrombosis of the limbs and pelvis.
3. Acute pulmonary embolism.
4. Clot in arteriovenous shunts.

The literature gives also other indications, such as acute myocardial infarction, thrombosis of the central retinal vein and artery, cerebral thrombosis, priapism and shock (for references, see Schmutzler, 1969).
1. According to Schmutzler (1969), acute *arterial occlusions* in the limbs may be treated either by vascular surgery or with a thrombolytic agent. Emergency surgery of the vessel provides the possibility of removing the occluding thrombus, while thrombolytic treatment may require one or more days to dissolve an arterial thrombus, and this delay may increase the risk of irreversible tissue damage. The shorter the interval between arterial occlusion and treatment, the easier it is to dissolve the obstructing thrombus, and arterial emboli are much easier to dissolve than arterial thrombi (Schmutzler 1969). According to Schmutzler, moderate ischaemia and an arterial occlusion below the origin of the superficial and the deep femoral artery are indications for thrombolytic treatment, whether it is a question of embolism, thrombosis or multiple embolism.
2. The possibility of successful thrombolytic treatment of acute *deep venous thrombosis* of the limbs depends largely on the length of the interval between the onset and treatment. The more recent the thrombus the easier it is to dissolve it (see Schmutzler, 1968). It is, as a rule, easy to estimate the age of postoperative thrombi because they usually begin to form during the operation (Flanc, Kakkar and Clarke, 1968). The onset of spontaneous thrombi is often difficult to date. In practice, it may be justified to relate the age of the thrombus to the onset of symptoms of thrombosis. Moreover, diagnostic phlebography can often reveal whether the thrombus is recent, subacute or old.

Also in venous thrombosis of the femoral and iliac veins one may be confronted with the choice between surgery (thrombectomy) and thrombolytic treatment. In such cases we have only exceptionally resorted to thrombectomy, while others use thrombectomy first and thrombolytic treatment only in the event of a recurrence.
3. It is naturally not difficult to date the onset of pulmonary emboli, at least not of large emboli, because they always produce acute symptoms,

which may, however, sometimes be difficult to distinguish from those of myocardial infarction. In recent years successful treatment of acute pulmonary embolism with thrombolytic agents has been reported (Hirsh, et al., 1970b). Since treatment of such cases is always urgent, Hirsh, et al., used a standardised method of treatment with streptokinase.

4. Three possibilities are available for treatment of occlusion of an arteriovenous shunt, *viz.*, heparin, streptokinase and change of the shunt, which one should avoid as long as possible. Heparin (injection and aspiration) usually has only a short-lived effect, probably because of residual thrombi and fibrin deposits (Gonzales and Cocke, 1971). Several investigations have, however, shown that thrombolytic therapy can prolong the life of the shunt (Arisz, et al., 1970; Gonzales and Cocke, 1971).

3. Remarks on thrombolytic therapy with streptokinase

Initial dose. As pointed out previously, no thrombolytic effect can be expected until after neutralisation of the streptokinase antibodies normally occurring in varying titre in the blood.

Many authors (e.g. Schmutzler, 1969) determine the individual initial dose before starting thrombolytic treatment. According to Schmutzler, the titrated initial dose should be given during a period of about 20 minutes followed once an hour by a maintenance dose corresponding to two-thirds of the initial dose. Only in the treatment of myocardial infarction, pulmonary embolism or shock, where thrombolytic treatment must be started immediately, does Schmutzler give a standardised initial streptokinase dose of 250.000 I.U. According to Schmutzler, the effect of treatment with a thrombolytic agent should be continually checked by determination of various fibrinolysis and coagulation parameters, such as one-stage prothrombin time, thrombin time, fibrinogen, euglobulin clot lysis time, and treatment should be adjusted accordingly.

Attempts have been made to devise standardised schedules not requiring laboratory control tests during treatment.

Table 20 shows that most patients (92–99 per cent) require an initial dose below 500.000–600.000 I.U. and according to Hirsh, et al. (1970b) and Robertson (1971b) 250.000–300.000 I.U. streptokinase should be sufficient to neutralise the streptokinase antibodies in more than 92 per cent of all patients with acute venous thrombo-embolism. In this conjunction it should also be recalled that though the titrated initial doses in different groups more of less agree, the determinations were made with different methods.

The following doses have been used as a standardised initial dose for thrombolytic treatment with streptokinase: 1.250.000 I.U. (Verstraete, et al., 1966). 600.000 I.U. (Olow, et al., 1970; Robertson, 1971b), 500.000 I.U. (Robertson, et al., 1970), 250.000 I.U. (Schmutzler, 1969; Hirsh, et al., 1970b). Since large initial doses, e.g. 1.250.000 I.U. often produce side-effects such as fever, pain in the loin and mild bronchospasm,

Author	Initial dose of SK	Patients with deep venous thrombosis with TID < initial dose of SK	Patients without deep venous thrombosis with TID < initial dose of SK
Verstraete, Vermylen, Amery & Vermylen (1966)	1.250.000		224 out of 231
Poliwoda (1967)	500.000	99 out of 100	95 out of 100
	250.000	92 out of 100	
Schmutzler (1968)	600.000	167 out of 170	
Hirsh, et al. (1970)	250.000	46 out of 50	

Table 20. Various initial doses and number of patients with TID less than the initial dose by different authors.

the dose ought to be kept reasonably low (Browse, Thomas and Pim, 1968).

Maintenance dose and duration of treatment. Opinions differ also on the size of the maintenance dose. As pointed out above, Schmutzler (1969) adjusts the maintenance dose according to the size of the initial dose (maintenance dose/hour = two-thirds of the initial dose).

In three coded series where the patients with phlebographically verified acute spontaneous venous thrombosis were treated with streptokinase or heparin and where various maintenance doses of streptokinase and different periods of treatment were tried, we found a maintenance dose of 50.000 I.U. streptokinase per hour to be insufficient (Robertson, et al., 1967, 1968, 1970). When 100.000 I.U. streptokinase per hour were given as a maintenance dose for 72 hours, streptokinase had three times as good an effect as heparin, as judged from the clinical and phlebographic findings. (Fig. 55).

Most authors now use a standardised maintenance dose of 100.000–150.000 I.U. streptokinase per hour. Some have treated their patients for 72–96 hours, while others have continued treatment for several days until control phlebography had shown that the thrombus had been dissolved. It is now generally agreed that treatment with a thrombolytic agent should be continued until the thrombus has dissolved, or for five or six days.

Corticosteroids and diuretics. To counteract febrile, and possibly also allergic reactions to treatment with streptokinase, corticosteroids are often given immediately before and during thrombolytic treatment (Kakkar, et al., 1969a; Hirsh, et al., 1970b; Olow, et al., 1970; Robertson, et al., 1970).

Acute thrombosis of the legs is characterised by simultaneous local swelling of varying degree. Thrombosis of the lower leg is often associated with such severe subfascial oedema that the deep subfascial veins in the lower legs are compressed and not demonstrable at phlebography (Robertson, et al., 1967, 1970). The venous return in the lower leg can therefore hardly pass through these deep veins and is forced through extrafascial veins. This probably means a further difficulty for streptokinase to reach subfascial thrombi in the affected segment of the vein.

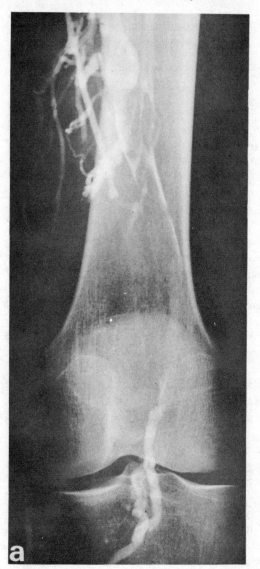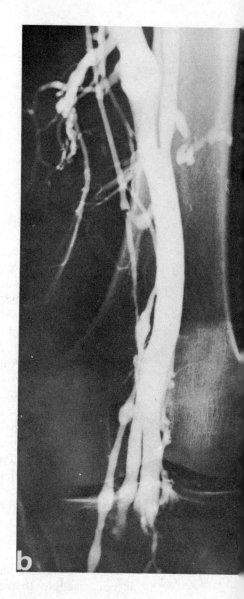

Fig 55. a.Femoral ascending phlebography of a patient with acute deep thrombosis of popliteal vein and femoral vein up to level of adductor canal. Small amounts of contrast medium are seen around proximal part of the thrombus. b. Phlebography of same patient 72 hours later. Entire thrombus dissolved and venous valves preserved (Robertson, et al.).

If the oedema can be reduced by diuretics and raising of the foot of the bed, it will increase the possibility of streptokinase reaching and dissolving the thrombi.

Anticoagulants after treatment with streptokinase. After the end of thrombolytic treatment, the injury of the vessel wall will probably persist at the previous site of the thrombus and thereby imply a risk of a recurrence. Anticoagulant therapy with heparin or dicoumarol should therefore be given towards, or after, the end of thrombolytic treatment (Browse, et al., 1968; Schmutzler, 1969; Hirsh, et al., 1970b; Olow, et al., 1970; Robertson, et al., 1970). Such anticoagulant therapy should be continued for 3–6 months or longer if necessary.

4. Complications

1. *Haemorrhage.* Haemorrhagic complications of thrombolytic treatment may occur during treatment with streptokinase or during or after anticoagulant therapy. The increased bleeding tendency is due not only to increased fibrinolytic activity with the breakdown of fibrinogen, Factor V and Factor VIII, but also to fibrin/fibrinogen degradation products, which inhibit polymerisation of fibrin.

Hirsh, et al. (1970b) studied different variables such as fibrinolytic status, coagulation defect and the nature and severity of bleeding episodes during and after thrombolytic treatment. They found that the most important cause of bleeding was a combination of local vessel injury (usually iatrogenic) and fibrinolysis.

To decrease the risk of haemorrhagic complications, no subcutaneous or intramuscular injections should be given during thrombolytic treatment. Phlebographic examination before and after thrombolytic treatment should be performed with the ascending technique, and the puncture should definitely not be made in the groin. In diagnostic arteriography because of arterial occlusion one should, if possible, puncture the contralateral femoral artery so that application of a pressure bandage, if necessary, will not impair the circulation in the affected leg still more. Body temperature should not be measured in the rectum because it involves the risk of rectal bleeding. In an analysis of various groups, Hess (1967) found bleeding in 4 per cent (fatal in 0·5 per cent) of 175 patients treated with thrombolytics. Simultaneous treatment with streptokinase and heparin is inadvisable because it increases the risk of bleeding. Drugs affecting platelet function, such as salicylic acid derivatives, should not be given during treatment with streptokinase because they increase the risk of bleeding.

2. *Fever.* Treatment with streptokinase is often accompanied by a rise in body temperature. Hirsh, et al. (1970b) found that 40 per cent of the patients experienced a rise in body temperature 12–24 hours after the beginning of streptokinase therapy. As a rule, it did not last long and did not require interruption of treatment.

3. *Pulmonary embolism.* During thrombolytic treatment of a floating

venous thrombus part of the thrombus may break off and cause pulmonary embolism. But since treatment with streptokinase is a good method for dissolving a pulmonary embolus, treatment should be continued for at least a further 12–24 hours in such cases.

In an analysis Hess (1967) found that the frequency of pulmonary embolism during thrombolytic treatment was 4 per cent of 170, and that 1·1 per cent were fatal. We have found pulmonary embolism to appear most often during the third day of the infusion. At this time, passive movement of patients with thrombosis of a limb should be kept to a minimum. Patients receiving streptokinase treatment are usually kept in bed for 4 days from the beginning of the infusion.

4. *Allergic reactions.* Allergic reactions to streptokinase therapy are, as a rule, rare. But cases with perioral oedema, stridor, hoarseness and mild bronchial spasm in patients with no allergy in their history have been reported (Browse, et al., 1968; Hirsh, et al., 1970b).

5. Results of thrombolytic treatment

In 65 patients with *acute arterial occlusion*, in most of whom the condition had been verified by X-ray, Schmutzler (1969) found that treatment with streptokinase was successful in 23 of 31 patients with embolism (74 per cent); 21 of 34 with thrombosis (62 per cent). Similar results have been reported by other authors.

In this connection it might be mentioned that streptokinase has been tried mainly by Ehringer, et al. (1970) in the treatment of chronic arterial occlusions and stenosis. Of Ehringer's 66 cases of non-acute stenosis and occlusion, successful thrombolysis was noted in 23. The best results were obtained in the group where the occlusions and stenoses were 1–6 weeks old, and in these the treatment had the most beneficial effect on the changes in inter alia the iliac artery, followed by the femoral artery and the popliteal artery in the order given. Thrombi in the lower leg were insusceptible to treatment. Martin, et al. (1970) and Heinrich and Schmutzler (1972) have achieved similar results in their investigations on 170 and 96 patients, respectively.

In *acute venous thrombosis* Schmutzler (1969) reported complete dissolution of the thrombus in 70 per cent (35 of 50) with a history of thrombosis for at most 3 days and in 54 per cent (13 of 24) of those known to have had the thrombus for at most 5 days. These figures included also venous thrombosis of the arms and vena cava. We have found thrombolytic treatment of acute thrombosis of the arm less successful than of acute venous thrombosis of the leg.

Schmutzler (1969), who treated three cases of acute caval thrombosis with thrombolytics, found such treatment to have no effect. Neither did we find any effect in two cases treated in this way.

Pfeifer (1970) and Ludwig (1966), who had shown that streptokinase does not pass through the placental barrier, have treated deep venous thrombosis in pregnant women. Of 22 cases, mainly thrombosis of the femoral and pelvic veins, Ludwig judged the treatment as successful in 17, and Pfeifer, who had treated altogether 79 patients with deep venous thrombosis, including 12 who were pregnant, reported satisfactory results in 74 per cent.

Miller, et al. (1971) and Hirsh, et al. (1971) compared the effect of streptokinase and heparin on massive pulmonary emboli. Both reported a significantly quicker resolution by streptokinase. According to Miller, embolectomy is indicated only when an immediate haemodynamic improvement is required or when the patient has become worse after medical treatment. Embolectomy should also be considered in cases where streptokinase is inadvisable.

6. Recommended principles of thrombolytic treatment with streptokinase

On the basis of our experience (Robertson, et al., 1967, 1968, 1970) we recommend the following principles of treatment of acute venous thrombosis of the limbs with streptokinase. Relevant parts of the treatment hold also for the treatment of acute arterial occlusion and of pulmonary embolism.

Thrombolytic treatment of acute thrombosis should be *considered* if:
the thrombus is known to be less than 5 days old,
the thrombus involves veins of the lower leg, popliteal vein, femoral or iliac vein (effect on thrombosis of the vena cava is poor)
Thrombolytic therapy is inadvisable if:
the patient has undergone a major operation within the last 5 days, especially on the neck, stomach, colon, uterus or operation for hernia of an intervertebral disc,
the patient has recently had a bleeding episode (ulcer, cerebral haemorrhage),
the patient has a coagulation defect or thrombocytopenia,
the patient has severe hypertension, treated or untreated,
the patient is more than 70 years old (though no absolute limit),
the patient has received thrombolytic treatment with streptokinase within the last 6 months.

a. Thrombolytic treatment should not be started before the acute deep venous thrombosis has been verified objectively by *ascending phlebography* or the isotope method.

b. Before treatment with thrombolytics is started determinations should be made of the *platelet count, haemoglobin* and *prothrombin* (P&P, thrombotest). Blood samples should be obtained for *blood grouping*. No laboratory analyses are necessary during treatment with thrombolytics.

c. The *initial dose* now used consists of 250.000 I.U. streptokinase (SK). This initial dose is given during a period of 30 minutes. Afterwards a *maintenance dose* of 100.000 I.U. streptokinase per hour is given for 72 *hours* (1.200.000 I.U. streptokinase dissolved in 500 ml 0·9 per cent saline or isotonic glucose solution for 12 hours' infusion). An electronic control unit should, if possible, be used for securing a constant rate of infusion.

d. *Diuretics* should be given before and after infusion therapy. The *foot of the bed should be raised* at least 15 cm.

e. 15 mg prednisone may be given by mouth immediately before the beginning of the infusion and then 10 mg prednisone by mouth every 12th hour.

f. The patient's *temperature* should preferably be *measured* every sixth hour. Owing to the risk of haemorrhage attending measurement of the temperature per rectum, the axillary or oral temperature should be used.

g. All treatment with thrombolytics should be followed by *anticoagulant therapy. Heparin s.c.* can be started 4 hours after the end of infusion therapy in a dose of 12.500 I.U. every 12th hour and continued for 4–6 days.

Dicoumarol therapy is usually started on day 4 and continued for, as a rule, 3–6 months.

h. The patient is confined to bed during the infusion.

Before mobilisation an elastic bandage should be wrapped around the leg (Lohmann-Dauer or similar bandage) from the tip of the toe to the knee joint. The bandage is removed at night and is wrapped round the leg again before the patient gets up the following morning. Such a bandage is recommended to be used for 6 months after the end of treatment with thrombolytics.

i. *Phlebographic control* is done after the end of infusion treatment and may be done during anticoagulant therapy. If phlebography shows that the thrombus has not dissolved satisfactorily after 72 hours' treatment, treatment may be continued for a further 1–3 days.

To dissolve a clot in an arteriovenous shunt 100.000 units of streptokinase are dissolved in physiological saline. 10.000–25.000 units (10–25 ml) is deposited in the obstructed part of the shunt, after which the latter is sealed on the venous side with a forceps and on the arterial side with a sterile syringe, which serves as an air cushion against which the artery pulsates. The treatment is repeated after 30–45 minutes when necessary.

Acquired coagulation defects

ULLA HEDNER

I. Coagulation disorders in different types of blood diseases

Thrombocythaemia. In thrombocythaemia, whether secondary or essential, there is an increased tendency to both thrombosis and haemorrhage. Secondary thrombocythaemia occurs particularly in myeloid leukaemia, polycythaemia vera, myelofibrosis, cancer, Boeck's sarcoid and Hodgkin's disease. Temporary thrombocytosis is apt to occur also in the postoperative period after splenectomy. When thrombocythaemia is complicated by haemorrhage, the condition is referred to as haemorrhagic thrombocythaemia. The cause of the increased bleeding tendency is still obscure. In these patients the *bleeding time* is often *prolonged* and *platelet adhesiveness* is *reduced* (Cronberg, et al., 1965). According to Cronberg and coworkers the platelets aggregate normally on addition of ADP or collagen. They feel that the reduced adhesiveness is due to some disorder of cellular metabolism.

Periods of *fibrinolysis* have also been observed in thrombocythaemia (Webb, et al., 1963).

Leukaemia. The commonest cause of haemorrhage in acute leukaemia is *thrombocytopenia*. It is also well known that in acute leukaemia the *fibrinogen content* in some patients or during some periods is *reduced*. The low fibrinogen concentration is ascribed to a short survival of the fibrinogen, which may be due to increased fibrinolysis (Fisher, et al., 1960; Nilsson, Andersson and Björkman, 1966; Brakman, et al., 1970) or increased consumption of fibrinogen because of intravascular coagulation (Didisheim, et al., 1964; Verstraete, et al., 1965; Pittman, et al., 1966; Hirsh, et al., 1967). On the other hand, the low fibrinogen content is probably not due to diminished synthesis because of involvement of the liver, since Factor VII, Factor X and prothrombin are usually not reduced (Finkbiner, et al., 1959). Recently it has been pointed out that markedly low fibrinogen levels occur in association with treatment of acute leukaemia with 1-asparaginase (Gralnick and Henderson, 1971). The reduction of the level of the fibrinogen may be due either to defibrination initiated by the release of intraleukocytic enzymes during treatment with 1-asparaginase or to deficient synthesis of fibrinogen. The fibrinogen formed may also be defective.

Hedner and Nilsson (1971b) found *fibrin/fibrinogen degradation products* in 25 per cent of patients with leukaemia.

A *low fibrinogen content* in association with increased *fibrinolytic activity, prolonged thrombin time* and *low Factor V* appears to be common, particularly in acute promyelocytic leukaemia (Giraud, et al., 1954; Nilsson, Sjoerdsma and Waldenström, 1960; Cooperberg, 1967). Cooperberg (1967) felt that the abnormal promyelocytes form activators of plasminogen. Most authors believe that this form of leukaemia is associated with defibrination (Straub and Frick, 1967; Merskey, 1968). Treatment with heparin has proved to have no clinical effect.

II. Coagulation disorders in various forms of dysproteinaemia

Collagen diseases. Various changes occur in the coagulation system in collagen diseases. Thrombocytopenia is common and is often accompanied by nose-bleeding and other mucosal bleeding. Also changes of the type seen in reactive processes such as increased AHF, fibrinogen and inhibitors of plasminogen activation are not uncommon either. Fibrin/fibrinogen degradation products are frequently demonstrable in the serum if the disease is in an active phase. In collagen diseases with involvement of the urinary tract, FDP occur also in the urine.

A not uncommon complication of collagen diseases is the occurrence of *circulating anticoagulants* (Hemmkörperhaemophilie). Anticoagulants are most common in lupus erythematosus (SLE), in which there is an increased tendency to form auto-antibodies.

The appearance of anticoagulants is often the first sign of disease and may occur several years before any other manifestations. Anticoagulants may be directed against AHF, haemophilia B factor, Factors XI and XII as well as against thromboplastin (Margolius, et al., 1961; Green, 1968; Robboy, et al., 1970; Castro, et al., 1972; Åberg and Nilsson, 1972). It has been shown that the antibodies are most often IgG immunoglobulins (Shapiro, 1967; Shapiro and Carroll, 1968; Anderson and Terry, 1968). Antibodies may also occur in conditions other than collagen diseases, such as in drug allergy, particularly penicillin allergy, postpartum, psoriasis, pulmonary tuberculosis, syphilis, cancer and ulcerative colitis (see Nilsson, et al., 1958; Margolius, et al., 1961; Hougie, 1964; Green, 1968, 1971b; Mason, 1969; Marengo-Rowe, et al., 1972). Anticoagulants to Factor V have recently been found in patients with penicillin allergy (Nilsson, Hedner, Ekberg and Denneberg, 1973c).

The bleeding in Hemmkörperhaemophilie are severe and resemble those in haemophilia. Severe bleeding symptoms with bleeding in the muscles and internal organs are seen. Patients with anticoagulants to Factor XI and Factor XII, however, have no bleeding symptoms. Treatment with steroids has previously been tried but with doubtful results (Margolius, et al., 1961; Green, 1968). Occasionally regression of such an anticoagulant has, however, been recorded (Nilsson, et al., 1958). Green (1971b) described a woman with psoriasis and an inhibitor of Factor VIII. The inhibitor was suppressed by simultaneous intravenous administration of cyclophosphamide and a large dose of Factor VIII. The recommendations given for the treatment cf haemophilia with anticoagulants hold also for Hemmkörperhaemophilie (see page 85).

Myeloma. An abnormal bleeding tendency is relatively common in multiple myeloma. The increased bleeding tendency has been ascribed to *thrombocytopenia, qualitative thrombocyte defects, disturbance of the thrombin-fibrinogen reaction, inhibition of various coagulation factors* and *increased fibrinolytic activity* (see Niléhn and Nilsson, 1966; Josso, et al., 1966; Vigliano and Horowitz, 1967). An investigation of 36 patients with myeloma has recently been published in America. In that investigation the coagulation defects were related to the molecular structure of respective paraproteins (Perkins, et al., 1970). Patients with IgA myeloma were found to bleed more than patients with IgG myeloma. In that study no thrombocytopenia was found in any appreciable extent in the patients with IgG or IgA myeloma. A low platelet count was not associated with a bleeding tendency. Prolonged bleeding time, however, occurred in 50 per cent of the patients with IgA myeloma. Platelet adhesiveness was reduced in 67 per cent of the patients with IgA myeloma and only in 30 per cent of those with IgG myeloma. Marked reduction of platelet adhesiveness proved to be associated with a bleeding tendency. The various coagulation factors were generally normal, but, according to Perkins, et al., they were more often reduced in patients with an abnormal tendency to bleed. Niléhn and Nilsson (1966) found coagulation defects equally often in patients with bleeding symptoms as in those without. It is noteworthy that in the American investigation Factor VII was low only in patients with IgG myeloma, while low Factor VIII and Factor V values were found only in association with IgA myeloma. This may suggest a specific mode of reaction between the specific paraprotein and the coagulation factor in question. It has also been assumed that plasma cell infiltration of the liver can impair the synthesis of the K-vitamin dependent coagulation factors. In the same way a low AHF content might be caused by cellular infiltration of the bone marrow. In 1968 Weiss and Kochwa, on the other hand, found the AHF value to be increased in 8 of 11 patients with IgG myeloma and occasionally in patients with IgA myeloma.

An increased antithrombin titre has been found in patients with myeloma (Niléhn and Nilsson, 1966; Perkins, et al., 1970). But such an increased titre is not associated with an increased bleeding tendency. In Niléhn and Nilsson's group prolongation of the thrombin time was not correlated with the amount of fibrin/fibrinogen degradation products. Perry (1963) believes that myeloma proteins bind thrombin.

Niléhn and Nilsson (1966) found an increased fibrinolytic activity and/or increased content of FDP in 50 per cent of all the patients. Hedner and Nilsson (1971b), however, found FDP in only 10 per cent of 119 patients with myeloma.

A decreased content of inhibitors of activation of plasminogen may occur in myeloma (Hedner and Nilsson, 1971a).

Lackner, et al. (1970) described two patients with myeloma with signs of abnormal fibrin polymerisation with myeloma protein adherent to thin fibrin threads. This abnormality resulted in defective retraction of the fibrin clot.

The most common coagulation defects seen in myeloma are thus:
1) thrombocytopenia
2) prolonged bleeding time
3) reduced platelet adhesiveness
4) reduced P&P value
5) reduced or increased content of AHF
6) prolonged thrombin time
7) increased fibrinolytic activity
8) FDP in serum
9) reduced content of inhibitors of plasminogen activation.

Macroglobulinaemia Waldenström. In macroglobulinaemia Waldenström the paraprotein in question has a molecular weight of about 1.000.000. An increased bleeding tendency is relatively common in macroglobulinaemia and manifests itself in the form of bleeding from the teeth, from the nose, from the ocular fundi and profuse menstrual flow.

The coagulation defects in macroglobulinaemia are largely the same as those seen in IgA myeloma. A *prolonged bleeding time* is thus relatively common. Thrombocytopenia, on the other hand, is not common (Perkins, et al., 1970). A *reduced platelet adhesiveness* has been described by several authors (Doumenc, et al., 1966; Perkins, et al., 1970). The ability of platelets to aggregate in the presence of ADP is also reduced in macroglobulinaemia (Doumenc, et al., 1966). Also the release of platelet factor 3 from the platelets is often impaired in macroglobulinaemia (Pachter, et al., 1959). The defective function of the platelets has been ascribed to adsorption of paraprotein to the surface of the platelets (Pachter, et al., 1959; Doumenc, et al., 1966). *A reduction of AHF* has been demonstrated in macroglobulinaemia (Niléhn, 1962; Perkins, et al., 1970). In addition, in macroglobulinaemia the fibrinogen may be decreased, but it is most often *increased.* The occurrence of an abnormal fibrin has been demonstrated electronmicroscopically in fibrin clots in macroglobulinaemia by Bang (1967). The paraprotein is believed to combine with fibrinogen or to be polymerised with fibrin monomers and intermediary polymers. The conversion of fibrinogen to fibrin is thereby delayed.

Cryoglobulinaemia. In cryoglobulinaemia the abnormal globulin precipitates at temperatures below 37°C. This type of paraprotein usually occurs as a complication of chronic systemic diseases such as myeloma, lymphoma, SLE and leukaemia. The most obvious symptom of cryoglobulinaemia is a tendency to vascular occlusion in the limbs owing to precipitation of cryoglobulin on exposure to the cold. Gangrene may develop. Occasionally bleeding, particularly from the nose and petechiae may appear.

In these patients *thrombocytopenia* and *reduced platelet adhesiveness* may be demonstrated (Sirridge, 1960). *Capillary fragility* is then also fairly common.

Cryofibrinogenaemia. In cryofibrinogenaemia the fibrinogen is abnormal and precipitates at temperatures below 37°C. Like cryoglobulinaemia, cryofibrinogenaemia is a complication of other conditions. Degradation of the fibrinogen by plasmin results in the formation of intermediary products, which are partly coagulable with thrombin. These also form complexes with fibrinogen. A characteristic of these complexes is that, like cryofibrinogen, they precipitate at + 4°C (Lipinski, et al., 1967). In *fibrinolysis* and *defibrination* with secondary fibrinolysis cryofibrinogen may occur. Cryofibrinogen precipitates on addition of protamine sulphate (Lipinski and Worowski, 1968).

Cryofibrinogen has been demonstrated not only in fibrinolysis and defibrination, but also in immunohaemolytic disease with multiple thromboses and in one case of pulmonary carcinoma and multiple thromboses (Sirridge, 1960, Thomas and Wessler, 1964).

The symptoms of cryofibrinogenaemia are the same as those of cryoglobulinaemia.

III. Coagulation disorders in liver diseases

Patients with various types of liver diseases (liver cirrhosis, hepatitis etc.) have long been known to have a tendency to bleed. In such patients multiple coagulation changes are found.

Several authors (Owren, 1949; Hallén and Nilsson, 1964; Donaldson, et al., 1969) have reported a reduction of all factors belonging to the *prothrombin complex* (Factor VII, Factor IX, Factor X, prothrombin) and *Factor V* in liver disease. All these factors are synthesized in the liver. These changes manifest themselves by a prolonged thromboplastin time (one-stage prothrombin time) and low P&P (or thrombotest) values and reduced content of various factors in specific tests. Hallén and Nilsson (1964) have thus found a low P&P in 75 per cent and a low Factor V in 83 per cent of patients with liver cirrhosis. Owren (1949) showed that both P&P and Factor V activity decreased with increasing hepatocellular damage. He also pointed out that reduction of Factor V to less than 50 per cent is a sign of a poor prognosis.

It is remarkable that the *Factor VIII content* is normal or increased in liver diseases (Zetterqvist and v. Francken, 1963).

Rapaport, et al. (1960) have shown that *Factor XI (PTA)* may be decreased in liver diseases.

The *fibrinogen content* is most often normal in liver diseases (Hallén and Nilsson, 1964; Donaldson, et al., 1969). In very severe liver injury the fibrinogen content may be decreased, but the patients then often have coexisting fibrinolysis. A low fibrinogen level may also be secondary to defibrination or disseminated intravascular coagulation.

An *increased fibrinolysis* in liver diseases, especially liver cirrhosis, has been reported by several authors (Fletcher, et al., 1964; Tytgat, et al., 1968; Das and Cash, 1969). Hedner and Nilsson (1971b) found FDP in 25 per cent of patients with liver cirrhosis. In some of these patients the fibrinolytic activity in the blood was also demonstably increased. According to Fletcher, et al. (1964) the liver plays an important role in the clearing mechanism of plasminogen activators. They believe that the increased fibrinolysis in liver cirrhosis is due to prolonged clearance of activators from the circulation. Others (O'Connell, et al., 1964) believe that the main cause is a reduced content of inhibitors of fibrinolysis. In a group of 304 patients with different types of liver injury, however, Hedner and Nilsson (1971a) only occasionally found a reduced content of inhibitors of plasminogen activation, α_2-macroglobulin or antiplasmin.

Plasminogen is often reduced in severe liver injury, probably because plasminogen is formed in the liver. The plasminogen may also be low in patients with fibrinolysis.

Fibrin stabilising factor, F XIII (FSF) in liver diseases has been studied by Walls and Losowsky (1969) and others. They found a decreased content of FSF with the lowest levels in those patients in whom the liver disease was most advanced.

The *thrombin time* may be prolonged in liver diseases. Various possible causes of the prolonged thrombin time have been suggested. An increased content of antithrombin has not been demonstrated (Hallén and Nilsson, 1964; Abildgaard, et al., 1970). Instead it has been demonstrated that a *low content of antithrombin III* (AT III) is a characteristic finding in liver disorders (Abildgaard, et al., 1970; Hedner and Nilsson, 1972). FDP are not common in high concentrations in liver diseases and the prolonged thrombin time is therefore probably not due to FDP. Recently it has been suggested that the prolongation of the thrombin time is due to the presence of an abnormal fibrinogen (see page 109).

Liver diseases are sometimes attended by *thrombocytopenia,* which is probably due to hypersplenism and not to any qualitative platelet defect.

Coagulation disorders in liver diseases may therefore be ascribed mainly to deficiency of a variety of coagulation factors because of impaired synthesis. To this must be added thrombocytopenia and fibrinolysis. Some authors, however, claim that the bleeding defect in liver diseases is due primarily to intravascular coagulation (Bergström, et al., 1960; Zetterqvist and v. Francken, 1963; Verstraete, et al., 1965; Tytgat, et al., 1968; McKay, 1969a, b). If it is so the increased fibrinolytic activity would be secondary to the formation of multiple thrombi.

In patients with *acute hepatic necrosis and liver coma* the coagulation disorders are severe. Such patients thus have thrombocytopenia, and the value for Factor V and the factors involved in the prothrombin complex are very low. The fibrinogen level is usually extremely low and the FDP concentration is high. In some cases the fibrinolytic activity is increased. The Factor VIII level is often very high. Holmberg and Nilsson (1973c) have recently found that AHF related protein is also markedly increased

(> 1000 per cent). Severe haemorrhagic diathesis is common. Some workers (Rake, et al., 1971) believe that the haemorrhagic diathesis in acute hepatic necrosis is due mainly to intravascular coagulation and they have tried treatment with heparin. Other workers claim that the coagulation defects are due, above all, to the impaired liver cell function, and prefer not to use heparin, but mainly exchange blood transfusions (Böhmig, et al., 1971). We have recently seen two cases of acute hepatic necrosis in young women post-partum. The first patient was given heparin, which, however, resulted in fatal bleeding. In the second patient 20–60 per cent of the blood volume was exchanged daily for 3 weeks and normalised the coagulation pattern.

K-vitamin deficiency

The synthesis of Factors VII, IX, X, and prothrombin in the liver requires the presence of vitamin K. Vitamin K deficiency results in a decrease of these factors. Conditions with associated vitamin K deficiency are characterised by a decreased content of Factors VII, IX, X and prothrombin (prolonged one-stage prothrombin time, prolonged cephalin time, low P&P). Factor V is not vitamin K dependent and is normal in these conditions, in contrast with what is seen in liver diseases. It is important to recall that vitamin K deficiency occurs in patients nourished only parentally for some time. In these patients low P&P values often increase after administration of Konakion® .

IV. Coagulation disorders in renal diseases

In acute and chronic renal insufficiency there is a tendency to both thrombosis and bleeding. The bleeding tendency is often manifested by mucosal bleeding, e.g. nose-bleeding and gingival bleeding, haematuria, and gastro-intestinal bleeding.

In patients with both chronic or acute renal insufficiency with associated uraemia the bleeding time according to Ivy is often prolonged despite a normal platelet count (see Larsson, et al., 1971a, b). In addition, platelet adhesion and aggregation are often reduced in patients with uraemia (see Larsson, et al., 1971a, b), which probably explains the prolonged bleeding time. The decrease in adhesion and aggregation of the platelets varies with the severity of the disease, the changes thus being more pronounced in patients with high creatinine and urea levels (Larsson, et al., 1971a, b). Hellem, et al. (1964) found that the urea, but not the creatinine, causes a decrease in platelet adhesiveness and concluded that the increased urea content of the blood in uraemia was the cause of the above coagulation disorders. Others have found that guanidine succinic acid, a metabolite of urea, is the cause of the impairment of the platelet function (Horowitz, et al., 1967; Stein, et al., 1969). Recent findings, however, suggest that urea *per se* impairs platelet adhesion induced by ADP, epinephrine or collagen (Davis, et al., 1972).

In acute as well as in chronic uraemia, Factor VIII, fibrinogen and inhibitors of plasminogen activation are, as a rule, increased (see Larsson, et al., 1971a, b) which is often regarded as a link in a reactive process. The fibrinogen turnover has also been found to be increased in uraemia.

Elevated P&P values are relatively common in acute as well as chronic uraemia.

The values given for antithrombin III (AT III) in uraemia vary. In 49 patients with chronic uraemia we found the AT III content to be normal (Hedner and Nilsson, 1972).

The fibrinolytic activity in blood has proved to be very low in renal insufficiency (see Wardle and Taylor, 1968; Larsson, et al., 1971a, b). The cause of this reduction has been widely discussed. A decreased uro-kinase activity in the urine has been found in renal insufficiency (Vreeken, 1966; Carlsson, et al., 1970). But many investigations suggest that uro-kinase and blood activators are not identical, for which reason a decreased production of urokinase by the affected kidneys can hardly explain the low fibrinolytic activity. Isacson and Nilsson (1969) found that on venous occlusion, patients subjected to bilateral nephrectomy showed normal fibrinolytic activity and had a normal content of activators of fibrinolysis in the vessel walls on histochemical determination. Low fibrinolytic activity in circulating blood probably depends on the marked increase of inhibitors of plasminogen activation (Larsson, et al., 1971a).

In this connection it might be of interest to mention that Losowsky and Walls (1969) showed a markedly decreased content of *fibrin stabilising factor* in acute as well as in chronic renal insufficiency.

Fibrin/fibrinogen degradation products (*FDP*) have been demonstrated in the serum and urine in acute uraemia and chronic uraemia and in concentrated urine in early glomerulonephritis (see page 134).

In *chronic* as well as in *acute uraemia* the following disorders may be seen in the coagulation mechanism:
1) prolonged Ivy bleeding time
2) reduced platelet adhesiveness
3) high P&P values
4) high content of Factor VIII
5) high content of fibrinogen
6) high content of inhibitors of plasminogen activation
7) decreased fibrinolytic activity
8) in the serum and urine high molecular weight FDP, whose occurrence is correlated to the activity of the disease.

Methods

ULLA HEDNER AND INGA MARIE NILSSON

Screening tests and some of the methods used at the coagulation laboratory, Malmö, Sweden.

I. Material and reagents

Haemolets. For determining Duke bleeding time. Standardised 'Haemolets' supplied by Dade Reagent, Inc., Miami, Florida, U.S.A.

Surgical Blades. For determining Ivy bleeding time. Gillette Surgical Blade E.

Vein cannulae. Relatively wide cannula, with *short bias polished on inner side* in the same way as serum iron cannulae. We now use disposable cannulae. Suitable outer diameter for adults 1·4–1·8 mm.

Tubes

1. For collection of blood (plasma). Plastic or siliconised tubes. Plastic tubes 18 mm diameter, length 11 cm with marks at 5 and 10 ml.

2. For collection of blood (serum). Glass tubes, 15 mm in diameter, length 10 cm.

3. Glass tubes for various coagulation tests. Disposable tubes, 10 mm in diameter, length 10 cm.

4. Tubes for determination of coagulation time (disposable tubes), 8 mm in diameter, length 55 mm. Glass beads, 5 mm diameter.

Pipettes

1. Siliconised drop-pipette (Pasteur-pipette or the like) with suitable rubber bulb. Used for aspiration of plasma and serum. Should be resiliconised after each time it has been used.

2. For coagulation analysis. Biopette automatic pipette with disposable plastic tips (Schwarz/Mann).

Plastic patches

Parafilm. When being frozen the tubes should be covered with parafilm (Marathon Products, Neenah, Wisconsin).

Sodium citrate solution. 3·8 per cent trisodium citrate. 2 H_2O. Sterile or at any rate not contaminated.

Calcium chloride solution. 0·03 M $CaCl_2$ solution.

$BaSO_4$ 'Baker'.

Epsikapron®. EACA solution from A.B. Kabi, containing 0·1 g EACA/ml.

Thrombin. Topostasin Roche ampoules containing 3.000 NIH units thrombin.

Reptilase®. Pentapharm Ltd, Basle.

Brain thromboplastin. Human brain thromboplastin prepared according to Owren (1947) and Astrup, et al. (1951). A fresh human brain is thoroughly rinsed in distilled water to remove any traces of blood. Cerebellum and meninges are removed. It is then macerated in 0·9 per cent NaCl (40° C) in a Turmix master. The emulsion is centrifuged for 25 minutes at $600 \times g$ and the sediment discarded. The thromboplastin extract obtained is stored in disposable plastic tubes at −20° C. If facilities for preparing brain thromboplastin are lacking, Ortho Brain Thromboplastin can be used.

Fibrinogen. Human fibrinogen (A.B. Kabi) and bovine fibrinogen Grade A (A.B. Kabi).

Stypven. Russell viper venom, 'Stypven', from Burroughs Wellcome & Co, London.

Thrombofax. Cephalin solution. Obtained from Ortho. Instead of Thrombofax one may use kaolin-cephalin reagent. Kaolin suspension is prepared by suspension of 4 g kaolin per 100 ml 0·9 per cent NaCl. Afterwards equal volumes of kaolin suspension and Thrombofax are mixed.

Activated partial thromboplastin time (APTT). Kaolin-cephalin solution. Obtained from General Diagnostics.

P&P-plasma. Prothrombin free BaSO₄-adsorbed bovine oxalated plasma prepared according to Brodthagen (1953). The plasma is stored in separate tubes at $-20°$ C.

Adsorbed human plasma for normalisation test. Mix 1 part 2·5 per cent potassium oxalate solution with 9 parts of venous blood from normal persons. Centrifuge. Suck off plasma. Adsorb with 50 mg BaSO₄/ml plasma during stirring for 20 minutes at room temperature. Then centrifuge twice at $4000 \times g$ for 20 minutes each time. The adsorbed plasma is pipetted off and distributed among plastic tubes and frozen at $-20°$ C.

Plasma from patients with severe haemophilia A and haemophilia B for normalisation test. See under Technique for sampling of blood and preparation of plasma and serum samples.

Normal serum. For normalisation tests.

Barbiturate buffer according to Owren (1947) containing 0·74 per cent NaCl, pH 7·38 and ionic strength 0·15.

Tris buffer. 0·07 M, pH 7·8 and ionic strength 0·15.

Phosphate buffer for fibrinogen determination. 1·67 g Na_2HPO_4. $2H_2O$ + 6·94 g KH_2PO_4 + 4·27 g NaCl are dissolved in 1 l. of distilled water, pH 6·05 and ionic strength 0·15.

Acetic acid. 0·014 per cent.

Water bath and stop watches.

II. Sampling technique and preparation of plasma and serum samples

Extreme care must be exercised when obtaining blood samples for coagulation analysis and all instruments used should be siliconised. Wide, disposable cannulae with polished inner surfaces should be used. Admixture of tissue thromboplastin should be avoided; the first few millilitres of blood should therefore be discarded. Avoid undue venous stasis and contact with glass. We do not use a syringe. Instead the blood is allowed to flow directly into prepared tubes.

For preparation of *citrated plasma* use plastic tubes or siliconised glass tubes with a mark at the 5 ml level and containing 0·5 ml citrate solution or marked at the 10 ml level and containing 1 ml citrate solution. It is very important that every tube containing citrate, when filled to the 5 or 10 ml mark, be inverted 2 or 3 times with the mouth sealed by a piece of parafilm held in position with the finger. Since several coagulation factors are labile, the blood must be processed immediately after collection. After immediate centrifugation at $2000 \times g$ for 20 minutes the plasma is sucked off with a siliconised drop-pipette and transferred to plastic tubes that are covered with parafilm. The plastic tubes containing the plasma are frozen immediately at $-20°$ C to $-30°$ C and if possible at $-60°$ C.

For preparation of *serum* glass tubes should be used. The blood is allowed to stand at room temperature for 2 hours, after which it is centrifuged and the serum is separated off and frozen.

Tubes with citrate for determination of fibrinogen should contain 10 mg EACA/ml citrated blood to prevent *in vitro* fibrinolysis.

Blood for determination of fibrin/fibrinogen degradation products (FDP) in serum is obtained in the presence of thrombin (30 NIH units to 2–3 ml blood) and EACA (25 mg to 2–3 ml blood).

III. Methods

A. *Screening analysis for investigation of coagulation defects*

1. Platelet counting

The platelet count should be repeatedly determined. We use Björkman's method (Björkman, 1959) (see also page 11).

2. Bleeding time

The bleeding time is a measure of the reaction of the capillaries to injury and is dependent on the platelets, plasma factors, vessel endothelium and the contractility of the capillaries. Two methods are available for determining the bleeding time, *viz.*, the method of Duke and the method of Ivy.

a. *Duke's method* consists in pricking the lobe of the ear with a lancet and noting the duration of bleeding. To secure a standardised depth of the prick we use a 'Haemolet' as a lancet. We also carry out the test on both ears. Normal value 1–4 minutes.

b. *Ivy's method* is performed according to a modification by Borchgrevink and Waaler (Borchgrevink and Waaler, 1958; Nilsson, Magnusson and Borchgrevink, 1963). During stasis (40 mm Hg) three transverse cuts are made on the forearm with a surgical blade (Gillette Surgical Blade E) — the cuts should be 1 mm deep and 10–14 mm long—and the mean bleeding time of the three incisions is used. The normal value according to this method is 6–12 minutes.

We have used Duke's and Ivy's methods on patients with von Willebrand's disease and on patients with other haemorrhagic diathesis (Nilsson, Magnusson and Borchgrevink, 1963; Silwer and Nilsson, 1964). In patients with mild bleeding symptoms the Duke bleeding time was normal or only slightly prolonged, while the Ivy bleeding time was invariably prolonged. In patients with severe bleeding symptoms the bleeding time was definitely prolonged by both methods. In investigation of cases with haemorrhagic diathesis we start with Duke's method. If the bleeding time according to this method is normal or only slightly prolonged, the bleeding time is determined with the method of Ivy, which is more sensitive. If the Duke bleeding time is markedly prolonged, there is no reason to measure the bleeding time with the method of Ivy.

3. Capillary fragility

We perform the test as follows. A sphygmomanometer cuff is wrapped around the arm and inflated to a pressure midway between the systolic and diastolic pressure. The cuff is left in position for 10 minutes after which the arm is inspected for petechiae. A circle 5 cm in diameter is drawn below the elbowfold and the petechiae within the circle are counted. The normal number ranges between 10 and 15.

4. Coagulation time in glass tubes

The determination must be made on venous blood and venous puncture should be smooth. We use a modification of Hedenius' (1936) method with somewhat larger tubes, 55×8 mm. Determinations are always repeated. Our normal values range from 8–14 minutes. The duration of the coagulation time is a measure of the rate of formation of thromboplastin. A defect in the first phase of coagulation should thus be demonstrable by measuring the coagulation time. It is also possible in patients with severe defects. For example, a patient with severe haemophilia A has a prolonged coagulation time. A patient with moderate or mild haemophilia with 5–10 per cent AHF, on the other hand, may have a normal coagulation time. In other words, a long coagulation time always suggests a severe coagulation defect, while a normal coagulation time does not exclude moderate or mild defects. Determination of the coagulation time is thus a crude and less sensitive method.

5. Coagulation time in siliconised or plastic tubes

Determination of the coagulation time is made in parallel in siliconised tubes or in plastic tubes, which is more sensitive than determination in glass tubes. It is the exclusion of contact with glass that makes the method more sensitive. 2–3 ml blood is allowed to run directly into a siliconised tube or a plastic tube which is stored at room temperature and observed every 2–3 minutes. The normal value for the 'silicone clotting time' is 15–25 minutes. Determinations should be repeated. In patients with moderate and mild coagulation defects the coagulation time may thus be prolonged in plastic tubes but normal in glass tubes.

6. Cephalin time and kaolin-cephalin time

Cephalin time. The cephalin time or partial thromboplastin time has in recent years been widely used in a number of laboratories as a screening method. The cephalin time is given as a measure of the activity in the intrinsic system. In this test system there is an addition of platelet substitute (usually cephalin or a commercial lipid preparation, e.g. Thrombofax, Ortho) to eliminate sensitivity to variations in the platelet content of the plasma. The test is called 'partial thromboplastin time' (PTT), because the added lipid is an incomplete or partial thromboplastin. In this test, then, the coagulation time is determined for plasma incubated with cephalin or Thrombofax after addition of Ca^{2+} (Nye, Graham and Brinkhous, 1962).

The test can be performed in the following way. 0.2 ml of citrated plasma $+ 0.2$ ml Thrombofax reagent are incubated in a water bath at $37°C$ for 30 seconds. 0.2 ml of 0.03 M $CaCl_2$ is added and the coagulation time is determined. Citrated plasma must be tested immediately after thawing.

Normally the cephalin time determined in this way is 100 seconds or shorter. The cephalin time is abnormally long, i.e. more than 100 seconds, if the content of Factors XII, XI, IX, VIII, V or X are less than 20–30 per cent. If the values of the above factors exceed 20–30 per cent the defect cannot be determined with certainty with this screening test. In the presence of heparin and circulating anticoagulant the cephalin times will be prolonged. The cephalin time will also be prolonged if the values for prothrombin and fibrinogen are low. In deficiency of Factor VII the cephalin time will not be prolonged.

Kaolin-cephalin time. The cephalin system is sensitive to contact and it may be difficult to reproduce coagulation times with this test. Proctor and Rapaport (1961) described a modification of the cephalin time consisting of addition of kaolin to the test system. This standardises the amount of contact and the coagulation times are more reproducible. In this test use is made of a kaolin-cephalin suspension consisting of kaolin suspension (4 g kaolin/100 ml 0·9 per cent NaCl) and cephalin reagent in equal volumes. The test can be performed in the following way, 0·2 ml of citrated plasma +0·2 ml of kaolin-cephalin reagent are incubated for 6 minutes in a water bath at 37°C. Afterwards 0·2 ml of 0·03 M $CaCl_2$ is added and the coagulation time is read. Normal values 45 ±3 seconds. A kaolin-cephalin reagent (APTT, General Diagnostics) is now commericially available and can be used to advantage.

It is important to remember that this is a screening method and that mild defects cannot be detected with certainty with these systems.

Normalisation tests. In the cephalin system further information about the defects can be obtained by addition of adsorbed plasma or plasma from patients with severe haemophilia A and haemophilia B. In such normalisation tests the following test systems are used:

Coagulation system:
> 0·2 ml patient's plasma+
> 0·2 ml kaolin-cephalin reagent+
> 0·2 ml NaCl or adsorbed plasma diluted 1 in 10
> > or haemophilia A plasma diluted 1 in 10
> > or haemophilia B plasma diluted 1 in 10 +
> 0·2 ml 0·03 M $CaCl_2$.

In AHF deficiency the defect is corrected by adsorbed plasma and haemophilia B plasma. This also holds for Factor V deficiency, but this defect makes itself felt also in the extrinsic system. The defect in haemophilia B is not corrected by adsorbed plasma. This holds also for Factor X, but these defects can be differentiated by determination of the one-stage prothrombin time. In Factor XI deficiency and Factor XII deficiency the defects are corrected by adsorbed plasma, haemophilia A plasma, haemophilia B plasma as well as by serum.

7. Thromboplastin time (one-stage prothrombin time)

This test determines the coagulation time after addition of an optimal amount of thromboplastin and Ca^{2+} to citrated plasma.

The thromboplastin time is affected not only by prothrombin, but also by Factor V, Factor VII, Factor X, and fibrinogen. It is thus a good screening test for defects in the second phase of coagulation when it measures the sum of the factors in this phase.

The test can be performed as follows. 0·2 ml of citrated plasma + 0·2 ml human brain thromboplastin are incubated for 3 minutes in a water bath at 37°C. Thereafter 0·2 ml of 0·03 M $CaCl_2$ is added and the coagulation time is read. Citrated plasma should not be thawed and refrozen and should, if it is not frozen immediately, be tested within 2 hours after the sample has been obtained. The thromboplastin time is normally 14–16 seconds. The thromboplastin time is prolonged in deficiency of Factors V, VII, X and prothrombin and in patients with very low fibrinogen values. The thromboplastin time is also prolonged in patients receiving heparin and in the presence of circulating anticoagulants active in the second phase. In deficiencies in the intrinsic system the thromboplastin time is not prolonged. If the thromboplastin time is to be determined during heparin treatment, the sample is obtained about 6 hours after the previous injection of heparin. If the dose of heparin is conventional, the concentration of heparin at this time will be low and any residual heparin can be neutralised by thromboplastin.

In the thromboplastin system further information can be obtained about the defect by addition of adsorbed plasma and serum. In such normalisation tests the following system is used.

Coagulation system:

0·2 ml patient's plasma +

0·2 ml thromboplastin +

0·2 ml NaCl or adsorbed plasma diluted 1 in 10

or serum diluted 1 in 10 +

0·2 ml 0·03 M $CaCl_2$.

Normal plasma coagulates within 14–17 seconds in this system but the coagulation time is prolonged, as previously mentioned, in the presence of deficiency of Factors VII, X, V and prothrombin. If the patient has Factor VII deficiency, the defect will be completely corrected with serum, but not with adsorbed plasma. In Factor X deficiency the same result will be obtained. It is, however, possible to distinguish Factor VII deficiency from Factor X deficiency by determining the Stypven time. In Factor VII deficiency the Stypven time is normal, while it is prolonged in Factor X deficiency. Determination of the Stypven time is performed in essentially the same way as determination of the thromboplastin time but brain thromboplastin is replaced by Stypven solution (1 ampoule of Stypven is dissolved in 5 ml of distilled water and this solution is afterwards used directly in the test). The Stypven time is normally 13–15 seconds. In Factor V deficiency correction is obtained with adsorbed plasma but not with serum. In prothrombin deficiency serum will produce partial correction (containing small amounts of prothrombin) and no correction will be obtained with adsorbed plasma.

This test system can also be used for testing whether there is any anticoagulant active in the extrinsic system.

Coagulation system:
> 0·2 ml normal plasma or patient's plasma +
> 0·2 ml thromboplastin +
> 0·2 ml NaCl or normal plasma diluted 1 in 10
>   or patient's plasma diluted 1 in 10 +
> 0·2 ml 0·03 M $CaCl_2$.

If the prolonged coagulation time is not normalised by diluted normal plasma and if the thromboplastin time of normal plasma is prolonged on addition of the patient's diluted plasma, this suggests an anticoagulant.

8. Owren's P&P test, thrombotest, normotest and Simplastin A-test

Owren's *P&P test system* (Owren and Aas, 1951) is such that it contains all factors in excess except those to be determined. $BaSO_4$-adsorbed bovine oxalated plasma is used as a test base. This supplies fibrinogen and a large amount of Factor V to the system. The bovine plasma contains 5–10 times as much Factor V as human plasma. $BaSO_4$-adsorbed plasma, on the other hand, contains no prothrombin, Factor VII or Factor X. Human brain thromboplastin is also added. The plasma to be tested is then added diluted 1/10 or 1/20 and finally $CaCl_2$. Pooled normal plasma serves as 100 per cent standard. This method measures the sum of prothrombin, Factor VII and Factor X.

The normal range of Owren's P&P method is 80–120 per cent. P&P is a stable and sensitive test system which is extremely useful for regulating dicoumarol therapy and for diagnosing impaired synthesis of factors of the prothrombin complex, e.g. in liver diseases. In the investigation of haemorrhagic diathesis P&P is a valuable supplement to the thromboplastin time. If the thromboplastin time is prolonged and the P&P is normal it suggests that the Factor V content is decreased. P&P is decreased in liver diseases and in conditions with vitamin K deficiency, e.g. malabsorption or obstructive jaundice. In systemic diseases and malignant diseases the P&P is often low. In intravascular coagulation P&P may be low. It is high during pregnancy, in women using P-pills and often in severe renal insufficiency.

Owren's *thrombotest and normotest systems* are similar and are well known at most routine laboratories.

Simplastin A-test (Warner-Chilcott, U.S.A.) is a new test which has proved to be a sensitive one-stage method for determining prothrombin.

Five different thromboplastin preparations and plasma for standardisation are now available from the Division of Biological Standards, National Institute for Medical Research, Mill Hill, London N.W.7, England.

9. Fibrinogen

The most reliable method for measuring fibrinogen is based on Morrison's (1947) syneresis method. According to this method, the plasma sample is coagulated with thrombin. After some hours the clot is taken up on a piece of cloth placed on filter paper and is to undergo syneresis. The fibrin is afterwards thoroughly washed with physiological saline and dissolved in urea or NaOH. The protein content of the dissolved clot is then determined by measurement of the extinction at 280 nm in Beckman DU spectrophotometer.

The method has been modified and improved (Jacobsson, 1955; Blombäck, B. and Blombäck, M., 1956; Nilsson and Olow, 1962b) and is now regarded as the most reliable method for determining fibrinogen.

At the coagulation laboratory in Malmö the fibrinogen is determined by the method described by Nilsson and Olow (1962b). To avoid false low fibrinogen values owing to activation of the fibrinolytic system after sampling, an inhibitor of fibrinolysis, EACA (10 mg/ml blood), is added to the test tube before determination of the fibrinogen.

1 ml of plasma is clotted with 0·1 ml thrombin solution (300 NIH units/ml) in 2 ml of phosphate buffer. The tube is then allowed to stand for 2 hours at room temperature and the clot is transferred to a piece of gauze and allowed to retract for 5 minutes. The clot is then washed in 0·9 per cent NaCl containing EACA and in alcoholic acetone, after which it is dissolved in 10 ml of 0·1 N NaOH in a boiling water bath for about 15 minutes. The extinction value is read in a Beckman DU spectrophotometer at 280 nm, and the fibrinogen content is calculated. The fibrinogen content is normally 0·20–0·40 g/100 ml.

The fibrinogen is increased in all reactive processes and high values are therefore common in patients with acquired diseases. The fibrinogen level may be low in patients with increased fibrinolytic activity and in intravascular coagulation.

As a quick test for determination of fibrinogen one may use Schneider's method for determining the fibrin titre (see page 217). The fibrinogen may also be determined immunologically according to Laurell's rocket method.

B. *Screening methods for acute bleeding conditions*

1. Platelet counting (see page 211)

2. Owren's P&P test, thrombotest, normotest and Simplastin A-test (see page 215).

3. Fibrinolysis tests

a) *Whole blood lysis test* is performed immediately after the sample has been obtained. Whole blood is allowed to clot in a glass tube. Immediately after the sample has been collected thrombin (150 NIH units to 2–3 ml whole blood) is added to accelerate coagulation. The clot is incubated at 37°C (water bath) and the time necessary for the clot to dissolve is noted.

Normally the clot is not dissolved within 24 hours. *Severe fibrinolysis* will, however, result in the dissolution of the clot within 5–10 minutes and *moderate fibrinolysis* within 1–2 hours. This method cannot be used for demonstrating abnormally low fibrinolytic activity.

b) *Euglobulin clot lysis time* gives a better impression of fibrinolysis, if any, than whole blood lysis time. In this test the so called euglobulin fraction (containing fibrinogen, plasminogen, plasmin etc.) is precipitated at pH 5·4 by 0·014 per cent acetic acid. The euglobulin fraction is dissolved in buffer and coagulated with thrombin and the time necessary for the clot to dissolve is noted. Normally this time for the euglobulin fraction is much shorter than for whole blood because the major part of the inhibitors of fibrinolysis is not precipitated together with the euglobulin fraction.

To 0·5 ml of citrated plasma is added 9·5 ml 0·014 per cent acetic acid. The tube is inverted and allowed to stand for 10 minutes in the refrigerator. It is afterwards centrifuged for 5 minutes, the supernatant is separated off and the precipitate is dissolved in 0·5 ml of 0·01 M Owren's buffer. It is incubated for 10 minutes at 37°C after which 0·5 ml of thrombin solution (2 NIH units/ml) is added and the stop watch is started. A clot is formed and the time necessary for it to dissolve is noted.

Normal range. 100–300 minutes. Short dissolution times are obtained if the patient has fibrinolysis or a low fibrinogen value (< 0.05 g/100 ml). A lysis time of 30 minutes or less is considered to be of pathological significance.

4. Quick test for fibrinogen

This can be performed with *Schneider's test*. The lowest plasma concentration which causes coagulation on addition of thrombin is a semi-quantitative measure of the amount of fibrinogen in the plasma. At the same time the fibrin titre in normal plasma is determined and used for reference.

The degree of fibrinolysis is estimated from the time it takes clots in the various plasma dilutions to dissolve at 37°C. If the fibrin titre alone is to be determined, citrated plasma obtained with addition of about 10 mg EACA/ml blood is used. In the determination of fibrinolysis citrated plasma is used without addition of EACA. Pooled plasma from ten normal persons is used as reference. In an acute situation venous blood from a healthy person, e.g. the examiner himself, may be obtained in the same way as that described above and used as reference plasma.

The test is performed as follows. Two series of seven glass tubes are set up in two rows. Into the first two tubes are pipetted 1·8 ml of 0·9 per cent NaCl and respectively 0·2 ml citrated plasma from the patient and 0·2 ml of control plasma. In the remaining tubes 1 ml of 0·9 per cent

NaCl is deposited. The dilution series are then set up by transferring 1 ml from tube No 1 to tube No 2 and then 1 ml from tube No 2 to tube No 3, etc. The dilutions in the different rows will then be 1/10, 1/20, 1/40, 1/80, 1/160, 1/320, 1/640. 0·1 ml of thrombin solution (50 NIH units/ml but if the patient has received heparin one must use a thrombin solution of 300 NIH units/ml) is added to each tube and the tubes are inverted and stop watches are started. The test is performed in a water bath at 37°C. The results of the test are read after 15, 60 and 120 minutes. The last tube in the series made with plasma with added EACA in which a clot appears within 15 minutes denotes the fibrin titre, this is reported as the dilution number.

In the estimation of fibrinolysis, the clot in the plasma obtained without addition of EACA is examined after 15, 60 and 120 minutes. The state of the clots is noted as follows:

$$+ \;=\; \text{firm clot}$$
$$(+) \;=\; \text{clot}$$
$$(-) \;=\; \text{clot floating free}$$
$$- \;=\; \text{no clot}$$

In the presence of fibrinolysis the clots in the patient's plasma will be dissolved quicker than in normal plasma.

Normal values for fibrin titre: clot occurs in dilutions up to 1/80–1/320.

5. Thrombin time

The thrombin time depends on the content of fibrinogen and partly on any substances which inhibit the effects of thrombin such as fibrin/fibrinogen degradation products (FDP).

0·2 ml citrated plasma is pipetted into tubes and placed at 37°C for 3 minutes. 0·1 ml of thrombin solution of different concentrations is then added. (A dissolved ampoule thrombin should always be stored in the refrigerator and never for more than 24 hours.)

    I 30 NIH units/ml: 1 ml of stock solution (300 NIH units/ml) + 9 ml Tris buffer

    II 6 NIH units/ml: 2 ml of I + 8 ml Tris buffer

    III 3 NIH units/ml: 1 ml of I + 9 ml Tris buffer

The coagulation time is determined. Plasma from the patient and normal plasma are always tested simultaneously. Repeat determinations are always made simultaneously of all thrombin concentrations in normal plasma. The thrombin time of the patient's plasma is determined first with 3 NIH units thrombin/ml. If this time is normal, i.e. does not deviate substantially from the value found for normal plasma, determinations with other thrombin dilutions are unnecessary.

 Normal value. 6 NIH units thrombin/ml give a normal coagulation time of 12–15 seconds, 3 NIH units thrombin/ml 18–20 seconds. The thrombin time is regarded as definitively prolonged if it is more than 4 seconds longer than that for normal plasma. *Prolongation* of the thrombin time occurs if 1) the fibrinogen content is very low (< 0·10 g/100 ml) (this can be controlled by repeating the test after addition of 0·4 per cent solution of human fibrinogen or normal plasma), 2) high content of FDP, 3) increased content of antithrombin, mainly in myeloma, 4) heparin in the blood, 5) dysfibrinogenaemia, 6) liver disease in which the thrombin time is often for some unknown reason prolonged.

6. Reptilase time

This is dependent on content and properties of fibrinogen and of FDP.

0·2 ml of citrated plasma is pipetted into tubes and placed at 37°C for 3 minutes. 0·1 ml of Reptilase is then added after which the coagulation time is measured. The patient's plasma and normal plasma are always tested simultaneously. Repeat determinations are made.

Normal value. The coagulation time for normal plasma is 18 seconds. The Reptilase time is regarded as prolonged if the clotting time is more than 4 seconds longer than that of normal plasma.

Prolongation of Reptilase time is present when 1) the fibrinogen content is very low (< 0·10 g/100 ml), 2) dysfibrinogenaemia exists, 3) there is a high content of FDP. In patients treated with heparin, however, the Reptilase time is normal while the thrombin time is markedly prolonged.

7. Quick test for determining fibrin/fibrinogen degradation products

At the coagulation laboratory in Malmö we use a latex agglutination inhibition test (Allington, 1971; Svanberg, et al., 1973). The method is based on the fact that high molecular weight degradation products and fragments D and E have antigenic determinants common to fibrinogen and thus react with antifibrinogen. Fibrinogen-coated latex particles can be obtained from A.B. Kabi.

Equal parts (0·1 ml) of a serum (diluted 1/1)—or urine sample (diluted 1/1)—and antifibrinogen (0·1 ml) are incubated at room temperature for more than 2 minutes.

0·1 ml of this mixture + 0·1 ml of fibrinogen-coated latex is then placed on a black glass plate and the sample is carefully rocked for 2 minutes. If the sample contains no FDP, all antifibrinogen will persist after incubation and react with the fibrinogen on the latex particles with clear agglutination as a result. But if the specimen contains FDP, the antifibrinogen will be neutralised during the incubation time and then no agglutination will occur on addition of fibrinogen-coated latex. In our modification the test is adjusted so that agglutination is inhibited if the specimen contains FDP in amounts larger than 10 μg/ml.

Sampling. Blood is obtained in tubes containing thrombin (30 NIH units per 3 ml blood) and EACA (25 mg per 3 ml blood).

Normal values. Provided the blood sample is obtained in tubes containing thrombin and EACA, normal serum will contain no demonstrable FDP.

A direct latex agglutination test is now available (Thrombo-Wellcotest).

8. Fibrin monomers

These can be determined with the ethanol gelation test according to Godal, et al. (1971). This test utilises the ability of ethanol to induce a quick end-to-end aggregation of fibrin, which gives rise to a transparent gel. This reaction has been said to be specific to fibrin and a positive reaction is thus obtained if the plasma contains dissolved fibrin derivatives. Ordinary citrated plasma is generally used for the test within 2 hours after sampling. Frozen plasma cannot be used.

0·5 ml of plasma is incubated for 3 minutes in a water bath ($20°C$) after which 0·15 ml of 50 per cent ethanol is added. The tube is thoroughly shaken and allowed to stand untouched at $20°C$ for 10 minutes. After exactly 10 minutes the test is read by carefully tilting the tube. Only samples in which a clear gel has been forced are regarded as positive. Positive results according to Godal, et al., are seen in general defibrination. False positive results may be obtained if the fibrinogen level is abnormally high.

C. *Other analyses*

1. Specific determination of coagulation factors

In the specific determination of coagulation factors either so called one-stage systems or two-stage systems can be used. The latter are used in some laboratories for measuring the factors in the first phase of coagulation and are based on the thromboplastin generation test (see page 227). One-stage methods, however, are easier and therefore most widely used.

A one-stage test system should contain optimal amounts of all the clotting factors except the one to be determined, whose concentration should be nil. The best test substrate is plasma from patients with a severe deficiency of the factor to be tested. Pooled normal plasma from 10–20 normal persons is generally used as standard. A standard curve is plotted on semilogarithmic or logarithmic paper by plotting the coagulation times on the ordinate and the concentrations of the standard plasma on the abscissa. The curve for an ideal testing system should not be flat, for such a curve allows demonstration of only large differences in the content of the factor. The greater the slope of the curve, the more sensitive the method. The curve must be stable and not drift in the course of the experiment. On the other hand, if the coagulation times are markedly prolonged, the error of the method will be greater. It is therefore important that the method be well standardised so that the error of the method can be kept as small as possible. Fig. 56 shows a typical standard curve on squared paper for a one-stage system. It is seen that roughly the same coagulation time is noted for dilution 1/1 (= 100 per cent) as for dilution 1/10 (= 10 per cent) of the standard plasma. This holds for practically all one-stage coagulation systems. It is the rule to start the standard curve with a 1/10 dilution of standard plasma and regard this dilution as 100 per cent. The standard plasma is tested in dilutions 1/10, 1/20, 1/50, 1/100, 1/200, 1/500, 1/1000.

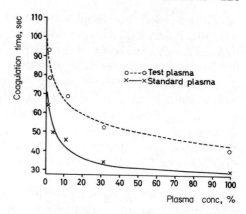

Fig 56. Standard curve for determination of coagulation factors.

The plasma to be determined is usually tested in dilutions 1/10, 1/20, 1/50 and 1/100. After reading the standard curve, the values obtained are multiplied by 1, 2, 5 and 10, respectively. An unknown sample is nearly always tested in two dilutions and the mean of the values for the different dilutions is given.

AHF and B factor determination. Haemophilia A and B factor activities are usually determined in one-stage recalcification systems as described above. The ability of a patient's plasma to correct the defect of haemophilia A or B plasma is compared with that of normal standard plasma. Such a test for determining AHF was first described by Langdell, et al. (1953) and was based on the partial thromboplastin time. Various modifications of the procedure have been worked out (Nilsson, et al., 1957; Waaler, 1959; Egeberg, 1961). Hardisty and Macpherson (1962) and Veltkamp (1968) added a kaolin suspension to standardise contact activation. Similar test systems are used also for determining B factor.

At the coagulation laboratory in Malmö the following one-stage methods are used (Nilsson, et al., 1957; Nilsson, et al., 1959).

Preparation of plasma
1. *Haemophilia A-plasma or haemophilia B-plasma.* From a patient with haemophilia A with < 0·1 per cent AHF or haemophilia B with < 0·1 per cent Factor IX citrated blood is obtained in the following way. 750 ml blood is collected in a plastic bag (Fenwal) containing 50 ml sodium citrate solution. By plasmapheresis it is possible to double the amount of plasma obtainable from one donor. The blood is immediately centrifuged at $200 \times g$ and at $+ 4°C$ for 10 minutes. The plasma is removed and properly mixed. The platelet count in the plasma is then determined. It should not be less than 150.000 per mm^3. The plasma is then distributed among small plastic tubes (4–5 ml/tube) and frozen at $-60°C$.

If haemophilia plasma is to be used as a test base, it should have a recalcification time of at least 480 seconds. It should also have a normal one-stage prothrombin time and normal P&P value. One should also check that the haemophilia plasma has no inhibitory effect (due to anticoagulant against AHF, for example).
2. *Plasma samples for testing.* The determinations are made on citrated plasma prepared from blood carefully obtained so that it is not contami-

nated with tissue thromboplastin and allowed to run directly into the test tube. If the blood does not flow but only drip into the tube, it cannot be used for determination of the AHF. Citrated blood is centrifuged at $2000 \times g$ for 20 minutes. The plasma is sucked off with a siliconised drop-pipette and distributed among 2–3 small plastic tubes and covered with a parafilm (about 2 ml plasma/tube) and frozen immediately at $-60°C$. The plasma should not be thawed until immediately before the determination. It is thawed in a water bath. Plasma samples that have been thawed and refrozen, or plasma that has been thawed and allowed to stand open for at least 1 hour, cannot be used for determination of the AHF.

3. *Standard plasma.* As standard plasma pooled citrated plasma from 10–20 normal persons is used (blood from women using P-pills or menopausal should not be used). The standard plasma should be handled and treated in the same way as plasma samples for testing.

Performance
The haemophilia test base, the patient's plasma and the standard plasma are thawed at 37°C immediately before the test is started. After it has been thawed all the tubes are inverted against a piece of plastic film. The haemophilia test base is placed in a beaker of ice and the remaining plasma samples are kept at room temperature. The standard plasma is then immediately *diluted* (1/10, 1/20, 1/50, 1/100, 1/200, 1/400, 1/500 and 1/1000) and the patient's plasma (1/10, 1/20, 1/50, 1/100, 1/200) in *plastic tubes* in 0·9 per cent NaCl or Tris buffer (0·07 M, pH 7·4). After the dilution has been prepared a plastic film is held tight against the mouth of the tube with the finger, and inverted.

To 0·2 ml of haemophilia test base is added 0·2 ml of various dilutions to be tested. The tubes are placed in a water bath at 37°C and incubated for 3 minutes. 0·2 ml of 0·03 M $CaCl_2$ solution is then added and a stop watch is started. The coagulation time is determined. The tubes should be shaken at least once a minute, as well as during the entire last minute before the calculated end of the test. About eight test tubes can be dealt with at a time. It is the rule first to test all the dilutions and the blank in the standard curve. When dilutions of the patient's plasma are afterwards tested it is necessary continuously to take samples from the standard curve to check that it has not shifted.

The patient's plasma is tested, if the AHF content or B factor content is not suspected of being very low, in dilution 1/50 and 1/100. If short times are obtained compared with the standard curve the plasma is tested also in a dilution of 1/200. In the event of signs of severe deficiency the samples are tested in dilution 1/10 and 1/20. Concentrates of AHF and B factor are tested in dilution 1/500 and 1/1000. The standard curve is drawn on squared paper (mm) beginning from the left—the times on the ordinate and concentration of the abscissa—so that 0–10 per cent corresponds to two 1 cm squares.

In a series of normal adults we have found the AHF content to vary between 60–160 per cent with a standard deviation of $\pm 17\cdot5$ per cent. The mean error of the method for various AHF values have been calculated as follows:

AHF content (%)	Standard error
$0\cdot1$ – 1	$\pm\ 0\cdot1$ – $\pm\ 0\cdot3$
2 – 3	$\pm\ 0\cdot6$
4 – 6	$\pm\ 1\cdot4$
15 – 25	$\pm\ 4\cdot5$
30 – 40	$\pm\ 5\cdot2$

The normal values for B factor lie between 60–140 per cent.

Shorter clotting times can be obtained by addition of cephalin or diluted thromboplastin dilutions. Such an addition simplifies the technical performance of the test, but the standard curve will be flat.

AHF and B factor can also be determined with a two-stage method based on the thromboplastin generation test (TGT) (see Pitney, 1956; Biggs, 1957; Pool and Robinson, 1959; Sen, et al., 1967). The ability of the patient's plasma and serum to form intrinsic thromboplastin is compared with that of normal plasma and normal serum respectively.

Factor XI and Factor XII determinations. As previously mentioned, several one-stage methods have been described for the determination of Factor XI. In these test systems determinations are made of the ability of the plasma to correct the coagulation defect in Celite adsorbed plasma, which does not contain Factor XI + Factor XII, in a cephalin recalcification system. In these test systems it is not possible to determine Factor XI separately. We use a modification of the methods of Soulier and Prou-Wartelle (1959) and Horowitz, et al. (1963). Normal plasma is adsorbed with 30 mg of Celite per ml plasma and Thrombofax is used as cephalin.

For qualitative diagnosis TGT may also be used.

If congenital Hageman deficiency plasma and plasma from a patient with severe Factor XI deficiency are available, these factors can be determined satisfactorily in one-stage systems similar to those used for the determination of AHF.

Factor V determination. The best test base for determining Factor V is plasma from a patient with congenital deficiency of Factor V (Owren, 1947). Since congenital Factor V deficiency is extremely rare, such a test base can be used only exceptionally. It is therefore the rule to determine the ability of the plasma to correct the prolonged thromboplastin time of stored human oxalated plasma. During storage of oxalated plasma Factor V is inactivated.

For determining Factor V we use a modification of Wolf's method (1953). The test system is as follows.

$0\cdot2$ ml of stored oxalated plasma (human oxalated plasma stored at 37°C until the thromboplastin time is at least 70 seconds, pH corrected to 7·4) + 0·2 ml of standard citrated plasma in different dilutions or 0·2 ml of the plasma sample to be tested in dilution 1/10 and 1/20 + 0·2 ml thromboplastin + 0·2 ml 0·03 M $CaCl_2$. Citrated plasma should be thawed immediately before the test.

Factor V content is normally 80–120 per cent. The values are lower in the presence of liver disease and certain systemic diseases such as advanced cancer, leukaemia. Low Factor V values occur in patients with fibrinolysis and defibrination.

Factor VII determination. For isolated determination of Factor VII activity we prefer to use plasma from patients with severe congenital Factor VII deficiency as a test base. The test system is otherwise made up in the same way as for the P&P test with thromboplastin. The Factor VII content is normally 80–120 per cent.

The Factor VII values will be low in congenital deficiency, in liver diseases, vitamin K deficiency and during treatment with dicoumarol. Raised Factor VII values are seen in pregnancy, in association with the use of P-pills and also in renal diseases.

Factor X determination. For isolated determination of Factor X activity plasma from a patient with severe Factor X deficiency is best (congenital or acquired in e.g. amyloidosis). The test system is the same as that for Factor VII.

Factor X content is normally 80–120 per cent. Isolated low values can be seen in congenital deficiencies and in amyloidosis. Otherwise Factor X is low in liver diseases, vitamin K deficiency and during dicoumarol therapy.

Prothrombin (Factor II) determination. It is difficult to determine prothrombin separately. The most reliable and sensitive methods are presumably modifications of the original two-stage method by Warner, Brinkhous and Smith (1936). In principle it consists of an incubation mixture made up of brain emulsion, Ca^{2+} and plasma or prothrombin preparation in high dilution. At different intervals after addition of Ca^{2+}, samples are obtained and their thrombin activity is determined on fibrinogen solution. Thrombin is used as a standard. The total amount of thrombin that can form is determined. The method is laborious and has not found wide clinical use. In normal plasma 200–300 NIH units thrombin/ml is formed.

For specific determination of prothrombin, Hjort, Rapaport and Owren (1955) modified Owren's P&P system. Instead of using brain thromboplastin they used Stypven and cephalin, which have the same effect as Factor VII. Serum is used as a source of Factor X. The standard curve is flat.

An immunochemical method for determining prothrombin has been worked out by Ganrot and Niléhn (1968b). The method is based on Laurell's electrophoretic technique (Laurell, 1966). To avoid coagulation of the samples, $10\mu l$ of the sample is applied to an agarose gel in barbiturate buffer, but without calcium lactate and the electrophoresis is run at 20 V/cm. When the coloured albumin (bromphenol blue) has migrated 3 cm the electrophoresis is stopped and the gel above the albumin is changed against a new agarose gel containing specific antibodies against prothrombin, after which the electrophoresis is allowed to continue but then in barbiturate buffer containing calcium lactate. Precipitation peaks are obtained and their height is measured and related to a standard for normal plasma.

As pointed out by Ganrot and Niléhn (1968b), this method determines the prothrombin protein but not the activity, which is obvious from a poor correlation between the P&P method and the immunochemical method. The same authors (Niléhn and Ganrot, 1968; Stenflo, 1972a, b) have also shown the formation of a pathological prothrombin molecule in association with treatment with dicoumarol, which still has the same immunological determinant, but not the same properties as the normal prothrombin.

Fibrin stabilising factor (Factor XIII). Deficiency of Factor XIII is rare. The defect may be suspected if the history reveals abnormal bleeding and poor wound healing. Factor XIII is a transamidating enzyme, which catalyses the cross-linking of fibrin. The determination of Factor XIII is based on its ability to incorporate fluorescent synthetic amines in casein (Lorand, et al., 1969, Lorand, 1973; personal communication).

After activation of Factor XIII in the plasma sample by Ca^{2+} and thrombin dansylcadaverine is incorporated in casein, which is then precipitated with trichloroacetic acid. The fluorescence of the precipitate is a measure of incorporated dansylcadaverine and the amount of Factor XIII in the plasma sample.

Citrated plasma is obtained in the usual way. 0·2 ml plasma and 50 μl 50 per cent glycerol are incubated at $56°C$ for 4 minutes. The tube is cooled and 50 μl 0·2 M dithiothreitol and 0·2 ml thrombin solution, 125 NIH units/ml, are added. After 20 minutes at room temperature 0·5 ml monodansylcadaverine (2mM in 0·05 M Tris buffer, pH 7·5) and 1·0 ml of 0·4 per cent casein in a glycerol-Tris-calcium chloride solution are added. The tube is left for exactly 30 minutes at room temperature. The casein is then precipitated with 2 ml 10 per cent trichloroacetic acid and washed 4 times, dried and dissolved in 1 ml 0·1 per cent NH_4HCO_3 containing 5 μl trypsin (10 mg/ml). After 12 hours, 2 ml of a urea-(8 M) Tris solution and 10 mg sodium dodecylsulphate are added to each sample. The fluorescence is read on a fluorometer and the result is calculated according to a formula given by Lorand, et al. (1969) and expressed in FSF units per ml.

Earlier methods for determining Factor XIII were based on the fact that normal plasma clots are insoluble in 5 M urea or 1 per cent monochloroacetic acid while clots that have formed in the absence of Factor XIII are soluble in 5 M urea or 1 per cent monochloroacetic acid (Lorand and Dickenman, 1955; Josso, et al., 1964). The method of Josso, et al., is as follows. The determination is made in citrated plasma from patients and normal persons. A series of tubes is set up, each containing 0·5 ml of the patient's plasma or 0·5 ml normal plasma, and one tube in which the patient's plasma and normal plasma have been mixed in the proportion 95 parts patient's plasma and 5 parts normal plasma. The contents of these tubes are recalcified with equal volumes of 0·03 M CaCl$_2$ solution. The tubes are allowed to stand in a water bath for about 20 minutes, after which the clot is carefully separated and transferred to other tubes containing 5 ml 5 M urea solution. These tubes are left at room temperature and are inspected at different intervals to see whether the clot has dissolved or not. In the event of Factor XIII deficiency, the clot will dissolve within 2–3 hours, while control plasma and mixtures of patient's plasma and normal plasma will remain undissolved for more than 24 hours. 1 per cent Factor XIII is sufficient to render the clot insolvable in 5 M urea.

2. Recalcification time of plasma

The recalcification time of plasma is the coagulation time of citrated plasma after addition of Ca^{2+}. To 0·2 ml plasma, incubated at 37°C for 3 minutes, is added 0·2 ml 0·03 M CaCl$_2$ solution. The recalcification time is normally 120–180 seconds. This test is very sensitive to contact and to maltreatment of the blood and, as a rule, does not give any information over and above that of the whole blood clotting time.

3. Prothrombin consumption test

The prothrombin consumption test is a test which gives a measure of the amount of prothrombin remaining in the serum for a certain time after coagulation has begun. After 1 hour's incubation of the blood sample at 37°C at most 30 per cent should persist in the serum after the beginning of coagulation. If the content of any of the factors in the first phase is low, the coagulation rate will be decreased and the prothrombin will thus not be consumed so rapidly as normally. We use a modification of Biggs and Macfarlane's method (1962). The amount of prothrombin in plasma and serum from the patient (serum separated exactly 1 hour after coagulation of the blood after incubation at 37°C) is determined in a one-stage system with addition of brain thromboplastin and fibrinogen. Division of the coagulation time of plasma by the coagulation time of serum and multiplying the quotient by 100 gives the prothrombin consumption index. *Normal value 0–30.*

Abnormal prothrombin consumption occurs in thrombocytopenia, in patients with platelet defects and with coagulopathies in the first phase of coagulation. The prothrombin consumption test is not a very sensitive method even though it is more sensible than determination of the coagulation time. A normal prothrombin consumption test thus need not mean that the content of the various factors in the first phase are normal. The prothrombin consumption test will, however, usually be abnormal in the presence of severe coagulation defects.

4. Thromboplastin generation test (TGT)

This test, which was elaborated by Biggs, Douglas and Macfarlane (1953a, b) is widely used for studying the course of reaction in the first phase of coagulation and for determining the various clotting defects in the first phase.

In TGT the incubation mixture consists of:
1) platelets or cephalin
2) adsorbed plasma, usually $BaSO_4$-adsorbed plasma containing AHF, Factors, V, XI and XII
3) serum containing Factors VII, IX, X, XI and XII
4) $CaCl_2$

After addition of $CaCl_2$ the mixture is incubated at 37°C. This results in the formation of plasma thromboplastin. At 1 minute intervals samples are taken and added to normal platelet-free plasma, which is then recalcified. The coagulation time at optimal incubation time (usually 10 minutes) is a measure of the amount of plasma thromboplastin formed. By successive replacement of the reagents included in the incubation mixture it is possible to form an opinion of the nature of the defect.

5. Circulating anticoagulants

The mechanism of coagulation can, though rarely, be inhibited by abnormal anticoagulants in the circulation. The coagulation time is then usually prolonged. It is technically easy to demonstrate the occurrence of circulating anticoagulants. But it is much more difficult to ascertain the target of the abnormal anticoagulant, its amount and properties.

To demonstrate the presence of circulating anticoagulants one may add the patient's plasma in different dilutions to a normal plasma and determine whether the patient's plasma prolongs the coagulation time of normal plasma. At the same time one should check whether the prolongation of the coagulation time of the patient's plasma disappears or not by addition of normal plasma in dilution. If the prolonged coagulation time is due to deficiency of one or more factors, the coagulation time will become normal on addition of normal plasma in dilution. If the patient has an anticoagulant it will not. The following test systems can be used for demonstrating the presence of an anticoagulant.

I. *Recalcification system*
0·2 ml normal citrated plasma +
0·2 ml normal citrated plasma diluted 1/10 (control) or
0·2 ml patient citrated plasma diluted 1/10 +
0·2 ml 0·03 M $CaCl_2$

If the patient's plasma prolongs the coagulation time it suggests the presence of an anticoagulant. The next step is to determine the highest dilution of the patient's plasma that prolongs the clotting time in order to decide on the activity of the anticoagulant.

Normalisation tests are performed in the same way but with the patient's plasma as a test base.

II. *Cephalin system*

0·2 ml normal citrated plasma +
0·2 ml normal citrated plasma diluted 1/10 (control) or
0·2 ml patient citrated plasma diluted 1/10 +
0·2 ml Thrombofax (incubated for 3 minutes) +
0·2 ml 0·03 M CaCl$_2$

This test system is positive if the anticoagulant is active in the first phase of the coagulation process.

III. *Thromboplastin system*

0·2 ml normal citrated plasma +
0·2 ml normal citrated plasma diluted 1/10 (control) or
0·2 ml patient citrated plasma diluted 1/10 +
0·2 ml brain thromboplastin (incubated 3 minutes) +
0·2 ml 0·03 M CaCl$_2$

This test system is positive if the anticoagulant is active against thromboplastin and the factors in the second phase of the coagulation process.

IV. *Refined test for anticoagulant against AHF*

Acquired anticoagulants are often directed against AHF. The following test system can be used for determining anti-AHF activity. 1 part of AHF concentrate (containing about 3 units AHF per ml) is incubated with 3 parts of patient's plasma for 2 hours at 37°C. As a control, haemophilia A plasma without an anticoagulant is used. The AHF content is determined both before and after incubation. If the patient has a high content of anticoagulant, it is necessary to dilute the plasma. The number of units of AHF inactivated by 1 ml of the patient's plasma can then be calculated directly. This test is most suitable for determination of anticoagulants in patients with haemophilia A.

V. *Refined test for anticoagulant against haemophilia B factor*

This test is the same as the refined test for anticoagulant against AHF, but with the use of B factor concentrate.

6. Fibrin plate method

The fibrin plate method of Astrup and Müllertz (1952) is convenient, accurate, and sensitive. In the fibrin plate method measured amounts of fibrinolytically active solutions are placed as drops on the surface of a layer of fibrin, which is then incubated and the areas of lysed zones produced are measured. The fibrin is contaminated by plasminogen. During the incubation time the activator content of the sample activates the plasminogen contained in the fibrin film to plasmin with fibrinolysis as a result. If the sample also contains plasmin, this effect will be added to that of the activator activity. By parallel testing on heated plates (Lassen, 1952), which measure only the plasmin activity, it is possible to assess to what extent the activity measured is due to activator. However, the fibrin is partly denatured by heating and less sensitive to plasmin (Lassen, 1952).

In Malmö we use the fibrin plate method as modified by Nilsson and Olow (1962a) with Plexiglass dishes of our own design. These are absolutely plane, which is important. We use bovine fibrinogen (Kabi) prepared principally according to the glycine method of Blombäck and Blombäck (1956). Undiluted citrated plasma and resuspended euglobulin precipitate from plasma are used as test solutions for the assay of the patients. It is very important that the plasma samples to be examined for activity are added to plates within at most 30 minutes of collection of the blood sample. As mentioned, the activator is labile. Neither can the sample be tested after having been frozen. Freezing and thawing of the sample is followed by a considerable loss of activity. For the assays, exactly 30 μl of the active solution is placed on the surface of the fibrin layer with a Carlsberg pipette. The activities are determined in triplicate. The sensitivity of the plates is checked with a standard preparation of urokinase and/or pigheart activator (see Albrechtsen, 1957) parallel with the test solutions. The circular area of the lysed zones produced after 18 hours of incubation is a measure of the activity. This is arbitrarily expressed as the product, in square millimeters, of two perpendicular diameters. The mean of three such areas is used. Readings are made with an accuracy of 0·5 mm. Details of the method as used at this time at the coagulation laboratory in Malmö is given in Table 21.

In our laboratory the spontaneous lytic activity on unheated fibrin plates of plasma from 832 normal subjects varied from 0–159 mm^2 with a mean value of 22·5 mm^2 and a standard deviation of 31 mm^2. The lytic activity of resuspended euglobulin precipitate from 332 normal subjects varied from 0–230 mm^2 with a mean value of 74 mm^2 and a standard deviation of 42 mm^2.

7. Fibrin/fibrinogen degradation products

Methods for determining FDP have been described on page 130. At the coagulation laboratory in Malmö we use Niléhn's immunochemical method for determining FDP (Niléhn, 1967b). This method is based on Laurell's technique (Laurell, 1966), according to which a glass plate is covered with agarose gel containing specific antibodies to the D fraction of FDP. With the aid of an electric current the antigen, 10 μl (serum 1/1 or urine 1/1), is forced into the gel. If the sample contains FDP, they will produce precipitation peaks, whose height is proportional to the concentration of the antigen. The height of these peaks is measured and related to a standard of high molecular weight degradation products. It is important that the serum samples for measuring FDP are collected in tubes containing EACA (about 25 mg per 3 ml blood) and thrombin (30 NIH units to 3 ml blood) to avoid *in vitro* fibrinolysis and to remove residual coagulable fibrinogen.

With this method it is possible to determine FDP in concentrations

Table 21. *Fibrin plates*

1. Plexiglass plates (II cm in diam) with 5 numbered circles in the bottom.
2. 28 ml of 0·1 per cent bovine fibrinogen (Kabi) in Tris buffer at pH 7·8 and ionic strength 0·15.
3. Coagulate with 150 μl thrombin (100 NIH units/ml).
4. Let the plate set for 30 minutes on plane support.
5. Place 30 μl of test solution (usually plasma and resuspended euglobulin precipitate) in each circle (3 samples from each test solution). It is important that the plasma sample be placed on the plate within at most 30 minutes of collection of the blood sample.
6. Incubate the plates for 18 hours at 37°C. The shelves must be plane and horizontal.

Record the lytic activity as the product of two perpendicular diameters in mm^2 of the lysed zones (mean of three determinations).

down to 5 μg/ml. Healthy volunteers have, according to our results, <5 μg FDP/ml in the serum and in urine, so that a positive result of the test may be regarded as abnormal.

FDP in serum is seen above all in chronic renal diseases in the active phase, acute renal diseases, in cancer, septic or postoperative haemorrhagic shock, collagen diseases in the active phase, and in women with complications of pregnancy, particularly toxicosis and hepatosis. If a patient has FDP in the serum or urine, it should indicate the investigation of the patient's state of health (see also page 133).

8. Plasminogen

Plasminogen is determined in Malmö using the direct immunological method described by Ganrot and Niléhn (1968a) and modified by Ekelund, Hedner and Nilsson (1970). The determination is based on Laurell's technique with electrophoresis in agarose gel containing specific antiserum to human plasminogen (1/200 in 1 per cent agarose in barbiturate buffer, ionic strength 0·07, pH 8·6 containing 2 mM calcium lactate). 10 μl of the serum samples (1/5) is applied and the electrophoresis is run for 4 hours at 20 V/cm. The height of the peaks is a measure of the amount of plasminogen. Their height is measured and related to a standard of mixed serum from 25 normals.

Samples for determination of the plasminogen should be collected in tubes containing EACA (about 25 mg per 3 ml blood) to avoid *in vitro* fibrinolysis.

The normal values according to this method are 70–130 per cent. The values are reduced in fibrinolysis and in liver disease.

The plasminogen may also be determined indirectly by activating the plasminogen to plasmin and allowing it to digest casein or bovine fibrin. The casein method is the one used most, usually with various modifications (see Müllertz, 1956; Hedner and Nilsson, 1965; Johnson, et al., 1969b).

9. Inhibitors of fibrinolysis

1) *Inhibitors of plasminogen activation* can be measured by their capacity

to inhibit urokinase-induced fibrinolysis (urokinase inhibitors), on which several methods are based. In Malmö *a clot lysis method* (Paraskevas, et al., 1962) is used. The test system includes fibrinogen, plasminogen, urokinase and thrombin. To these are added the serum to be tested in varying dilution and its inhibiting effect on the activation of plasminogen by urokinase is determined. The activity is expressed as a percentage of that found for pooled normal serum from 25 persons. This method determines not only the inhibitors of activation of plasminogen, but also partially the antiplasmin activity. This must be borne in mind in the evaluation of the results. It has, however, been shown that differences in the antiplasmin content must be large before they affect the results and that the inhibitors of the activation vary independently of the antiplasmin activity (Bennett, 1967; Hedner and Nilsson, 1971a).

The normal value for this method is 80–120 per cent. Low values are sometimes seen in patients with myeloma. Increased values occur in all reactive processes, renal insufficiency and after renal transplantation.

The inhibitors of plasminogen activation can also be determined with *a caseinolytic method* devised by Lauritsen (1968) and modified somewhat by Hedner, Nilsson and Jacobsen (1970). The test system in this method consists of porcine plasminogen, which is activated by urokinase. After a certain period the activation is stopped by addition of EACA and the plasmin activity is determined caseinolytically. The difference between inhibition by addition of serum to the system before activation of the plasminogen and the inhibition by addition of serum after activation is a measure of the activating inhibitors in human serum. The results are expressed as the difference in extinction values.

Normal values in this method are 0·022–0·056.

2) α_2-*macroglobulin* (immediately reacting antiplasmin) is determined with an esterolytic method described by Ganrot (1966). The normal values are 80–120 per cent. The values are low during treatment with thrombolytics. Raised values occur in nephrosis, and slightly raised levels are seen in diabetes and during pregnancy. The normal values are higher in children than in adults.

3) *The antiplasmin activity* is determined with methods in which plasmin is added in excess to serum. After a certain incubation period, residual plasmin is determined with a caseinolytic method or with the fibrin plate method (Shamash and Rimon, 1964; Ekelund, et al., 1970). These methods determine the sum of α_2M and α_1-antiplasmin.

10. Histochemistry of plasminogen activator (fibrin slide technique)

The method was originally described by Todd (1959). Pandolfi, et al. (1967, 1968, 1972) have modified the method to permit quantitation of the fibrinolytic activity in tissues. The modification of the method used routinely at this laboratory for assaying the fibrinolytic activity of superficial arm veins is described below.

Biopsy specimens of the distal part of a hand vein, a 0·5–1·0 cm long segment, are obtained under local anaesthesia (0·5 per cent Carbocain). The specimens are packed hermetically and quickly frozen with carbon dioxide.

Bovine fibrinogen, prepared essentially according to Brakman's modification of the double ammonium sulphate precipitation method of Astrup and Müllertz (Brakman, 1965) is used as substrate in a 1 per cent solution in Sörensen's phosphate buffer, pH 7·8.

Thrombin Topostasin Roche, 20 NIH units/ml unbuffered saline.

Sections 6–8 μm thick are cut on an International Harris' cryostat and collected on glass slides. They are then covered with a mixture of 0·06 ml of fibrinogen and 0·01 ml of thrombin, spread over an area of 10 cm². In this way a fibrin film about 0·07 mm thick is obtained. The fibrin is allowed to stabilise at room temperature (21°-24°C) for 30 minutes in a moist chamber. The slides are afterwards transferred to another moist chamber at 37°C and incubated for different periods. After incubation the sections are fixed in 10 per cent formaldehyde (formalin) and stained together with the fibrin film with Harris' haematoxylin. Areas of fibrinolysis at the sites of active cells in the sections appear as defects in the fibrin film.

Evaluation of fibrinolytic activity. We prepare a series of 4 slides for each specimen and incubate them for progressively increasing periods (0, 10, 20, 30 minutes). To each slide are then allotted 1 point for small punctate areas of lysis in the majority of the sections, 2 points for larger, confluent areas of lysis, and 3 for massive fibrin digestion. 1·5 and 2·5 points are allotted for intermediate degrees of lysis 1–2 and 2–3, respectively. The sum of the points scored by each set of slides is taken as a direct measure of the fibrinolytic activity of the specimen. In this way the potential score of each vein biopsy can vary between 0 and 12. Fifty vein biopsy specimens of hand veins from apparently healthy subjects gave values ranging from 7 to 11.

11. Platelet adhesiveness

Platelet adhesiveness can be determined with Hellem's, Salzman's or Bowie's method.

In *Hellem's method* for whole blood, citrated blood is passed through specially manufactured plastic tubes containing glass beads. During their passage, some of the platelets adhere to the glass beads and the difference between the number of platelets in the blood before and after passage through the plastic tube is calculated. It is important that the blood sample be allowed to stand 45 minutes to 1 hour after sampling before being used for the test. Blood tested immediately after collection gives a very low value and after 2 hours the adhesiveness decreases again. The method requires a special apparatus with automatic injection, stand and siliconised glass syringe. To the siliconised glass syringe ('Summit') is fastened a short plastic tube through which 6 ml of blood is sucked up. The blood must be sucked up by a single pull in order to avoid injury to the platelets.

The glass tube is fastened to the holder of the injection apparatus and the apparatus is started. In a plastic tube filled with 10 ml of 3·8 per cent sodium citrate solution blood is collected for exactly 26 *seconds*. During this time exactly 1 ml of blood is collected. (It is important that the collection period be very exact. Even a small error in this respect will cause a disproportionately large error of the final result. Since it takes a varying time after the apparatus has been started until the blood begins to drip out of the plastic tube, it is advisable to discard the first few drops and immediately afterwards start a stop watch and, after exactly 26 seconds, stop the apparatus and include any drop still hanging from the tube). The plastic tube is then sealed with parafilm and inverted a few times. The plastic tube is removed from the glass syringe as soon as possible and coupled to the special aggregate of glass beads, and afterwards placed upright in a stand. The apparatus is started and the blood is allowed to pass through a plastic tube containing 19 ml of 3·8 per cent sodium citrate solution and collected for 26 seconds. (After the apparatus has been started and the blood has begun to rise in the aggregate, the apparatus is not stopped before all the blood has been collected. The collection period must be very precise. Since the end-tube of the aggregate is narrower and since the machine feeds the blood for a long time at a steady rate, one may very well start the stop watch as soon as the blood reaches the end of the tube and then switch off the machine after exactly 26 seconds, including any drop still hanging from the tube.) Check that the aggregate does not leak, otherwise the results would be wrong. The plastic tube should be inverted as soon as possible. A parafilm is used as a lid. (No further platelet adhesion to the plastic tube occurs in this high citrate concentration. On the other hand, it is important that the two collections of blood be made in quick succession to prevent the platelets from fastening to the wall of the glass syringe, should the latter be inadequately siliconised.)

The samples with 1 ml blood +19 ml 3·8 per cent sodium citrate solution are then allowed to stand for one or more hours so that the erythrocytes may sediment, after which the platelets in the control tube and the 'aggregate tube' are counted. One drop of the supernatant fluid is then transferred to a Bürker counting chamber and after incubation for 30 minutes in a moist chamber the platelets are counted in a phase contrast microscope. Platelet adhesiveness is measured in terms of the difference between the number of platelets in the control blood and in the blood that has passed through the aggregate of glass beads. *Normal values* 17–35 per cent. Low values occur in thrombasthenia, thrombocytopenia and in uraemia.

When determining platelet adhesiveness according to *Salzman* the blood is run directly through a filter with glass beads and the platelets that become attached are numbered. The filters are manufactured in accordance with Salzman (1963). The glass bead filter is attached to a Vacutainer® which contains EDTA and has a capacity of 7 ml of blood. When sampling, blood is allowed to flow directly through a glass filter and also through a control tube, where it flows directly down into a glass tube containing EDTA. 1 ml of the sample and 1 ml of the control blood are transferred to 19 ml of a dilution fluid (we use that described by Björkman and containing potassium rhodanide and sulphuric acid), after which the platelets are counted in a Bürker counting chamber. The method has certain technical difficulties and requires practice. The results vary from one occasion to another in one and the same person and the normal range of variation is wide.

Normal values about 30 per cent. Values below 20 per cent are seen mainly in von Willebrand's disease, thrombasthenia and other conditions with a prolonged bleeding time. The method is used mainly in the investigation of patients with suspected von Willebrand's disease, especially in family studies.

Determination of platelet adhesiveness according to *Bowie* (1969) may also be valuable in the diagnosis of von Willebrand's disease. As originally described the test only measures decreased adhesiveness. Blood is drawn in heparin (4 units/ml blood) and is then passed through a glass bead column by means of a pump. The 4th and the 5th ml expelled from the tube are collected. A good discrimination between normals and von Willebrand's disease has been reported, but the test is sensitive to careless handling of the sample and it is not very reproducible.

12. Clot retraction

Clot retraction is, above all, a measure of platelet function. In thrombasthenia the platelets are non-adhesive and lack the contractile mechanism. In thrombasthenia, therefore, there is no clot retraction. In thrombocytopenia clot retraction is inadequate at platelet counts below 100.000 per mm^3. In the determination of clot retraction we use a modification of the method described by Hartmann and Conley (1953). The test is performed in the investigation of haemorrhagic diseases with a prolonged bleeding time.

The method requires both *platelet-rich citrated plasma* ($=$PRP, citrated blood is centrifuged at $185 \times g$ for 10 minutes) and *platelet-poor citrated plasma* ($=$PPP, citrated blood is centrifuged first at $2000 \times g$ for 20 minutes, afterwards the plasma is sucked off and recentrifuged at $16.000 \times g$ for 20 minutes at $+4°C$). The test should be performed about 2 hours after the blood sample has been collected, for otherwise the values will be too low.

Dilutions containing 200.000 platelets/mm^3, 100.000 platelets/mm^3 and 50.000 platelets/mm^3 are made of platelet-rich plasma with the platelet-poor plasma. To 0·9 ml of the respective dilutions is added 0·1 ml thrombin (20 NIH units/ml) and the tubes are immediately inverted twice. PPP is used as a control. After incubation for 60 minutes at 37°C the clot is removed and the serum volume is measured. The amount of serum is a measure of clot retraction during 60 minutes' incubation and is converted to a percentage of the total volume.

Normal value. Clot retraction is 80–85 per cent for dilutions containing 100.000 platelets/mm^3, 65–75 per cent for dilutions containing 50.000 platelets/mm^3 and 35–55 per cent for dilutions containing 25.000 platelets/mm^3.

References

ABILDGAARD, CH. F.: Recognition and treatment of intravascular coagulation. J. Pediat. 74 (1969) p 163.

ABILDGAARD, CH. F., CORNET, J. A., FORT, E. & SCHULMAN, I.: The in vivo longevity of antihaemophilic factor (factor VIII). Brit. J. Haematol. 10 (1964) p 225.

ABILDGAARD, CH. F., SIMONE, J. V., COR-RIGAN, J. J., SEELER, R. A., EDELSTEIN, G., VANDERHEIDEN, J. & SCHULMAN, J.: Treatment of hemophilia with glycineprecipitated factor VIII. New Engl. J. Med. 275 (1966) p 471.

ABILDGAARD, CH. F., SIMONE, J. V., HONIG, G. R., NORMAN, E. N., JOHNSON, CH. A. & SEELER, R. A.: von Willebrand's disease: A comparative study of diagnostic tests. J. Pediat. 73 (1968) p 355.

ABILDGAARD, U.: a. Inhibition of the thrombin-fibrinogen reaction by antithrombin III, studied by N-terminal analysis. Scand. J. Clin. Lab. Invest. 20 (1967) p 205.

ABILDGAARD, U.: b. Purification of two progressive antithrombins of human plasma. Scand. J. Clin. Lab. Invest. 19 (1967) p 190.

ABILDGAARD, U.: Highly purified antithrombin III with heparin cofactor activity prepared by disc electrophoresis. Scand. J. Clin. Lab. Invest. 21 (1968) p 89.

ABILDGAARD, U.: a. Inhibition of the thrombin-fibrinogen reaction by α_2-macroglobulin, studied by N-terminal analysis. Thromb. Diath. Haemorrh. 21 (1969) p 173.

ABILDGAARD, U.: b. Binding of thrombin to antithrombin III. Scand. J. Clin. Lab. Invest. 24 (1969) p 23.

ABILDGAARD, U., FAGERHOL, M. K. & EGEBERG, O.: Comparison of progressive antithrombin activity and the concentrations of three thrombin inhibitors in human plasma. Scand. J. Clin. Lab. Invest. 26 (1970) p 349.

ABRAHAMSEN, A. F.: Platelet survival studies in man. Scand. J. Haematol. Suppl. 3 (1968) p 1.

ACHENBACH, W.: Angiohämophilie. Ergeb. Inn. Med. Kinderheilk. 14 (1960) p 68.

ADELSON, E., RHEINGOLD, J. J., PARKER, O., BUENAVENTURA, A. & CROSBY, W. H.: Platelet and fibrinogen survival in normal and abnormal states of coagulation. Blood 17 (1961) p 267.

AGGELER, P. M.: von Willebrand's disease. Editorial. Calif. Med. 111 (1969) p 143.

AHLBERG, Å.: Haemophilia in Sweden. VII. Incidence, treatment and prophylaxis of arthropathy and other musculo-skeletal manifestations of haemophilia A and B. Acta Orthop. Scand. Suppl. 77 (1965).

AHLBERG, Å.: Radioactive gold in treatment of chronic synovial effusion in haemophilia. VIIth Congress of the World Federation of Haemophilia, Tehran-Iran, May (1971) p 84.

AHLBERG, Å., NYLANDER, G., ROBERTSON, B., CRONBERG, S. & NILSSON, I. M.: Dextran in prophylaxis of thrombosis in fractures of the hip. Acta Chir. Scand. Suppl. 387 (1968) p 83.

ALAMI, S. Y., HAMPTON, J. W., RACE, G. J. & SPEER, R.: The relationship of plasma fibrinogen (factor I) level to fibrin stabilizing factor (factor XIII) activity. Blood 31 (1968) p 93.

ALBRECHTSEN, O. K.: The fibrinolytic activity of human tissues. Brit. J. Haematol. 3 (1957) p 284.

ALBRECHTSEN, O. K.: The fibrinolytic agents in saline extracts of human tissues. Scand. J. Clin. Lab. Invest. 10 (1958) p 91.

ALKJAERSIG, N.: The purification and properties of human plasminogen. Biochem. J. 93 (1964) p 171.

ALKJAERSIG, N., FLETCHER, A. P. & SHERRY, S.: a. The mechanism of clot dissolution by plasmin. J. Clin. Invest. 38 (1959) p 1086.

ALKJAERSIG, N., FLETCHER, A. P. & SHERRY, S.: b. ε-aminocaproic acid: an inhibitor of plasminogen activation. J. Biol. Chem. 234 (1959) p 832.

ALLANBY, K. D., HUNTSMAN, R. G. & SAKKER, L. S.: Thrombotic microangiopathy. Recovery of a case after heparin and magnesium therapy. Lancet I (1966) p 237.

ALLINGTON, M. J.: Detection of fibrin (ogen) degradation products by a latex clumping method. Scand. J. Haematol. Suppl. 13 (1971) p 115.

ALMÉR, L. O., HEDNER, U. & NILSSON, I. M.: Fibrin degradation products in the early differential diagnosis of acute myocardial infarction. Thromb. Res. 1 (1972) p 59.

AMBRUS, J. L. & MARKUS, G.: Plasminantiplasmin complex as reservoir of fibrinolytic enzyme. Amer. J. Physiol. 199 (1960) p 491.

AMERY, A., MAES, H., VERMYLEN, J. & VERSTRAETE, M.: The streptokinase reactivity test. I. Standardization. Thromb. Diath. Haemorrh. 9 (1963) p 175.

ANDÉN, N. E., HENNING, M. & OBIANWU, H.: Effect of epsilon amino caproic acid on adrenergic nerve function and tissue monoamine levels. Acta Pharmacol. Toxicol. 26 (1968) p 113.

ANDERSEN, B. R. & TERRY, W. D.: Gamma G4-globulin antibody causing inhibition of clotting factor VIII. Nature 217 (1968) p 174.

ANDERSEN, B. R. & TROUP, S. B.: Inhibition of human factor VIII (AGH) caused by a γG antibody. Fed. Proc. 26 (1967) p 532.

ANDERSEN, B. R. & TROUP, S. B.: γG-antibody to human anti-hemophilic globulin (factor VIII). J. Immunol. 100 (1968) p 175.

ANDERSSON, L.: Treatment of so-called essential haematuria with fibrinolytic inhibitor (epsilon-aminocaproic acid). Acta Chir. Scand. 124 (1962) p 355.

ANDERSSON, L.: Antifibrinolytic treatment with epsilon-amino-caproic acid in connection with prostatectomy. Acta Chir. Scand. 127 (1964) p 552.

ANDERSSON, L., NILSSON, I. M., COLLEEN, S., GRANSTRAND, B. & MELANDER, B.: Role of urokinase and tissue activator in sustaining bleeding and the management thereof with EACA and AMCA. Ann. N. Y. Acad. Sci. 146 (1968) p 642.

ANDERSSON, L., NILSSON, I. M., LIEDBERG, G., NILSSON, L., RYBO, G., ERIKSSON, O., GRANSTRAND, B. & MELANDER, B.: Antifibrinolytica. Vergleichende Untersuchungen von trans-4-(Aminomethyl)-cyclohexancarbonsäure, Aminocapronsäure und p-Aminomethylbenzoesäure. Arzneim-Forsch. (Drug. Res.) 21 (1971) p 424.

ANDERSSON, L., NILSSON, I. M., NILÉHN, J.-E., HEDNER, U., GRANSTRAND, B. & MELANDER, B.: Experimental and clinical studies on AMCA, the antifibrinolytically active isomer of p-aminomethyl cyclohexane carboxylic acid. Scand. J. Haematol. 2 (1965) p 230.

ANDERSSON, L.-O., BORG, H. & MILLER-ANDERSSON, M.: Purification of factor IX by affinity chromatography. IVth International Congress on Thrombosis and Haemostasis, Vienna (1973) p 142.

ANTOINE, B., NEVEU, T. & WARD, P. D.: Fibrinuria during renal transplantation. Transplantation 8 (1969) p 98.

AOKI, N. & von KAULLA, K. N.: a. The extraction of vascular plasminogen activator from human cadavers and a description of some of its properties. Amer. J. Clin. Path. 55 (1971) p 171.

AOKI, N. & von KAULLA, K. N.: b. Dissimilarity of human vascular plasminogen activator and human urokinase. J. Lab. Clin. Med. 78 (1971) p 354.

AOKI, N. & von KAULLA, K. N.: c. Human serum plasminogen antiactivator: its distinction from antiplasmin. Amer. J. Physiol. 220 (1971) p 1137.

ARISZ, L., TEGZESS, A. M., JORDANS, J. G. M. & van der HEM, G. K.: Fibrinolytic agents in the treatment of thrombosed arteriovenous shunt. Ned. T. Geneesk. 114 (1970) p 1484.

AROCHA-PINANGO, C. L.: A comparison of the TRCHII and latex-particle tests for the titration of FR-antigen. J. Clin. Path. 25 (1972) p 757.

ARONSON, D. L.: Purification and properties of normal and abnormal factor IX. IVth International Congress on Thrombosis and Haemostasis, Vienna (1973) p 16.

ARONSON, D. L., MUSTAFA, A. J. & MUSHINSKI, J. F.: Purification of human factor X and comparison of peptide maps of human factor X and prothrombin. Biochim. Biophys. Acta 188 (1969) p 25.

ARONSON, D. L., PREISS, J. W. & MOSESSON, M. W.: Molecular weights of factor VIII (AHF) and factor IX (PTC) by electron irradiation. Thromb. Diath. Haemorrh. 8 (1962) p 270.

ASTER, R. H. & JANDL, J. H.: Platelet sequestration in man. I. Methods. J. Clin. Invest. 43 (1964) p 843.

ASTRUP, T.: Fibrinolysis in the organism. Blood 11 (1956) p 781.

ASTRUP, T.: Tissue activators of plasminogen. Fed. Proc. 25 (1966) p 42.

ASTRUP, T. & MÜLLERTZ, S.: The fibrin plate method for estimating fibrinolytic activity. Arch. Biochem. 40 (1952) p 346.

ASTRUP, T., MÜLLERTZ, S. & HANSEN, J. R.: The value of Owren's method of estimating prothrombin. Scand. J. Clin. Lab. Invest. 3 (1951) p 209.

ASTRUP, T. & THORSEN, S.: The physiology of fibrinolysis. Med. Clin. N. Amer. 56 (1972) p 153.

ATTAR, S., HANASHIRO, P., MANSBERGER, A., MCLAUGHLIN, J., FIRMINGER, H. & COWLEY, R. A.: Intravascular coagulation—reality or myth? Surgery 68 (1970) p 27.

AZIZ, M. A. & SIDDIQUI, A. R.: Congenital deficiency of fibrin-stabilizing factor (factor XIII): A report of four cases (two families) and family members. Blood 40 (1972) p 11.

BAEHNER, R. L. & STRAUSS, H. S.: Hemophilia in the first year of life. New Engl. J. Med. 275 (1966) p 524.

BAILEY, K. & BETTELHEIM, F. R.: The nature of the fibrinogen-thrombin reaction. Brit. Med. Bull. 11 (1955) p 50.

BALL, A. P., HILL, R. L. & McKEE, P. A.: The number of crosslink sites per subunit in fully crosslinked fibrin. International Soc. of Thrombosis and Haemostasis, Washington (1972).

BANG, N. U.: Ultrastructure of the fibrin clot. Blood Clotting Enzymology, Ed. W. H. Seegers, Academic Press, New York and London (1967) p 488.

BANG, N. U & CLIFFTON, E. E.: The effect of alimentary hyperlipemia on thrombolysis in vivo. Thromb. Diath. Haemorrh. 4 (1960) p 149.

BARLOW, G. H., SUMMARIA, L. & ROBBINS, K. C.: Molecular weight studies on human plasminogen at the microgram level. J. Biol. Chem. 244 (1969) p 1138.

BARNHART, M. I.: Cellular site for prothrombin synthesis. Amer. J. Physiol. 199 (1960) p 360.

BARNHART, M. & RIDDLE, J. M.: Cellular localization of profibrinolysin (plasminogen). Blood 21 (1963) p 306.

BARROW, E. M. & GRAHAM, J. B.: von Willebrand's disease. Progr. Haematol. 4 (1964) p 203.

BARROW, E. M. & GRAHAM, J. B.: Anti-hemophilic factor activity isolated from kidneys of normal and hemophilic dogs. Amer. J. Physiol. 220 (1971) p 1020.

BARTH, P., MOMMERELL, B. & BECKMAN, U.: Isolierung des Kontakt-aktivierungsproduktes des Gerinnungssystems aus Schweineplasma. Thromb. Diath. Haemorrh. 21 (1969) p 500.

BARTON, P. G., JACKSON, C. M. & HANAHAN, D. J.: Relationship between factor V and activated factor X in the generation of prothrombinase. Nature 214 (1967) p 923.

BAUER, G.: Clinical experiences of a surgeon in the use of heparin. Amer. J. Cardiol. 14 (1964) p 29.

BAUMANN, R. & STRAUB, P. W.: Familien-untersuchung bei kongenitalen Mangel an Hage-man-Faktor (Gerinnungsfaktor XII). Schweiz. med. Wochenschr. 98 (1968) p 1653.

BECK, E.: Hypofibrinogenemia and dysfibrino-genemia. VIIth Congress of the World Federation of Haemophilia, Tehran-Iran, May (1971) p 38.

BECK, E., CHARACHE, P. & JACKSON, D. P.: A new inherited coagulation disorder caused by an abnormal fibrinogen ("fibrinogen Baltimore"). Nature 208 (1965) p 143.

BECK, E., DUCKERT, F. & ERNST, M.: The influence of fibrin stabilizing factor on the growth of fibroblasts in vitro and wound healing. Thromb. Diath. Haemorrh. 6 (1961) p 485.

BECK, P., GIDDINGS, J. C. & BLOOM, A. L.: Inhibitor of factor VIII in mild haemophilia. Brit. J. Haematol. 17 (1969) p 283.

BECKER, J.: The relation of platelet adhesiveness to postoperative venous thrombosis of the legs. Acta Chir. Scand. 138 (1972) p 781.

BECKER, J., BORGSTRÖM, S. & SALTZMAN, G. F.: Occurrence and course of thrombosis following prostatectomy. A. phlebographic investigation. Acta Radiol. 10 (1970) p 513.

BEHNKE, O.: Further studies on microtubules. J. Ultrastruct. Res. 13 (1965) p 469.

BEHNKE, O.: Electron microscopic observations on the membrane systems of the rat blood platelet. Anat, Rec. 158 (1967) p 121.

BELL, W. R., BOLTON, G. & PITNEY, W. R.: a. The effect of Arvin on blood coagulation factors. Brit. J. Haematol. 15 (1968) p 589.

BELL, W. R., PITNEY, W. R. & GOODWIN, J. F.: b. Therapeutic defibrination in the treatment of thrombotic disease. Lancet I (1968) p. 490.

BENNETT, B. & RATNOFF, O. D.: Studies on the response of patients with classic hemophilia to transfusion with concentrates of antihemophilic factor. A difference in the half-life of antihemophilic factor as measured by procoagulant and immunologic techniques. J. Clin. Invest. 51 (1972) p 2593.

BENNETT, E. & DORMANDY, K.: Pool's cryoprecipitate and exhausted plasma in the treatment of von Willebrand's disease and factor XI-deficiency. Lancet II (1966) p 731.

BENNETT, E. & HUEHNS, E. R.: Immunological differentiation of three types of haemophilia and identification of some female carriers, Lancet II (1970) p 956.

BENNETT, N. B.: A method for the quantitative assay of inhibitor of plasminogen activation in human serum. Thromb. Diath. Haemorrh. 17 (1967) p 12.

BERG, W. & KORSAN-BENGTSEN, K.: Separation of human fibrinogen and plasminogen by means of gel filtration. Thromb. Diath. Haemorrh. 9 (1963) p 151.

BERGSTRÖM, K., BLOMBÄCK, B. & KLEEN, G.: Studies on plasma fibrinolytic activity in a case of liver cirrhosis. Acta Med. Scand. 168 (1960) p 291.

BERGSTRÖM, K. & WALLÉN, P.: Removal of contaminating plasminogen from purified bovine fibrinogen. Arkiv Kemi 17 (1961) p 503.

BERNARD, J., DELOBEL, J., SOFTIC, I. V. & CAEN, J.: Remarques cliniques et étiologiques sur 341 cas personnels. Actualités hématologique. Masson, Paris 4 (1970) p 3.

BERNARD, J. & SOULIER, J. P.: Sur une nouvelle variété de dystrophie thrombocytaire hémorragipare congénitale. Sémaine Hop. Paris 24 (1948) p 3217.

BETTEX-GALLAND, M. & LÜSCHER, E. F.: Thrombosthenin—a contractile protein from thrombocytes. Its extraction from human blood platelets and some of its properties. Biochim. Biophys. Acta (Amst.) 49 (1961) p 536.

BIDWELL, E.: The purification of bovine antihaemophilic globulin. Brit. J. Haematol. 1 (1955) p 35.

BIDWELL, E.: Acquired inhibitors of coagulants. Ann. Rev. Med. 20 (1969) p 63.

BIDWELL, E., BOOTH, J. M., DIKE, G. W. R. & DENSON, K. W. E.: The preparation for therapeutic use of a concentrate of factor IX containing also factors II, VII and X. Brit. J. Haematol. 13 (1967) p 568.

BIDWELL, E., DENSON, K. W. E., DIKE, G. W. R., AUGUSTIN, R. & LLOYD, G. M.: b. Antibody nature of the inhibitor to antihaemophilic globulin (factor VIII). Nature 210 (1966) p 746.

BIDWELL, E., DIKE, G. W. R. & DENSON, K. W. E.: a. Experiments with factor VIII separated from fibrinogen by electrophoresis in free buffer film. Brit. J. Haematol. 12 (1966) p 583.

BIGGS, R.: Assay of antihaemophilic globulin in treatment of haemophilic patients. Lancet II (1957) p. 311.

BIGGS, R.: The detection of defects in blood coagulation. Brit. J. Haematol. 15 (1968) p 115.

BIGGS, R.: Clinical experience with factor IX concentrate of Bidwell. Hemophilia and New Hemorrhagic States, International Symposium, New York. Ed. K. M. Brinkhous. The University of North Carolina Press, Chapel Hill (1970) p 31.

BIGGS, R. & DENSON, K. W. E.: The fate of prothrombin and factors VIII, IX and X transfused to patients deficient in these factors. Brit. J. Haematol. 9 (1963) p 532.

BIGGS, R., DENSON, K. W. E., AKMAN, N., BORRETT, R. & HADDEN, M.: Antithrombin III, antifactor Xa and heparin. Brit. J. Haematol. 19 (1970) p 283.

BIGGS. R., DENSON, K. W. E., RIESENBERG, D. & MCINTYRE, C.: The coagulant activity of platelets. Brit. J. Haematol. 15 (1968) p 283.

BIGGS, R., DOUGLAS, A. S. & MACFARLANE, R. G.: a. The formation of thromboplastin in human blood. J. Physiol. 119 (1953) p 89.

BIGGS, R., DOUGLAS, A. S. & MACFARLANE, R. G.: b. The initial stages of blood coagulation. J. Physiol. 122 (1953) p 538.

BIGGS, R. & MACFARLANE, R. G.: Human blood coagulation and its disorders. 3rd Ed. Blackwell, Oxford (1962).

BIGGS, R. & MACFARLANE, R. G. (eds.): Treatment of haemophilia and other coagulation disorders. Blackwell, Oxford (1966).

BIGGS, R. & MATTHEWS, J. M.: The treatment of haemorrhage in von Willebrand's disease and the blood level of factor VIII (AHG). Brit. J. Haematol. 9 (1963) p 203.

BITHELL, T. C., PIZARRO, A. & DIARMID, W. D.: Variant of factor IX deficiency in female with 45, X Turner's syndrome. Blood 36 (1970) p 169.

BJÖRKMAN, S. E.: A new method for enumeration of platelets. Acta Haematol. 22 (1959) p 377.

BJÖRLIN, G. & NILSSON, I. M.: Tooth extractions in haemophiliacs after administration of a single dose of factor VIII or factor IX concentrate supplemented with AMCA. Oral Surg, Oral Med, Oral Path 36 (1973) p. 482.

BLATTNER, R. J.: Recent developments in the management of hemophilia with particular reference to intracranial bleeding. J. Pediat. 70 (1967) p 449.

BLOMBÄCK, B.: Fibrinogen to fibrin transformation. Blood Clotting Enzymology. Ed. W. H. Seegers. Academic Press, New York and London (1967) p 143.

BLOMBÄCK, B.: The N-terminal disulphide knot of human fibrinogen. Brit. J. Haematol. 17 (1969) p 145.

BLOMBÄCK, B.: Subunit structure of fibrinogen. Scand. J. Haemat. Suppl 13 (1971) p 71.

BLOMBÄCK, B. & BLOMBÄCK, M.: Purification of human and bovine fibrinogen. Arkiv Kemi 10 (1956) p 415.

BLOMBÄCK, B. & BLOMBÄCK, M.: Purification

and stabilization of factor V. Nature 198 (1963) p 886.

BLOMBÄCK, B. & BLOMBÄCK, M.: The molecular structure of fibrinogen. Ann. N. Y. Acad. Sci. 202 (1972) p 77.

BLOMBÄCK, B., BLOMBÄCK. M. & NILSSON, I. M.: Note on the purification of human antihemophilic globulin. Acta Chem. Scand. 12 (1958) p 1878.

BLOMBÄCK, B., CARLSSON, L. A., FRANZÉN, S. & ZETTERQVIST, E.: Turnover of ^{131}I-labelled fibrinogen in man studies in normal subjects, in congenital coagulation factor deficiency states, in liver cirrhosis, in polycytemia vera and in epidermolysis bullosa. Acta Med. Scand. 179 (1966) p 557.

BLOMBÄCK, M.: Purification of antihemophilic globulin. Arkiv Kemi 12 (1958) p 387.

BLOMBÄCK, M.: Molecular structure of fibrinogen. Internat. Soc. on Thrombosis and Haemostasis. Washington (1972).

BLOMBÄCK, M., BLOMBÄCK, B., JORPES, E. & NILSSON, I. M.: On the preparation of human antihaemophilic globulin (AHG). Proc. 7th Congr, Europ. Soc. Haemat., London 1959; Part II (1960) p 587.

BLOMBÄCK, M., BLOMBÄCK, B., MAMMEN, E. F. & PRASAD, A. S.: Fibrinogen Detroit—a molecular defect in the N-terminal disulphide knot of human fibrinogen? Nature 218 (1968) p 134.

BLOMBÄCK, M., EGBERG, N., GRUDER, E., JOHANSSON, S.-A., JOHNSON, H., NILSSON, S. E. G. & BLOMBÄCK, B.: Treatment of thrombotic disorders with Reptilase. Thromb. Diath. Haemorrh. Suppl 45 (1971) p 51.

BLOMBÄCK, M., JORPES, E. & NILSSON, I. M.: von Willebrand's disease. Amer. J. Med. 34 (1963) p 236.

BLOMBÄCK, M. & NILSSON, I. M.: Treatment of hemophilia A with human antihemophilic globulin. Acta Med. Scand. 161 (1958) p 301.

BLOOM, A. L., GIDDINGS, J. C., BEVAN, B., LETTON, M. & DRUMMOND, R. J.: Comparison of quick and low thaw methods of producing cryoprecipitate antihaemophilic factor from fresh and 24-hour-old blood. J. Clin. Path. 22 (1969) p 447.

BOBEK, K. & CEPELAK, V.: Laboratory diagnosis of venous thrombosis. Acta Med. Scand. 160 (1958) p 121.

BOHN, H.: Isolierung und Charakterisierung des Fibrinstabilisierenden Faktors aus menschlichen Thrombozyten. Thromb. Diath. Haemorrh. 23 (1970) p 445.

BOHN, H. & HAUPT, H.: Eine quantitative

Bestimmung von Faktor XIII mit Anti-Faktor-XIII-Serum. Thromb. Diath. Haemorrh. 19 (1968) p 309.

BOIJSEN, E. & EIRIKSSON, E.: Plethysmographic and phlebographic findings in venous thrombosis of the leg. Acta Chir. Scand. Suppl. 398 (1968) p 43.

BOMMER, W., KÜNZER, W. & SCHRÖER, H.: Kongenitale Afibrinogenämie. Ann. Paediat. 200 (1963) p 46.

BONNAR, J. & CRAWFORD, J. M.: Haemorrhagie diathesis due to abruptio placentae treated by fibrinogen, ε-aminocaproic acid, and hysterotomy. Lancet I (1965) p 241.

BONNAR, J., DAVIDSON, J. F., PIDGEON, C. F., MCNICOL, G. P. & DOUGLAS, A. S.: Fibrin degradation products in normal and abnormal pregnancy and parturition. Brit. Med. J. 3 (1969) p 137.

BORCHGREVINK, C. F. & WAALER, B. A.: The secondary bleeding time. A new method for differentiation of hemorrhagic diseases. Acta Med. Scand. 162 (1958) p 361.

BORN, G. V. R.: Aggregation of blood platelets by adenosine diphosphate and its reversal. Nature 194 (1962) p 927.

BOUHASIN, J. D., MONTELEONE, P. & ALTAY, C.: Role of lymphocyte in antihemophilic globulin production: A rise in antihemophilic globulin levels in a hemophilic subject with acute lymphoblastic leukemia. J. Lab. Clin. Med. 78 (1971) p 122.

BOUMA, B. N.: The results of a comparison of the tanned red cell haemagglutination inhibition immunoassay with an immunochemical method for the determination of split products. Scand. J. Haematol. Suppl. 13 (1971) p 111.

BOUMA, B. N., HEDNER, U. & NILSSON, I. M.: Typing of fibrinogen degradation products in urine in various clinical disorders. Scand. J. Clin. Lab. Invest. 27 (1971) p 331.

BRECKENRIDGE, R. T. & RATNOFF, O. D.: The activation of proaccelerin by bovine thrombokinase. Blood 27 (1966) p 527.

BREDDIN, K. & BAUKE, J.: Thrombozytenagglutination und Gefässkrankheiten. Blut 11 (1965) p 144.

BREDDIN, K. & BÜRCK, K. H.: Zur Klinik der Thrombozytenfunktionsstörungen unter besonderer Berücksichtigung der Ausbreitungsfähigkeit der Thrombozyten an silikonisierten Glasflächen. Thromb. Diath. Haemorrh. 9 (1963) p 525.

BREEN, F. A. JR & TULLIS, J. L.: Prothrombin concentrates in treatment of Christmas disease and allied disorders. J. Amer. Med. Ass. 208 (1969) p. 1853.

BRINKHOUS, K. M.: Hemophilia—Pathophysiologic studies and the evolution of transfusion therapy. Amer. J. Clin. Pathol. 41 (1964) p 342.

BRINKHOUS, K. M.: The development of our knowledge of hemophilia A and B. Ser. Haematol. 7 (1965) p 1.

BRINKHOUS, K. M. & GRAHAM, J. H.: Hemophilia and the hemophilioid states. Blood 9 (1954) p 254.

BRINKHOUS, K. M., PENICK, G. D., LANGDELL, R. D., WAGNER, R. H. & GRAHAM, J. B.: Physiologic basis of transfusion therapy in hemophilia. A.M.A. Arch. Pathol. 61 (1956) p 6.

BRINKHOUS, K. M., ROBERTS, H. R. & WEISS, A. E.: Prevalence of inhibitors in hemophilia A and B. Thromb. Diath. Haemorrh. Suppl 51 (1972) p 315.

BRINKHOUS, K. M., SHANBROM, E., ROBERTS, H. R., WEBSTER, W. P., FEKETE, L. & WAGNER, R. H.: A new high potency glycine-precipitated antihemophilic factor (AHF) concentrate: Treatment of classical hemophilia and hemophilia with inhibitors. J. Amer. Med. Ass. 250 (1968) p 613.

BRITTEN, A. & GROVE-RASMUSSEN, M.: Stability of factor VIII in the frozen state. Transfusion 6 (1966) p 230.

BRODTHAGEN, H.: The preparation of prothrombin-free ox plasma in the estimation of prothrombin. Scand. J. Clin. Lab. Invest. 5 (1953) p 376.

BOUMA, B. N., WIEGERINCK, Y., SIXMA, J. J., van MOURIK, J. A. & MOCHTAR, I. A.: Immunological characterization of purified antihaemophilic factor A (factor VIII) which corrects abnormal platelet retention in von Willebrand's disease. Nature New Biol. 236 (1972) p 104.

BOWIE, E. J. W., OWEN, CH. A. JR, THOMPSON, J. H. JR & DIDISHEIM, P.: Platelet adhesiveness in von Willebrand's disease. Amer. J. Clin. Path. 52 (1969) p 69.

BOWIE, E. J. W., THOMPSON, J. H. JR, DIDISHEIM, P. & OWEN, CH. A. JR: Disappearance rates of coagulation factors: Transfusion studies in factor-deficient patients. Transfusion 7 (1967) p 174.

BRAIN, M. C., BAKER, L. R. I., MCBRIDE, J. A., RUDENBERG, M. L. & DACIE, J. V.: Treatment of patients with microangiopathic haemolytic anaemia with heparin. Brit. J. Haematol. 15 (1968) p 603.

BRAIN, M. C. & HOURIHANE, D. O'B.: Microangiopathic haemolytic anaemia: The occurrence of haemolysis in experimentally produced vascular disease. Brit. J. Haematol. 13 (1967) p 135.

BRAKMAN, P.: Bovine fibrinogen without detectable plasminogen. Anal. Biochem. 11 (1965) p 149.

BRAKMAN, P., MOHLER, E. R. & ASTRUP, T.: A group of patients with impaired plasma fibrinolytic system and selective inhibition of tissue activator-induced fibrinolysis. Scand. J. Haematol. 3 (1966) p 389.

BRAKMAN, P., SNYDER, J., HENDERSSON, E. S. & ASTRUP, T.: Blood coagulation and fibrinolysis in acute leukaemia. Brit. J. Haematol. 18 (1970) p 135.

BRAUN, W. E. & MERRILL, J. P.: Urine fibrinogen fragments in human renal allografts. New Engl. J. Med. 278 (1968) p 1366.

BRECHER, G. & CRONKITE, E. P.: Morphology and enumeration of human blood platelets. J. Appl. Physiol. 3 (1950) p 365.

BROWN, D. L., HARDISTY, R. M., KOSOY, M. H. & BRACKEN, C.: Antihaemophilic globulin: Preparation by an improved cryoprecipitation method and clinical use. Brit. Med. J. 2 (1967) p 79.

BROWN, P. E., HOUGIE, C. & ROBERTS, H. R.: The genetic heterogeneity of hemophilia B. New Engl. J. Med. 283 (1970) p 61.

BROWSE, N.: Deep vein thrombosis: Diagnosis. Brit. Med. J. 4 (1969) p 676.

BROWSE, N. L., THOMAS, M. & PIM, H. P.: Streptokinase and deep vein thrombosis. Brit. Med. J. 3 (1968) p 717.

BRUNING, P. F., SWART, A. C. W., VELTKAMP, J. J., HEMKER, H. C. & LOELIGER, E. A.: Factor IX concentrate: Preparation by a simple method and clinical use. Hemophilia and new Hemorrhagic States. International Symposium New York. Ed. K. M. Brinkhous. The University of North Carolina Press, Chapel Hill (1970) p 3.

BRÜSTER, H., RINGLER, W., GLASSNER, K., RIECH, P.-CHR. & HIMMELBACH, E.: Colonresektion bei schwerer Hämophilie A unter dem Schutz von antihämophilen Kryopräzipitaten. Deut. med. Wochenschr. 94 (1969) p 1799.

BULL, B. S., SCHNEIDERMAN, M. A. & BRECHER, G.: Platelet counts with the Coulter Counter. Amer. J. Clin. Path. 44 (1965) p 678.

BULUK, K., JANUSZKO, T. & OLBROMSKI, J.: Conversion of fibrin to desmofibrin. Nature 191 (1961) p 1093.

BYGDEMAN, S, (Ed.): Thrombotic diseases with reference to the use of dextrans. Acta Chir. Scand. Suppl. 387 (1968).

BYGDEMAN, S., ELIASSON, R. & GULLBRING, B.: Effect of dextran infusion on the adenosine diphosphate induced adhesiveness and the spreading capacity of human blood platelets. Thromb. Diath. Haemorrh. 15 (1966) p 451.

BYGDEMAN, S. & WELLS, R.: Studies on platelet adhesiveness, blood viscosity and the microcirculation in patients with thrombotic disease. J. Atheroscler. Res. 10 (1969) p 33.

BÖHMIG, H. J., ABOUNA, G. M. & DIEZ-PARDO, J. A.: Coagulation studies in acute hepatic necrosis. Effects on coagulation of extra-corporeal liver perfusion and exchange blood transfusion. Thromb. Diath. Haemorrh. 26 (1971) p 341.

CAEN, J., CASTALDI, P. & INCEMAN, S.: Le rôle du fibrinogène dans l'hémostase primaire. Nouv. Rev. Franc. Hématol. 5 (1965) p 327.

CAEN, J. P., CRONBERG, S., LEVY-TOLE-DANO, S., KUBISZ, P. & PINKHAS, J. P.: New data in Glanzmann's thrombasthenia. Proc. Soc. Exp. Biol. Med. 136 (1971) p 1082.

CAEN, J., LEGRAND, Y., SULTAN, Y., CRON-BERG, S., JEANNEU, C. & PIGNAUD, G.: Allongement du temps de saignement et anomalies du collagène. Nouv. Rev. Franc. Hématol. 10 (1970) p 426.

CAEN, J. P., SULTAN, Y. & LARRIEU, M. J.: A new familial platelet disease. Lancet I (1968) p 203.

CARLSSON, S.: Fibrinogen degradation products in serum from patients with cancer. Acta Chir. Scand. 139 (1973) p. 499.

CARLSSON, S., HEDNER, U., NILSSON, I. M., BERGANTZ. S. E. & LJUNGQVIST, U.: Kidney transplantation and fibrinolytic split products in serum and urine. Transplantation 10 (1970) p 366.

CARROLL, H. J. & TICE, D. A.: The effect of epsilon amino-caproic acid upon potassium metabolism in the dog. Metabolism 15 (1966) p 449.

CASH, J. D. & ALLAN, A. G.: The fibrinolytic response to moderate exercise and intravenous adrenaline in the same subjects. Brit. J. Haematol. 13 (1967) p 376.

CASH, J. D., DAS, P. C. & RUCKLEY, V. A.: Serum fibrin/fibrinogen degradation products associated with post-operative pulmonary embolus and venous thrombosis. Scand. J. Haematol. Suppl. 13 (1971) p 323.

CASTRO, O., FARBER, L. R. & CLYNE, L. P.: Circulating anticoagulants against factors IX and XI in systemic lupus erythematosus. Ann. Intern. Med. 77 (1972) p 543.

CATT, K. J., HIRSH, J., CASTELAN, D. J., NIALL, H. D. & TREGEAR, G. W.: Radioimmunoassay of fibrinogen and its proteolysis products. Thromb. Diath. Haemorrh. 20 (1968) p 1.

CETINGIL, A. I., ULUTIN, O. N. & KARACA, M.: A platelet defect in a case of scurvy. Brit. J. Haematol. 4 (1958) p 350.

CHAKRABARTI, R., EVANS, J. F. & FEARN-LEY, G. R.: Effects on platelet stickness and fibrinolysis of phenformin combined with ethyloestrenol or stanozolol. Lancet I (1970) p 591.

CHAKRABARTI, R., FEARNLEY, G. R. & EVANS, J. F.: Effects of clofibrate on fibrinolysis, platelet stickiness, plasma-fibrinogen, and serum-cholesterol. Lancet II (1968) p 1007.

de la CHAPELLE, A., IKKALA, E. & NE-VANLINNA, H. R.: Haemophilia A in a girl. Lancet II (1961) p 578.

CHIRAWONG, PH., SINGH NANRA, R. & KINCAID-SMITH, P.: Fibrin degradation products and the role of coagulation in "persistent" glomerulonephritis. Ann. Intern. Med. 74 (1971) p 853.

CLARKE, R. L., ORANDI, A. & CLIFFTON, E. E.: Induction of fibrinolysis by venous obstruction. Angiology 11 (1960) p 367.

CLARKSON, A. R., MACDONALD, M. K., PETRIE, J. J. B., CASH, J. D. & ROBSON, J. S.: Serum and urinary fibrin/fibrinogen degradation products in glomerulonephritis. Brit. Med. J. 3 (1971) p 447.

CLARKSON, A. R., MORTON, J. B. & CASH, J. D.: Urinary fibrin/fibrinogen degradation products after renal homotransplantation. Lancet II (1970) p 1220.

CLIFFTON, E. E. & GROSSI, C. E.: Fibrinolytic activity of human tumors as measured by the fibrin-plate method. Cancer 8 (1955) p 1146.

COHEN, P. & GARDNER, F.: Thrombocytopenia as laboratory sign and complication of gram-negative bacteremic infection. Arch. Intern. Med. 117 (1966) p 113.

COLE, E. R., KOPPEL, J. L. & OLWIN, J. H.: Phospholipid-protein interactions in the formation of prothrombin activator. Thromb. Diath. Haemorrh. 14 (1965) p 431.

COLLEN, D., TYTGAT, G. N., CLAEYS, H. & PIESSENS, R.: a. Metabolism and distribution of fibrinogen. I. Fibrinogen turnover in physiological conditions in humans. Brit. J. Haemat. 22 (1972) p 681.

COLLEN, D., TYTGAT, D., CLAEYS, H. & WALLÉN, P.: b. Metabolism of plasminogen in healthy subjects: effect of tranexamic acid. J. Clin. Invest. 51 (1972) p 1310.

COLLER, B. S. & ZUCKER, M. B.: Reversible decrease in platelet retention by glass bead columns (adhesiveness) induced by disturbing the blood. Proc. Soc. Exp. Biol. Med. 136 (1971) p 769.

COLMAN, R. W.: The effect of proteolytic enzymes

on bovine factor V. II. Kinetics of activation and inactivation by papain, plasmin, and other proteolytic enzymes. Biochemistry 8 (1969) p 1445.

COLMAN, R. W., MEYERS, A. R., BLOCH, K. J., NIEWIAROWSKI, S. & THOMAS, D. P.: Patterns of fibrinogen degradation products in human disease: A comparative study of three assays. XIII. Int. Congr. Hematol., Munich (1970) p 253.

COLMAN, R. W., MORAN, J. & PHILIP, G.: Kinetic properties and molecular size of thrombin-activated factor V. J. Biol. Chem. 245 (1970) p 5941.

COLMAN, R. W., ROBBOY, S. J. & MINNA, J. D.: Disseminated intravascular coagulation (DIC): An approach. Amer. J. Med. 52 (1972) p 679.

CONRAD, F. G., BRENEMAN, W. L. & GRISHAM, D. B.: A clinical evaluation of plasma thromboplastin antecedent (PTA) deficiency. Ann. Intern. Med. 62 (1965) p 885.

COOKE, J. V., HOLLAND, P. V. & SHULMAN, N. R.: Cryoprecipitate concentrates of factor VIII for surgery in hemophiliacs. Ann. Intern. Med. 68 (1968) p 39.

COOPERBERG, A. A.: Acute promyelocytic leukemia. Canad. Med. Ass. J. 97 (1967) p 57.

CORNU, P., LARRIEU, M. J., CAEN, J. & BERNARD, J.: Maladie de Willebrand: Etude clinique, génétique et biologique. Nouv. Rev. Franc. Hématol. 1 (1961) p 231.

CORRIGAN, J.: Oral bleeding in hemophilia: Treatment with epsilon aminocaproic acid and replacement therapy. J. Pediat. 80 (1972) p 124.

CORRIGAN, J. J. JR & JORDAN, CH. M.: Heparin therapy in septicemia with disseminated intravascular coagulation. Effect on mortality and on correction of hemostatic defects. New Engl. J. Med. 283 (1970) p 778.

CORRIGAN, J. J. JR, RAY, W. L. & MAY, N.: Changes in the blood coagulation system associated with septicemia. New Engl. J. Med. 279 (1968) p 851.

COX, H. T., POLLER, L. & THOMSON, J. M.: Gastric fibrinolysis. A possible aetiological link with peptic ulcer. Lancet I (1967) p 1300.

van CREVELD, S.: Prophylaxis of joint haemorrhages in haemophilia. Acta. Haemat. 45 (1971) p 120.

van CREVELD, S. & MOCHTAR, I. A.: von Willebrand's disease—a plasma deficiency cause of the prolonged bleeding time. Ann. Paediat. 194 (1960) p 37.

van CREVELD, S., PASCHA, C. H. & VEDER, H. A.: The separation of AHF from fibrinogen. Thromb. Diath. Haemorrh. 6 (1961) p 282.

CRONBERG, S.: Investigations in haemorrhagic disorders with prolonged bleeding time but normal number of platelets. With special reference to platelet adhesiveness. Acta Med. Scand. Suppl. 486 (1968).

CRONBERG, S.: Evaluation of platelet aggregation. Coagulation 3 (1970) p 139.

CRONBERG, S.: Abnormal behaviour of platelets. In Caen, J. P. (ed.) Platelet aggregation. Masson, Paris (1971).

CRONBERG, S. & CAEN, J. P.: a. Release reaction in washed platelet suspensions induced by kaolin and other particles. Scand. J. Haematol. 8 (1971) p 151.

CRONBERG, S. & CAEN, J. P.: b. Platelet aggregation in washed suspensions. Scand. J. Haematol. 8 (1971) p 161.

CRONBERG, S., KUBISZ, P. & CAEN, J. P.: Demonstration of a plasmatic cofactor different from fibrinogen necessary for platelet release by ADP and adrenaline. Thromb. Diath. Haemorrh. 24 (1970) p 409.

CRONBERG, S. & NILSSON, I. M.: Coagulation studies after administration of a fat emulsion, Intralipid. Thromb. Diath. Haemorrh. 18 (1967) p 664.

CRONBERG, S. & NILSSON, I. M.: a. Investigations in a family with thrombasthenia of moderately severe type with 16 affected members. Scand. J. Haematol. 5 (1968) p 17.

CRONBERG, S. & NILSSON, I. M.: b. Investigations of patients with mild thrombasthenia—a haemorrhagic disorder with prolonged bleeding time probably due to a primary platelet defect. Acta Med. Scand. 183 (1968) p 163.

CRONBERG, S. & NILSSON, I. M.: Pneumococcal sepsis with generalized Shwartzman reaction. Acta Med. Scand. 188 (1970) p 293.

CRONBERG, S., NILSSON, I. M. & GYDELL, K.: Haemorrhagic thrombocythaemia due to defective platelet adhesiveness. Scand. J. Haematol. 2 (1965) p 208.

CRONBERG, S., NILSSON, I. M. & SILWER, J.: Studies on the platelet adhesiveness in von Willebrand's disease. Acta Med. Scand. 180 (1966) p 43.

CRONBERG, S., ROBERTSON, B., NILSSON, I. M. & NILÉHN, J.-E.: Suppressive effect of dextran on platelet adhesiveness. Thromb. Diath. Haemorrh. 16 (1966) p 384.

CUMMINGS, J. R. & WELTER, A. N.: Cardiovascular studies on aminocaproic acid. Toxicol. Appl. Pharmacol. 9 (1966) p 57.

DAS, P. C., ALLAN, A. G. E., WOODFIELD, D. G. & CASH, J. D.: Fibrin degradation products in sera of normal subjects. Brit. Med. J. 4 (1967) p 718.

DAS, P. C. & CASH, J. D.: Fibrinolysis at rest and after exercise in hepatic cirrhosis. Brit. J. Haematol. 17 (1969) p 431.

DAVEY, M. G.: The survival and destruction of human platelets. Bibl. Haematol. 22 (1966) p 137.

DAVIDSON, J. F., LOCHHEAD, M., MC-DONALD, G. A. & MCNICOL, G. P.: Fibrinolytic enhancement by stanozolol: A double blind trial. Brit. J. Haemat. 22 (1972) p 543.

DAVIE, E. W. & RATNOFF, O. D.: Waterfall sequence for intrinsic blood clotting. Science 145 (1964) p 1310.

DAVIS, J. W., MCFIELD, J. R., PHILLIPS, Ph. E. & GRAHAM, B. A.: Guanidinosuccinic acid on human platelet effects of exogenous urea, creatinine, and aggregation in vitro. Blood 39 (1972) p 388.

DAY, H. J., HOLMSEN, H. & HOVIG, T.: Subcellular particles of human platelets. Scand. J. Haematol. Suppl. 7 (1969) p 3.

DAY, W. C. & BARTON, P.: Studies on the stability of bovine plasma factor V. Biochim. Biophys. Acta 261 (1972) p 457.

DEGGELLER, K. & VREEKEN, J.: The human prothrombin-activating enzyme. Thromb. Diath. Haemorrh. 22 (1969) p 45.

DENSON, K. W. E.: Electrophoretic studies of the Prower factor; a blood coagulation factor which differs from factor VII. Brit. J. Haematol. 4 (1958) p 313.

DENSON, K. W. E.: The use of antibodies in the study of blood coagulation. Blackwell, Oxford (1967).

DENSON, K. W. E., BIGGS, R., HADDON, M. E., BORRETT, R. & COBB, K.: Two types of haemophilia (A^+ and A^-): A study of 48 cases. Brit. J. Haematol. 17 (1969) p 163.

DENSON, K. W. E., BIGGS, R. & MANNUCCI, P. M.: An investigation of three patients with Christmas disease due to an abnormal type of factor IX. J. Clin. Pathol. 21 (1968) p 160.

DENSON, K. W. E., CONARD, J. & SAMAMA, M.: Genetic variants of factor VII. Lancet I (1972) p 1234.

DENSON, K. W. E., LURIE, A., DE CATALDO, F. & MANNUCCI, P. M.: The factor-X defect: Recognition of abnormal forms of factor X. Brit. J. Haematol. 18 (1970) p 317.

DEUTSCH, E.: Die Bedeutung des zirkulierenden Plasminogens und Plasmin im Verlauf einer thrombolytischen Therapie. In H. Hess (ed): Thrombolytische Therapie. Symposion der Deutschen Gesellschaft für Angiologie, München, Oktober 1966, p. 35. F. K. Schattauer-Verlag, Stuttgart (1967).

DEUTSCH, E. & FISCHER, M.: The effect of intravenously administrated streptokinase on fibrinolysis and blood coagulation. Thromb. Diath. Haemorrh. 4 (1960) p 482.

DEUTSCH, E., IRSIGLER, K. & LOMOSCHITZ, H.: Studien über Gewebethromboplastin. 1. Reinigung. chemische Charakterisierung und Trennung in einen Eiweiss- und Lipoidanteil. Thromb. Diath. Haemorrh. 12 (1964) p 12.

DIDISHEIM, P., BOWIE, E. J. & OWEN, C. A. JR: Intravascular coagulation-fibrinolysis (ICF) syndrome and malignancy: Historical review and report of two cases with metastatic carcinoid and with acute myelomonocytic leukemia. Thromb. Diath. Haemorrh. Suppl. 36 (1969) p 215.

DIDISHEIM, P., TROMBOLD, J. S., VANDERVOORT, R. L. E. & MIBASHAN, R. S.: Acute promyelocytic leukemia with fibrinogen and factor V deficiencies. Blood 23 (1964) p 717.

DIKE, G. W. R., BIDWELL. E. & RIZZA, C. R.: The preparation and clinical use of a new concentrate containing factor IX, prothrombin and factor X and of a separate concentrate containing factor VII. Brit. J. Haemat. 22 (1972) p 469.

DODDS, W. J., RAYMOND, S. L., MOYNIHAN, A. C. & FENTON, J. W.: Independent stimulators regulating the production of coagulation factors VIII and IX in perfused spleens. J. Lab. Clin. Med. 79 (1972) p 770.

DONALDSON, G. W. K., DAVIES, S. H., DARG, A. & RICHMOND, J.: Coagulation factors in chronic liver disease. J. Clin. Pathol. 22 (1969) p 199.

DONATI, M. B., VERMYLEN, J. & VERSTRAETE, M.: The staphylococcal clumping test for detection of fibrinogen-like material. Scand. J. Haematol. Suppl. 13 (1971) p 137.

DOOLITTLE, R. F., CASSMAN, K. G., CHEN, R., SHARP, J. J. & WOODING, G. L.: Correlation of the mode of fibrin polymerization with the pattern of cross-linking. Ann. N. Y. Acad. Sci. 202 (1972) p 114.

DOUGHTEN, R. M. & PEARSON, H. A.: Disseminated intravascular coagulation associated with Aspergillus endocarditis. J. Pediat. 73 (1968) p 576.

DOUGLAS, A. S.: Current status of anticoagulant treatment. In Recent Advances in Blood coagulation. Edited by L. Poller. Churchill, London (1969).

DOUMENC, J., PROST, R. J., SAMAMA, M. & BOUSSER, J.: Anomalie de l'aggrégation plaquettaire au cours de la maladie de Waldenström (A propos 3 cas.) Nouv. Rev. Franc. Hematol. 6 (1966) p 734.

DUCKERT, F., FLÜCKIGER, P., MATTER, M. & KOLLER, F.: Clotting factor X. Physiologic and physico-chemical properties. Proc. Soc. Exp. Biol. Med. 90 (1955) p 17.

DUCKERT, F., JUNG, E. & SHMERLING, D. H.: A hitherto undescribed congenital haemorrhagic diathesis probably due to fibrin stabilizing factor deficiency. Thromb. Diath. Haemorrh. 5 (1960) p 179.

EBBE, S.: Megakaryocytopoiesis and platelet turnover. Ser. Haematol. I, 2 (1968) p 65.

EDSON, J. R., WHITE, J. G. & KRIVIT, W.: The enigma of severe factor XI deficiency without hemorrhagic symptoms. Distinction from Hageman factor and "Fletcher factor" deficiency; family study; and problems of diagnosis. Thromb. Diath. Haemorrh. 18 (1967) p 342.

EGEBERG, O.: Assay of antihemophilic A, B and C factors by one-stage cephalin systems. Scand. J. Clin. Lab. Invest. 13 (1961) p 140.

EGEBERG, O.: a. A family with antihemophilic C factor (AHC-plasma thromboplastin antecedent) deficiency without bleeding tendency. Scand. J. Clin. Lab. Invest. 14 (1962) p 478.

EGEBERG, O.: b. Changes in the coagulation system following major surgical operations. Acta Med. Scand. 171 (1962) p 679.

EGEBERG, O.: The effect of muscular exercise on hemostasis in von Willebrand's disease. Scand. J. Clin. Lab. Invest. 15 (1963) p 273.

EGEBERG, O.: a. Thrombophilia caused by inheritable deficiency of blood antithrombin. Scand. J. Clin. Lab. Invest. 17 (1965) p 92.

EGEBERG, O.: b. An inherited hemorrhagic trait with characteristic resembling both mild hemophilia of type A and von Willebrand's disease. Scand. J. Clin. Lab. Invest. Suppl 84 (1965) p 25.

EHRICH, C., WOODS, K. R. & THILL, W.: Production of cryoprecipitate and AHF-concentrate at the New York Blood Center. Thromb. Diath. Haemorrh. Suppl. 43 (1971) p 175.

EHRINGER, H., FISCHER, M., LECHNER, K. & MAYRHOFER, E.: Thrombolytische Therapie nicht akuter arterieller Verschlüsse. Dtsch. Med. Wschr. 95 (1970) p 610.

EIKA, C. & ABILDGAARD, U.: Inhibition of thrombin induced aggregation of human platelets by antithrombin III. Scand. J. Haemat. 7 (1970) p 460.

EKELUND, H., HEDNER, U. & NILSSON, I. M.: Fibrinolysis in newborns. Acta Paediat. Scand. 59 (1970) p 33.

EKERT, H., BARRATT, T. M., CHANTLER, C. & TURNER, M. W.: Immunologically reactive equivalents of fibrinogen in sera and urine of children with renal disease. Arch. Dis. Childh. 47 (1972) p 90.

ELLISON, R. C. & BROWN, J.: Fibrinolysis in pulmonary vascular disease. Lancet I (1965) p 786.

EMMONS, P. R. & MITCHELL, J. R. A.: Postoperative changes in platelet-clumping activity. Lancet I (1965) p 71.

ENEROTH, G. & GRANT, C. A.: Epsilon aminocaproic acid and reduction in fertility of male rats. Acta Pharm. Suecica 3 (1966) p 115.

ENGELBERG, H.: Heparin, Metabolism, Physiology and Clinical Application. Thomas, Springfield (1963).

ENGSTRÖM, K., LUNDQUIST, A. & SÖDERSTRÖM, N.: Periodic thrombocytopenia or tidal platelet dysgenesis in a man. Scand. J. Haematol. 3 (1966) p 290.

ERICHSON, R. B.: The hypercoagulable state. N. Y. State J. Med. 65 (1965) p 1091.

ERIKSSON, A. W.: Eine neue Blutersippe mit v. Willebrand-Jürgens'scher Krankheit (erbliche Thrombopathie) auf Åland (Finnland). Ac. Ge. Med. Ge. 10 (1961) p 157.

ESNOUF, M. P.: Biochemical aspects of blood coagulation. Proc. Roy. Soc., Ser. B 173 (1969) p 269.

ESNOUF, M. P. & JOBIN, F.: The isolation of factor V from bovine plasma. Biochem. J. 102 (1967) p 660.

ESNOUF, M. P. & TUNNAH, G. W.: The isolation and properties of the thrombin-like activity from ancistrodon rhodostoma venom. Brit. J. Haematol. 13 (1967) p 581.

ESNOUF, M. P. & WILLIAMS, W. J.: The isolation and purification of a bovine-plasma protein which is a substrate for the coagulant fraction of Russell's-viper venom. Biochem. J. 84 (1962) p 62.

EVENSEN, S. A. & HJORT, P. F.: Pathogenesis of disseminated intravascular coagulation. XIII. Int. Congr. Hematol., Plenary Sessions Munich (1970) p 109.

EVENSEN, S. A. & JEREMIC, M.: Platelets and the triggering mechanism of intravascular coagulation. Brit. J. Haematol. 19 (1970) p 33.

FAGERHOL, M. K. & ABILDGAARD, U.: Immunological studies on human antithrombin III. Influence of age, sex and use of oral contraceptives on serum concentration. Scand. J. Haematol. 7 (1970) p 10.

FEARNLEY, G. R.: Fibrinolysis. Arnold, London (1965).

FEARNLEY, G. R., CHAKRABARTI, R. & EVANS, J. F.: Fibrinolytic and defibrinating effect of phenformin plus ethyloestrenol in vivo. Lancet I (1969) p 910.

FEINSTEIN, D. I., RAPAPORT, S. I. & CHONG, M. N. Y.: Immunologic characterization of 12 factor VIII inhibitors. Blood 34 (1969) p 85.

von FELTEN, A., STRAUB, P. W. & FRICK, P. G.: Dysfibrinogenemia in a patient with primary hepatoma. New Engl. J. Med. 280 (1969) p 405.

FINKBINER, R. B., MCGOVERN, J. J., GOLD-STEIN, R. & BUNKER, J. P.: Coagulation defects in liver disease and response to transfusion during surgery. Amer. J. Med. 26 (1959) p 199.

FISHER, SH., FLETCHER, A. P., ALKJAERSIG, N. & SHERRY, S., Immunoelectrophoretic characterization of plasma fibrinogen derivatives in patients with pathological plasma proteolysis. J. Lab. Clin. Med. 70 (1967) p 903.

FISHER, S., RAMOT, B. & KREISLER, B.: Fibrinolysis in acute leukemia: A case report. Israel Med. J. 19 (1960) p 195.

FLANC, C., KAKKAR, V. V. & CLARKE, M. B.: The detection of venous thrombosis of the legs using 125 I-labelled fibrinogen. Brit. J. Surg. 55 (1968) p 742.

FLETCHER, A. P.: Pathological fibrinolysis. Fed. Proc. 25 (1966) p 84.

FLETCHER, A. P. & ALKJAERSIG, N.: Plasma fibrinogen and hemostatic functions (pathological and genetic disorders). Progr. Haematol. 5 (1966) p 246.

FLETCHER, A. P., ALKJAERSIG, N. & O'BRIEN, J.: Blood hypercoagulability and thrombosis. XIII. Intern. Congress Hematol. Munich. August (1970) Abstract volume p 244.

FLETCHER, A. P., ALKJAERSIG, N. & SHERRY, S.: The maintenance of a sustained thrombolytic state in man. I. Induction and effects. J. Clin. Invest. 38 (1959) p 1096.

FLETCHER, A. P., ALKJAERSIG, N. & SHERRY, S.: Pathogenesis of the coagulation defect developing during pathological plasma proteolytic ("fibrinolytic") states. I. The significance of fibrinogen proteolysis and circulating fibrinogen breakdown products. J. Clin. Invest. 41 (1962) p 896.

FLETCHER, A. P., BIEDERMAN, O., MOORE, D., ALKJAERSIG, N. & SHERRY, S.: Abnormal plasminogen-plasmin system activity (fibrinolysis) in patients with hepatic cirrhosis: its cause and consequences. J. Clin. Invest. 43 (1964) p 681.

FORBES, C. D., HUNTER, J., BARR, R. D., DAVIDSON, J. F., SHORT, D. W., MC-DONALD, G. A., MCNICOL, G. P., WALLACE, J. & DOUGLAS. A. S.: Cryoprecipitate therapy in haemophilia, Scot. Med. J. 14 (1969) p 1.

FORMAN, W. B. & BARNHART, M. I.: Cellular site for fibrinogen synthesis. J. Amer. Med. Ass. 187 (1964) p 128.

FRANK, M., SERGENT, J., KANE, M. &

ALLING, D. W.: Epsilon aminocaproic acid therapy on hereditary angioneurotic edema. New Engl. J. Med. 286 (1972) p 808.

FRANKLIN, W. A., SIMON, N. M., POTTER, E. W. & KRUMLOVSKY, F. A.: The hemolytic-uremic syndrome. Arch. Path. 94 (1972) p 230.

FURLAN, M. & BECK, E. A.: Plasmic degradation of human fibrinogen. I. Structural characterization of degradation products. Biochim. Biophys. Acta 263 (1972) p 631.

GAARDER, A., JONSEN, J., LALAND, S., HELLEM, A. & OWREN, P. A.: Adenosine diphosphate in red cells as a factor in the adhesiveness of human blood platelets. Nature 192 (1961) p 531.

GABRYELEWICZ, A., NIEWIAROWSKI, S., PROKOPOWICZ, J. & WOROWSKI, K.: Fibrinolytic system in hypotensive patients; with a special reference to the effect of epsilon-amino-caproic acid (EACA). Thromb. Diath. Haemorrh. 18 (1967) p 433.

de GAETANO, G., VERMYLEN, J. & VER-STRAETE, M.: Inhibition of platelet aggregation—its potential clinical usefulness: A review. Hematologic reviews. J. L. Ambrus (ed.). Marcel Dekker, New York 2 (1970) p 205.

GAFFNEY, J. & DOBOS, P.: A structural aspect of human fibrinogen suggested by its plasmin degradation. FEBS Letters 15 (1971) p 13.

GANROT, P. O.: Determination of α_2-macro-globulin as trypsin-protein esterase. Clin. Chim. Acta 14 (1966) p 493.

GANROT, P. O.: Studies on serum protease inhibitors with special reference to α_2-macro-globulin. Acta Univ. Lund II (1967) p 2.

GANROT, P. O. & NILÉHN, J.-E.: Competition between plasmin and thrombin for α_2-macro-globulin. Clin. Chim. Acta 17 (1967) p 511.

GANROT, P. O. & NILÉHN, J.-E.: a. Immuno-chemical determination of human plasminogen. Clin. Chim. Acta 22 (1968) p 335.

GANROT, P. O. & NILÉHN, J.-E.: b. Plasma prothrombin during treatment with dicumarol II. Demonstration of an abnormal prothrombin fraction. Scand. J. Clin. Lab. Invest. 22 (1968) p 23.

GANROT, P. O. & NILÉHN, J.-E.: Prothrombin fragmentation during coagulation of whole blood and plasma. Scand. J. Clin. Lab. Invest. 24 (1969) p 15.

GANROT, P. O. & STENFLO, J.: Prothrombin derivatives in human serum. Isolation and some properties of the non-thrombin fragments. Scand. J. Clin. Lab. Invest. 26 (1970) p 161.

GARDIKAS, C., BAKALOUDIS, P., HATZIO-ANNOU, J. & KOKKINOS, D.: The factor-VIII concentration of the hepatic venous blood. Brit. J. Haematol. 11 (1965) p 380.

GARRETT, J., SILVA, R. C. F. & MENDES-COUTO, M. N.: Diuretic activity of epsilon-aminocaproic acid. Pharmacology 1 (1968) p 43.

GARVEY, B. & BLACK, J. M.: The detection of fibrinogen/fibrin degradation products by means of a new antibody-coated latex particle. J. Clin. Path. 25 (1972) p 680.

GASTON, L. W.: Studies on a family with an elevated plasma level of factor V (proaccelerin) and a tendency to thrombosis. Pediatrics 68 (1966) p 367.

GAUTVIK, K. M. & RUGSTAD, H. E.: Kinin formation and kininogen depletion in rats after intravenous injection of ellagic acid. Brit. J. Pharmacol. Chemother. 31 (1967) p 390.

GERATZ, J. D. & GRAHAM, J. B.: Plasma thromboplastin component (Christmas factor, factor IX) levels in stored human blood and plasma. Thromb. Diath. Haemorrh. 4 (1960) p 376.

GILCHRIST, G. S., EKERT, H., SHANBROM, E. & HAMMOND, D.: Evaluation of a new concentrate for the treatment of factor IX deficiency. New Engl. J. Med. 280 (1969) p 291.

GILCHRIST, G. S., HAMMOND, D. & MELNYK, J.: Hemophilia A in a phenotypically normal female with XX/XO mosaicism. New Engl. J. Med. 273 (1965) p 1402.

GILCHRIST, G. S. & LIEBERMANN, E.: Haemo-lytic-uraemic syndrome and heparin therapy. Lancet II (1969) p 1069.

GIRAUD, G., CAZAL, P., LATOUR, H., IZ-NARU, P., LEVY, A., BARJON, P. & RIB-STEIN, M.: Syndrome hémorragique mortel par fibrinolyse aigue au cours d'une leucose myéloïde. Sang 25 (1954) p 628.

GIROLAMI, A.: Further studies on the ellagic acid induced hypercoagulable state. Lack of thrombosis in the dog after long term administration of the compound. Coagulation 2 (1969) p 263.

GIROLAMI, A., LAZZARIN, M., SCARPA, R. & BRUNETTI, A.: a. Congenital hypoprothrombinemia. A case report with some considerations on the behavior of the T. G. T. in this condition. Coagulation 3 (1970) p 45.

GIROLAMI, A., MOLARO, G., LAZZARIN, M., SCARPA, R. & BRUNETTI, A.: b. A "new" congenital haemorrhagic condition due to the presence of an abnormal factor X (factor X Friuli): Study of a large kindred. Brit. J. Haematol. 19 (1970) p 179.

GIROMINI, M. & LAPERROUZA, C.: Prolonged survival after bilateral nephrectomy in an adult with haemolytic-uraemic syndrome. Lancet II (1969) p 169.

GLADHAUG, A. & PRYDZ, H.: Purification of the coagulation factors VII and X from human serum. Some properties of factor VII. Biochim. Biophys. Acta 215 (1970) p 105.

GODAL, H. C.: The assay of heparin in thrombin systems. Scand. J. Clin. Lab. Invest. 13 (1961) p 153.

GODAL, H. C. & ABILDGAARD, U.: Gelation of soluble fibrin in plasma by ethanol. Scand. J. Haematol. 3 (1966) p 342.

GODAL, H. C., ABILDGAARD, U. & KIERULF, P.: Ethanol gelation and fibrin monomers in plasma. Scand. J. Haematol. Suppl. 13 (1971) p 189.

GOLDFINE, I. D., SCHACHTER, H., BARC-LAY, W. R. & KINGDON, H. S.: Consumption coagulopathy in miliary tuberculosis. Ann. Intern. Med. 71 (1969) p 775.

GONZALES, F. M. & COCKE, T. B.: Use of streptokinase in occluded arteriovenous shunts. Thromb. Diath. Haemorrh. Suppl 47 (1971) p 201.

GORDON-SMITH, I. C., Le QUESNE, L. P., GRUNDY, D. J., NEWCOMBE, J. F. & BRAMBLE, F. J.: Controlled trial of two regimens of subcutaneous heparin in prevention of postoperative deep-vein thrombosis. Lancet. I (1972) p 1133.

GORMSEN, J. & LAURSEN, B.: Treatment of acute phlebothrombosis with streptase. Acta Med. Scand. 181 (1967) p 373.

GRAHAM, J. B., BARROW, E. M. & HOUGIE, C.: Stuart clotting defect. II. Genetic aspects of a "new" hemorrhagic state. J. Clin. Invest. 36 (1957) p 497.

GRALNICK, H. R. & FINLAYSON, J. S.: Congenital dysfibrinogenemias. Ann. Intern. Med. 77 (1972) p 471.

GRALNICK, H. R. & HENDERSON, E.: Hypofibrinogenemia and coagulation factor deficiencies with 1-asparaginase treatment. Cancer 27 (1971) p 1313.

GRAMMENS, G. L., PRASAD, A. S., MAMMEN, E. F., BARNHART, M. I. & SCHWANDT, V. F.: Physico-chemical and immunological properties of bovine Hageman factor. Thromb. Diath. Haemorrh. 25 (1971) p 405.

GRANSTRAND, B., et al.: Effect of tranexamic acid (AMCA) and aminocaproic acid (EACA) on the noradrenaline level of various organs of the rat. Paper presented at the XII Scand. Congr. Physiol., Abo, Finland August (1966).

GRAY, G. R., TEASDALE, J. M. & THOMAS, J. W.: Hemophilia B$_M$ Canad. Med. Ass. J. 98 (1968) p 552.

GREEN, D.: Spontaneous inhibitors of factor VIII. Brit. J. Haematol. 15 (1968) p 57.

GREEN, D.: a. A simple method for the purification of factor VIII (antihemophilic factor) employing snake venom. J. Lab. Clin. Med. 77 (1971) p 153.

GREEN, D.: b. Suppression of an antibody to factor VIII by a combination of factor VIII and cyclophosphamide. Blood 37 (1971) p 381.

GRETTE, K.: Studies on the mechanism of thrombin-catalyzed hemostatic reactions in blood platelets. Acta Physiol. Scand. Suppl. 195 (1962) p 56.

GRÖTTUM, K. A., HOVIG, T., HOLMSEN, H., ABRAHAMSEN, A. F., JEREMIC, M. & SEIP, M.: Wiskott-Aldrich syndrome: Qualitative platelet defects and short platelet survival. Brit. J. Haematol. 17 (1969) p 373.

GÅRDLUND, B., KOWALSKA-LOTH, B., GRÖNDAHL, N. & BLOMBÄCK, B.: Hydrophobic disulfide knots in human fibrinogen. International Soc. on Thrombosis and Haemostasis, Washington (1972).

HAANEN, C., HOMMES, F., BENRAAD, H. & MORSELT, G.: A case of Hageman factor deficiency and a method to purify the factor. Thromb. Diath. Haemorrh. 5 (1960) p 201.

HAANEN, C., MORSELT, G., SCHOENMAKERS, J., MATERS, M. & BRAAMS, R.: The molecular weight of factor XII (Hageman factor) estimated with ionizing radiation. Scand. J. Haematol. 2 (1965) p 248.

HABIB, R., COURTECNISSE, V., LECLERC, F., MATHIEW, H. & ROYER, P.: Etude anatomopathologigue de 35 observations de syndrome hemolytique et uremique de l'enfant. Arch. Franc. Pédiat. 26 (1969) p 391.

HALL, M.: Haemophilia complicated by an acquired circulating anticoagulant: a report of three cases. Brit. J. Haemat. 7 (1961) p 340.

HALLBERG, L., HÖGDAHL, A. M., NILSSON, L. & RYBO, G.: Menstrual blood loss—a population study. Acta Obstet. Gynecol. Scand. 45 (1966) p 25.

HALLÉN, A. & NILSSON, I. M.: Coagulation studies in liver disease. Thromb. Diath. Haemorrh. 11 (1964) p 51.

HARDAWAY, R. M.: Syndromes of Disseminated Intravascular Coagulation. Thomas, Springfield (1966).

HARDISTY, R. M.: A naturally occurring inhibitor of Christmas factor (factor IX). Thromb. Diath. Haemorrh. 8 (1962) p 67.

HARDISTY, R. M. & HUTTON, R. A.: The kaolin clotting time of platelet-rich plasma: a test of platelet factor-3 availability. Brit. J. Haematol. 11 (1965) p 258.

HARDISTY, R. M. & HUTTON, R. A.: Bleeding tendency associated with "new" abnormality of platelet behaviour. Lancet I (1967) p 983.

HARDISTY, R. M. & INGRAM. G. I. C.: Bleeding Disorders: Investigation and Management. Davis, Philadelphia (1965).

HARDISTY, R. M. & MACPHERSON, J. C.: A one-stage factor VIII (antihaemophilic globulin) assay and its use on venous and capillary plasma. With a note on the calculation of confidence limits by G. I. C. Ingram. Thromb. Diath. Haemorrh. 7 (1962) p 215.

HARTMANN, R. C. & CONLEY, C. L.: Clot retraction as a measure of platelet function. I. Effects of certain experimental conditions on platelets in vitro. Bull. Johns Hopkins Hosp. 93 (1953) p 355.

HASSELBACK, R., MARION, R. B. & THOMAS, J. W.: Congenital hypofibrinogenemia in five members of a family. Canad. Med. Ass. J. 88 (1963) p 19.

HATHAWAY, W. E., MULL, M. M., GITHENS, J. H., GROTH, C. G., MARCHIORO, T. L. & STARZI, T. E.: Attempted spleen transplant in classical hemophilia. Transplantation 7 (1969) p 73.

HAWIGER, J., NIEWIAROWSKI, S., GUREWICH, V. & THOMAS, D. P.: Measurement of fibrinogen and fibrin degradation products in serum by staphylococcal clumping test. J. Lab. Clin. Med. 75 (1970) p 93.

HEDENIUS, P.: An apparatus for determining the coagulation time of the blood. Acta Med. Scand. 88 (1936) p 440.

HEDLUND, P. O.: Antifibrinolytic therapy with cyklokapron in connection with prostatectomy. Scand. J. Urol. Nephrol. 3 (1969) p 177.

HEDNER, U.: Purification of an activator inhibitor in serum. International Society on Thrombosis and Haemostasis. II. Congress Oslo, Norway July (1971) p 120.

HEDNER, U.: Urinary fibrin/fibrinogen degradation products (FDP) in renal diseases and during thrombolytic therapy. Scand. J. Clin. Lab. Invest. 32 (1973) p 175.

HEDNER, U., EKBERG, M. & NILSSON, I. M.: Urinary fibrin (ogen) degradation products (FDP) and glomerulonephritis. Acta Med. Scand. In press (1973).

HEDNER, U. & NILSSON, I. M.: Determination of plasminogen in human plasma by a casein method. Thromb. Diath. Haemorrh. 14 (1965) p 545.

HEDNER, U. & NILSSON, I. M.: a. Urokinase inhibitors in serum in a clinical series. Acta Med. Scand. 189 (1971) p 185.

HEDNER, U. & NILSSON, I. M.: b. Clinical experience with determination of fibrinogen degradation products. Acta Med. Scand. 189 (1971) p 471.

HEDNER, U. & NILSSON, I. M.: Parallel determinations of FDP and fibrin monomers with various methods. Thromb. Diath. Haemorrh. 28 (1972) p 268.

HEDNER, U. & NILSSON, I. M.: Antithrombin III in a clinical material. Internat. Soc. on Thrombosis and Haemostasis. Washington (1972) p 398.

HEDNER, U., NILSSON, I. M., BERGENTZ, S. E. & CRONBERG, L.: Hyperactive connective tissue in seven patients with recurrent thrombotic occlusions. Haemostasis. 1 (1972/73) p 148.

HEDNER, U., NILSSON, I. M. & JACOBSEN, C. D.: Demonstration of low content of fibrinolytic inhibitors in individuals with high fibrinolytic capacity. Scand. J. Clin. Lab. Invest. 25 (1970) p 329.

HEDNER, U., NILSSON, I. M. & ROBERTSON, B.: Determination of plasminogen in clots and thrombi. Thromb. Diath. Haemorrh. 16 (1966) p 38.

HEDNER, U. & ÅSTEDT, B.: Fibrinolytic split products in serum and urine in pregnancy. Acta Obstet. Gynec. Scand. 49 (1970) p 363.

HEDWALL, P. R., MAITRE, L. & BRUNNER, H.: Influence of ω-amino-acids on blood pressure, catecholamine stores and the pressor response to physostigmine in the rat. J. Pharm. Pharmacol. 20 (1968) p 737.

HEIMBURGER, N.: Basic mechanism of action of streptokinase and urokinase. Thromb. Diath. Haemorrh. Suppl 47 (1971) p 21.

HEINRICH, F. & SCHMUTZLER, R.: Ergebnisse der Thrombolysebehandlung chronischer Gliedmassenarterienverschlüsse. Dtsch. Med. J. 23 (1972) p 351.

HELLEM, A. J.: The adhesiveness of human blood platelets in vitro. Scand. J. Clin. Lab. Invest. 12, Suppl. 51 (1960) p 117.

HELLEM, A. J.: Platelet adhesiveness. Ser. Haematol. I (1968) p 99.

HELLEM, A. J.: Platelet adhesiveness in von Willebrand's disease. Scand. J. Haematol. 7 (1970) p 374.

HEMKER, H. C., ESNOUF, M. P., HEMKER, P. W., SWART, A. C. W. & MACFARLANE, R. G.: Formation of prothrombin converting activity. Nature 215 (1967) p 248.

HEMKER, H. C. & KAHN, M. J. P.: Studies on blood coagulation factor V. VI. The inactivation

of factor V and prothrombinase. Thromb. Diath. Haemorrh. 27 (1972) p 33.

HEMKER, H. C., KAHN, M. J. P. & DEVILEE, P. P.: The adsorption of coagulation factors onto phospholipids—Its role in the reaction mechanism of blood coagulation. Thromb. Diath. Haemorrh. 24 (1970) p 214.

HENSCHEN, A.: a. Number and reactivity of disulfide bonds in fibrinogen and fibrin. Arkiv Kemi 22 (1964) p 355.

HENSCHEN, A.: b. Peptide chains in S-sulfo-fibrinogen and S-sulfo-fibrin: Isolation methods and general properties. Arkiv Kemi 22 (1964) p 375.

HERSCHLEIN, H. J. & STEICHELE, D. F.: Immunochemischer Nachweis von Fibrinogenderivaten im Urin bei Verbrauchskoagulopathien. Thromb. Diath. Haemorrh. 19 (1968) p 248.

HERSHGOLD, E. J., DAVISON, A. M. & JANSZEN, M. E.: a. Isolation and some chemical properties of human factor VIII (antihemophilic factor). J. Lab. Clin. Med. 77 (1971) p 185.

HERSHGOLD, E. J., DAVISON, A. M. & JANSZEN, M. E.: b. Human factor VIII (antihemophilic factor): Activation and inactivation by phospholipases. J. Lab. Clin. Med. 77 (1971) p 206.

HERSHGOLD, E., POOL, J. & PAPPENHAGEN, A.: The potent antihemophilic globulin concentrate derived from a cold insoluble fraction of human plasma; Characterization and further data on preparation and clinical trial. J. Lab. Clin. Med. 67 (1966) p 23.

HERSHGOLD, E., SILVERMAN, L., DAVISON, A. & JANSZEN, M.: Native and purified factor VIII: Molecular and electron microscopical properties and a comparison with hemophilic plasma. Fed. Proc. 26 (1967) p 488.

HERSHGOLD, E. J. & SPRAWLS, S.: Molecular properties of purified human, bovine and porcine anti-hemophilic globulins. Fed. Proc. 25 (1966) p 317.

HESS, H.: In H. Hess (ed.): Thrombolytische Therapie. Symposion der Deutschen Gesellschaft für Angiologie München. Oktober 1966. pp 141–143. Schattauer, Stuttgart (1967).

HESS, H., GROSSENS, U. & FROST, H.: Behandlung rezidivierender Embolien in Extremitätenarterien mit Streptokinase und Urokinase. Fortschr. Med. 84 (1966) p 296.

HIEMEYER, V.: Spontanlyse von arteriellen Verschlüssen. In H. Hess (ed.): Thrombolytische Therapie. Symposion der Deutschen Gesellschaft für Angiologie, München. Schattauer, Stuttgart (1967) p 66.

HIRSH, J., EKERT, H., TAFT, L. I., COLEBATCH, J. H. & SPENSLEY, J. C.: Hypofibrinogenaemia in acute leukaemia with extensive fibrinous pericarditis. Ann. Austr. Med. 16 (1967) p 333.

HIRSH, J. & MCBRIDE, J. A.: Increased platelet adhesiveness in recurrent venous thrombosis and pulmonary embolism. Brit. Med. J. 2 (1965) p 797.

HIRSH, J., MCDONALD, I. G., HALE, G. A., O'SULLIVAN, E. F. & JELINEK, V. M.: Comparison of the effects of streptokinase and heparin on the early rate of resolution of major pulmonary embolism. Can. Med. Ass. J. 104 (1971) p 488.

HIRSH, J., O'SULLIVAN, E. F., GALLUS, A. S. & MARTIN, M.: The activated partial thromboplastin time in the control of heparin treatment. Aust. Ann. Med. 4 (1970) p 334.

HIRSH, J., O'SULLIVAN, E. F. & MARTIN, M.: Evaluation of a standard dosage schedule with streptokinase. Blood 35 (1970) p 341.

HJORT, P. F., EGEBERG, O. & MIKKELSEN, S.: Turnover of prothrombin, factor VII and factor IX in a patient with hemophilia A. Scand. J. Clin. Lab. Invest. 13 (1961) p 668.

HJORT, P. F. & HASSELBACK, R.: A critical review of the evidence for a continuous hemostasis in vivo. Thromb. Diath. Haemorrh. 6 (1961) p 580.

HJORT, P. F., PERMAN, V. & CRONKITE, E. P.: Fresh, disintegrated platelets in radiation thrombocytopenia: Correction of prothrombin consumption without correction of bleeding. Proc. Soc. Exp. Biol. 102 (1959) p 31.

HJORT, P. F. & RAPAPORT, S. I.: The Shwartzman reaction: Pathogenetic mechanisms and clinical manifestations. Ann. Rev. Med. 16 (1965) p 135.

HJORT, P. F., RAPAPORT, S. I. & JÖRGENSEN, L.: Purpura fulminans. Report of a case successfully treated with heparin and hydrocortisone. Review of 50 cases from the literature. Scand. J. Haematol. 1 (1964) p 169.

HJORT, P., RAPAPORT, S. I. & OWREN, P. A.: A simple, specific one-stage prothrombin assay using Russell's viper venom in cephalin suspension. J. Lab. Clin. Med. 46 (1955) p 89.

HOAG, M. S., JOHNSON, F. J., ROBINSON, J. A. & AGGELER, P. M.: Treatment of hemophilia B with a new clotting-factor concentrate. New Engl. J. Med. 280 (1969) p 581.

HOAK, J. C., SWANSON, L. W., WARNER, E. D. & CONNER, W. E.: Myocardial infarction associated with severe factor-XII deficiency. Lancet II (1966) p 884.

HOLMBERG, L. & NILSSON, I. M.: Genetic variants of von Willebrand's disease. Brit. Med. J. 3 (1972) p 317.

HOLMBERG, L. & NILSSON, I. M.: a. Immunologic studies in haemophilia A. Scand. J. Haemat. 10 (1973) p 12.

HOLMBERG, L. & NILSSON, I. M.: b. Studies on two genetic variants of von Willebrand's disease. New Engl. J. Med. 288 (1973) p 595.

HOLMBERG, L. & NILSSON, I. M.: c. On the structure of the antihemophilic factor. IVth International Congress on Thrombosis and Haemostasis Vienna (1973) p 255.

HOLMSEN, H., DAY, H. J. & STORM, E.: Adenine nucleotide metabolism of blood platelets. VI. Subcellular localization of nucleotide pools with different functions in the platelet release reaction. Biochim. Biophys. Acta 186 (1969) p 254.

HOLMSEN, H., DAY, H. J. & STORMORKEN, H.: The blood platelet release reaction. Scand. J. Haematol. Suppl. 8 (1969) p 3.

HOLMSEN, H. & WEISS, H. J.: Hereditary defect in the platelet release reaction caused by a deficiency in the storage pool of platelet adenine nucleotides. Brit. J. Haemat. 19 (1970) p 643.

HONIG, G. R., FORMAN, E. N., JOHNSTON, C. A., SEELER, R. A., ABILDGAARD, CH. F. & SCHULMAN, I.: Administration of single doses of AHF (factor VIII) concentrates in the treatment of hemophilic hemarthroses. Pediatrics 43 (1969) p 26.

HORNE, C. H. W., WEIR, R. J., HOWIE, P. W. & GOUDIE, R. B.: Effect of combined oestrogenprogestogen oral contraceptives on serum-levels of α_2-macroglobulin, transferrin, albumin, and IgG. Lancet I (1970) p 49.

HOROWITZ, H. I., COHEN, B. D., MARTINEZ, P. & PAPAYOANOU, M.: Defective ADP-induced platelet factor 3 activation in uremia. Blood 30 (1967) p 331.

HOROWITZ, H. I., WILCOX, W. P. & FUJIMOTO, M. M.: Assay of plasma thromboplastin antecedent (PTA) with artificially depleted normal plasma. Blood 22 (1963) p 35.

HOUGIE, C.: Naturally occurring species specific inhibitor of human prothrombin in lupus erythematosus. Proc. Soc. Exp. Biol. Med. 116 (1964) p 359.

HOUGIE, C., BARROW, E. M. & GRÄHAM, J. B.: Stuart clotting defect. I. Segregation of an hereditary hemorrhagic state from the heterogeneous group heretofore called "stable factor" (SPCA proconvertin, factor VII) deficiency. J. Clin. Invest. 36 (1957) p 485.

HOUGIE, C. & TWOMEY, J. J.: Haemophilia B$_M$: A new type of factor-IX deficiency. Lancet I (1967) p 698.

HOVIG, T.: Release of a platelet-aggregating substance (adenosine diphosphate) from rabbit blood platelets induced by saline "extract" of tendons. Thromb. Diath. Haemorrh. 9 (1963) p 264.

HOVIG, T.: The ultrastructure of blood platelets in normal and abnormal states. Series Haematol. I (1968) p 3.

HOVIG, T.: Blood platelet surface and shape—a scanning electron microscopic study. Scand. J. Haematol. 7 (1970) p 420.

HOWELL, M.: Effects of plasma lipids on fibrinolysis. Brit. Med. Bull. 20 (1964) p 200.

HOYER, L. W. & BRECKENRIDGE, R. T.: Nonfunctional AHF-like material in patients with a genetic variant of hemophilia A. J. Lab. Clin. Med. 72 (1968) p 883.

HOYER, L. W. & BRECKENRIDGE, R. T.: Immunologic studies of antihemophilic factor (AHF, factor VIII). II. Properties of cross-reacting material. Blood 35 (1970) p 809.

HUGUES, J.: Accolement des plaquettes au collagène. Compt. Rend. Soc. Biol. 154 (1960) p 866.

HULME, B. & PITCHER, P. M.: Rapid latex-screening test for detection of fibrin/fibrinogen degradation products in urine after renal transplantation. Lancet I (1973) p 6.

HUMAIR, L., POTTER, E. V. & KWAAN, H. C.: The role of fibrinogen in renal disease. I. Production of experimental lesions in mice. J. Lab. Clin. Med 74 (1969) p 60.

HUME, M. & CHAN, Y. K.: Examination of the blood in the presence of venous thrombosis. J. Amer. Med. Ass. 200 (1967) p 747.

HUTCHISON, H. E., STARK, J. M. & CHAPMAN, J. A.: Platelet serotonin and normal haemostasis. J. Clin. Path. 12 (1959) p 265.

IATRIDIS, S. G. & FERGUSON, J. H.: Active Hageman factor: A plasma lysokinase of the human fibrinolytic system. J. Clin. Invest. 41 (1962) p 1277.

IKKALA, E., MYLLYLÄ, G. & NEVANLINNA, H. R.: Transfusion therapy in factor XIII (F.S.F.) deficiency. Scand. J. Haematol. I (1964) p 308.

IKKALA, E. & NEVANLINNA, H. R.: Congenital deficiency of fibrin stabilizing factor. Thromb. Diath. Haemorrh. 7 (1962) p 567.

IKKALA, E. & SIMONEN, O.: Factor VIII inhibitors and the use of blood products in patients with haemophilia A. Scand. J. Haemat. 8 (1971) p 16.

IMPERATO, C. & DETTORI, A. G.: Ipofibrinogenemia congenita con fibrinoastenia (Congenital hypofibrinogenemia with fibrinoasthenia). Helv. Paediat. Acta 13 (1958) p 380.

INCEMAN, S., CAEN, J. & BERNARD, J.: Aggregation, adhesion, and viscous metamorphosis of platelets in congenital fibrinogen deficiencies. J. Lab. Clin. Med. 68 (1966) p 21.

ISACSON, S.: Effect of prednisolone on the coagulation and fibrinolytic systems. Scand. J. Haematol. 7 (1970) p 212.

ISACSON, S. & NILSSON, I. M.: The kidneys and the fibrinolytic activity in the blood. Thromb. Diath. Haemorrh. 22 (1969) p 211.

ISACSON, S. & NILSSON, I. M.: Effect of treatment with combined phenformin and ethylo-estrenol on the coagulation and fibrinolytic system. Scand. J. Haematol. 7 (1970) p 404.

ISACSON, S. & NILSSON, I. M.: a. Coagulation and platelet adhesiveness in recurrent "idiopathic" venous thrombosis and thrombophlebitis. Acta Chir. Scand. 138 (1972) p 263.

ISACSON, S. & NILSSON, I. M.: b. Defective fibrinolysis in blood and vein walls in recurrent "idiopathic" venous thrombosis. Acta Chir. Scand. 138 (1972) p 313.

ISACSON, S. & NILSSON, I. M.: c. Coagulation and fibrinolysis in acute cholecystitis. Acta Chir. Scand. 138 (1972) p 179.

ISACSON, S. & NILSSON, I. M.: d. Antithrombotic effect of combined phenformin and ethyloestrenol. First International Conf. on Synthetic Fibrinolytic-Thrombolytic Agents Paris (1972).

ITO, T., NOWA, T. & MATSUI, E.: Fibrinolytic activity in renal disease. Clin. Chim. Acta 36 (1972) p 145.

JACKSON, D. P., BECK, E. A. & CHARACHE, P.: Congenital disorders of fibrinogen. Fed. Proc. 24 (1965) p 816.

JACOBSEN, C. D.: Proteolytic capacity in human plasma. II. Genetics and clinical study. Scand. J. Clin. Lab. Invest. 21 (1968) p 227.

JACOBSEN, C. D. & CHANDLER, A. B.: Thrombolysis in vitro. I. Method, comparison of various thrombolytic agents, and factors influencing thrombolysis. Scand. J. Clin. Lab. Invest. 17 (1965) p 209.

JACOBSSON, B.: a. Effect of vascular catheterisation on platelet adhesiveness. Europ. Surg. Res. I (1969) p 290.

JACOBSSON, B.: b. Effect of pretreatment with dextran 70 on platelet adhesiveness and thromboembolic complications following percutaneous arterial catheterisation. Acta Radiol. 8 (1969) p 289.

JACOBSSON, K.: Studies on fibrinogen. Scand. J. Clin. Lab. Invest. Suppl. 14: 7 (1955).

JAMIESON, G. A., URBAN, C. L. & BARBER,

A. J.: Enzymatic basis for platelet: collagen adhesion as the primary step in haemostasis. Nature New Biol. 234 (1971) p 5.

JANSEN, Hj.: Dextran as a prophylaxis against thromboembolism in general surgery. Acta Chir. Scand. Suppl. 387 (1968) p 86.

JERUSHALMY, Z. & ZUCKER, M. B.: Some effect of fibrinogen degradation products (FDP) on blood platelets. Thromb. Diath. Haemorrh. 15 (1966) p 413.

JIMENEZ, J. M. & PRITCHARD, J. A.: Pathogenesis and treatment of coagulation defects resulting from fetal death. Obstet. Gynecol. 32 (1968) p 449.

JOHNSON, A. J., KARPATKIN, M. H. & NEWMAN, J.: a. Preparation of and clinical experience with antihemophilic factor concentrates. Thromb. Diath. Haemorrh. Suppl. 35 (1969) p 49.

JOHNSON, A. J., KARPATKIN, M. H. & NEWMAN, J.: Clinical investigation of intermediate and high-purity antihaemophilic factor (factor VIII) concentrates. Brit. J. Haemat. 21 (1971) p 21.

JOHNSON, A. J., KLINE, D. L. & ALKJAERSIG, N.: b. Assay methods and standard preparations for plasmin, plasminogen and urokinase in purified systems 1967–1968. Thromb. Diath. Haemorrh. 21 (1969) p 259.

JOHNSON, A. J. & MERSKEY, C.: Diagnosis of diffuse intravascular clotting: its relation to secondary fibrinolysis and treatment with heparin. Thromb. Diath. Haemorrh. Suppl. 20 (1966) p 161.

JOHNSON, A. J. & MERSKEY, C.: Clinical and laboratory differentiation of fibrinolytic disease. Thromb. Diath. Haemorrh. Suppl. 39 (1970) p 229.

JOHNSON, A. J., NEWMAN, J., HOWELL, M. B. & PUSZKIN, S.: Two large-scale procedures for purification of human antihemophilic factor (AHF). Blood 28 (1966) p 1011.

JOHNSON, A. J., NEWMAN, J., HOWELL, M. B. & PUSZKIN, S.: Purification of antihaemophilic factor (AHF) for clinical and experimental use. Thromb. Diath. Haemorrh. Suppl. 26 (1967) p 377.

JOHNSON, A. J., SKOZA, L. & TSE, A. O.: Studies on plasmin inhibition and plasminogen activation and its inhibition. Thromb. Diath. Haemorrh. Suppl. 32 (1969) p 105.

JOHNSSON, S. R., BYGDEMAN, S. & ELIASSON, R.: Effect of dextran on postoperative thrombosis. Acta Chir. Scand. Suppl. 387 (1968) p 80.

JORPES, E.: Bibliography of K. P. Link. Proc. I. Intern. Conf. Thromb. Embolism. Basel 1954. Koller, Th. & Merz. W. R. (Ed.). Schwabe, Basel (1955) p 175.

JORPES, J. E.: Heparin, its chemistry, pharmacology and clinical use. Amer. J. Med. 33 (1962) p 692.

JORPES, J. E., BLOMBÄCK, B., BLOMBÄCK, M. & MAGNUSSON, S.: A pilot plant for the preparation of a human plasma fraction containing the human antihaemophilic factor A (factor VIII) and v. Willebrand's factor. Acta Med. Scand. Suppl. 379 (1962) p 7.

JOSSO, F., BOUSSEN, M., PROU-WARTELLE, O., PIGUET, H., SULTAN, Y. & BOUSSER, J.: Anomalies complexes de la coagulation dans deux de maladie de Kahler avec syndrome hémorrhagique. Signification du déficit en facteur Stuart au cours myélome. Nouv. Rev. Franc. Hematol. 6 (1966) p 739.

JOSSO, F., PROU-WARTELLE, O., ALAGILLE, D. & SOULIER, J. P.: Le déficit congénital en facteur stabilisant de la fibrine (facteur XIII). Etude de deux cas. Nouv. Rev. Franc. Hématol. 4 (1964) p 267.

JOSSO, F., STEINBUCH, M., MÉNACHÉ, D., BLATRIX, C. & SOULIER, J. P.: Preparation of Factor IX Concentrates, with Special Reference to the P.P.S.B. Fraction. Hemophilia and New Hemorrhagic States. International Symposium New York. Ed. K. M. Brinkhous. The University of North Carolina Press, Chapel Hill (1970) p 14.

JÜRGENS, J.: Zur Klinik der von Willebrand-Jürgens-Syndrome. Haemat. Bluttransf. 6 (1969) p 164.

JÜRGENS, R. & DEUTSCH, E. (Ed.): Hämorrhagische Diathesen. Internationales Symposion Wien 1955. Springer-Verlag, Wien (1955).

KAHN, M. J. P. & HEMKER, H. C.: Studies on blood coagulation factor V. IV. A partially purified factor V preparation from human plasma. Coagulation 3 (1970) p 63.

KAHN, M. J. P. & HEMKER, H. C.: Studies on Blood Coagulation factor V. V. Changes of molecular weight accompanying activation of factor V by thrombin and the procoagulant protein of Russell's viper venom. Thromb. Diath. Haemorrh. 27 (1972) p 25.

KAKKAR, V. V., FLANC, C., HOWE, C. T., O'SHEA, M. & FLUTE, P. T.: a. Treatment of deep vein thrombosis. A trial of heparin, streptokinase and Arvin. Brit. Med. J. 1 (1969) p 806.

KAKKAR, V. V., HOWE, C. T., FLANC, C. & CLARKE, M. B.: b. Natural history of postoperative deep-vein thrombosis. Lancet II (1969) p 230.

KAKKAR, V. V., NICOLAIDES, A. N., FIELD, E. S., FLUTE, P. T., WESSLER, S. & YIN, E. T.: Low doses of heparin in prevention of deep-vein thrombosis. Lancet II (1971) p 669.

KAKKAR, V. V., NICOLAIDES, A. N., RENNEY, J. T., FRIEND, J. R. & CLARKE, M. B.: 125 I-labelled fibrinogen test adapted for routine screening for deep-vein thrombosis. Lancet I (1970) p 540.

KAKKAR, V. V., SPINDLER, J., FLUTE, P. T., CORRIGAN, T., FOSSARD, D. P., CRELLIN, R. Q., WESSLER, S. & YIN, E. T.: Efficacy of low doses of heparin in prevention of deep-vein thrombosis after major surgery. A double-blind, randomised trial. Lancet II (1972) p 101.

KARACA, M., CRONBERG, L. & NILSSON, I. M.: Abnormal platelet-collagen reaction in Ehlers-Danlos syndrome. Scand. J. Haemat. 9 (1972) p 465.

KARACA, M. & NILSSON, I. M.: Fibrinolytic activity in hemiplegic patients. Acta Med. Scand. 189 (1971) p 325.

KARACA, M. & NILSSON, I. M.: PTA (factor XI) deficiency and prolonged bleeding time. Acta Med. Scand. 192 (1972) p 171.

KASPER, C. K., DIETRICH, S. L. & RAPAPORT, S. I.: Hemophilia prophylaxis with factor VIII concentrate. Arch. Intern. Med. 125 (1970) p 1004.

KATO, N., MORIMATSU, M., TANAKA, K. & HORIE, A.: Effects of trans-4-aminomethyl-cylohexane carboxylic acid as an antifibrinolytic agent on arterial wall and experimental atherosclerotic lesions in rabbits. Thromb. Diath. Haemorrh. 24 (1970) p 85.

KATTLOVE, H. E. & SPAET, T. H.: The effect of chromium on platelet function in vitro. Blood 35 (1970) p 659.

KATZ, J., LURIE, A. & KAPLAN, B.: Haemolytic-uraemic syndrome and heparin therapy. Lancet II (1969) p 700.

KATZ, J., LURIE, A., KAPLAN, B. S., KRAWITZ, S. & METZ, J.: Coagulation findings in the haemolytic-uraemic syndrome of infancy: similarity to hyperacute renal allograft rejection. J. Pediat. 78 (1971) p 426.

von KAULLA, K. N.: Chemistry of thrombolysis: Human fibrinolytic enzymes. Thomas. Springfield (1963).

von KAULLA, E. & von KAULLA, K. N.: Antithrombin III and diseases. Amer. J. Clin. Pathol. 48 (1967) p 69.

KEKWICK, R. A. & WOLF, P.: A concentrate of human antihaemophilic factor. Its use in six cases of haemophilia. Lancet I (1957) p 647.

KELLERMEYER, W. F. JR. & KELLERMEYER, R. W.: Hageman factor activation and kinin formation in human plasma induced by cellulose sulfate solutions. Proc. Soc. Exp. Biol. Med. 130 (1969) p 1310.

KERR, C. B.: Intracranial haemorrhage in haemo-philia. J. Neurol. Neurosurg. Psychiat. 27 (1964) p 166.

KIESSELBACH, T. H. & WAGNER, R. H.: Fibrin-stabilizing factor: a thrombin-labile platelet protein. Amer. J. Physiol. 211 (1966) p 1472.

KINCAID-SMITH, P.: a. Anticoagulants in renal disease. Amer. Heart J. 77 (1969) p 840.

KINCAID-SMITH, P.: b. Modification of the vascular lesions of rejection in cadaveric renal allografts by dipyridamole and anticoagulants. Lancet II (1969) p 920.

KINGDON, H. S., DAVIE, E. W. & RATNOFF, O. D.: The reaction between activated plasma thromboplastin antecedent and diisopropyl-phosphofluoridate. Biochem. 3 (1964) p 166.

KINGSLEY, C. S.: Familial factor V deficiency: the pattern of heredity. Quart. J. Med. 23 (1954) p 323.

KJELLMAN, H.: Data based on Noble F.: Toxicology findings with tranexamic acid in mammals. Cyanamid Interoffice Correspondence, January 12 (1972).

KLEINER, G. J., MERSKEY, C., JOHNSON, A. J. & MARKUS, W. B.: Defibrination in normal and abnormal parturition. Brit. J. Haematol. 19 (1970) p 159.

KLINE, D. L.: Purification and crystallization of plasminogen (profibrinolysin). J. Biol. Chem. 204 (1953) p 949.

KLINE, D. L.: Blood coagulation: Reactions leading to prothrombin activation. Ann. Rev. Physiol. 27 (1965) p 285.

KLINE, D. L. & FISHMAN, J. B.: Proactivator function of human plasmin as shown by lysine esterase assay. J. Biol. Chem. 236 (1961) p 2807.

KLOEZE, J.: Prostaglandins and platelet aggregation. In Platelets and vessel wall fibrin depositions. Ed. G. Schettler. Thieme, Stuttgart (1970) p 54.

KOFFLER, D. & PARONETTO, F.: Fibrinogen deposition in acute renal failure. Amer. J. Path. 49 (1966) p 383.

KOK, P. & ASTRUP, T.: Isolation and purification of a tissue plasminogen activator and its comparison with urokinase. Biochemistry 8 (1969) p 79.

KOK, P. & ASTRUP, T.: Differentiation between plasminogen activators by means of epsilon-aminocaproic acid. Thromb. Diath. Haemorrh. 27 (1972) p 77.

KORSAN-BENGTSEN, K.: Comparison between various methods used to control dicumarol therapy. Acta Med. Scand. 188 (1970) p 327.

KORSAN-BENGTSEN, K., YSANDER, L., BLOHMÉ, G. & TIBBLIN, E.: Extensive muscle necrosis after long-term treatment with aminocaproic acid (EACA) in a case of hereditary periodic edema. Acta Med. Scand. 185 (1969) p 341.

KOTILAINEN, M.: Platelet kinetics in normal subjects and in haematological disorders. Scand. J. Haematol. Suppl. 15 (1969).

KOWALSKI, E.: Fibrinogen derivatives and their biologic activities. Seminar Hematol. 5 (1968) p 45.

KUCINSKI, C. S., FLETCHER, A. P. & SHERRY, S.: Effect of urokinase antiserum on plasminogen activators. Demonstration of immunologic dissimilarity between plasma plasminogen activator and urokinase. J. Clin. Invest 47 (1968) p 1238.

KULLANDER, S. & NILSSON, I. M.: Human placental transfer of an antifibrinolytic agent (AMCA). Acta Obstet. Gynecol. Scand. 49 (1970) p 241.

KURZ, R., GLATZL, J., HOLZKNECHT, F. & SPÖTTL, F.: Isolierter familiärer Faktor-X-Mangel (Nachweis des recessiven Erbgangs). Schweiz. med. Wschr. 99 (1969) p 885.

KWAAN, H. C. & ASTRUP, T.: Fibrinolytic activity in thrombosed veins. Circulation Res. 17 (1965) p 477.

KWAAN, H. C., COCCO, A. & MENDELOFF, A. I.: Histologic demonstration of plasminogen activation in rectal biopsies from patients with active ulcerative colitis. J. Lab. Clin. Med. 64 (1964) p 877.

KWAAN, H. C. & FISCHER, S.: Localization of fibrinolytic activity in kidney tissues. Fed. Proc. 24, 2 (1965).

KÜNZER, W. & AALAM, F.: Zur Heparinbehandlung des akuten hämolytisch-urämischen Syndroms. Klin. Wochenschr. 42 (1964) p 820.

LACKNER, H., HUNT, V., ZUCKER, M. B. & PEARSON, J.: Abnormal fibrin ultrastructure, polymerization and clot retraction in multiple myeloma. Brit. J. Haematol. 18 (1970) p 625.

LAKI, K. (Ed.).: Fibrinogen. Marcel Dekker, New York (1968).

LANCHANTIN, G. F., PLESSET, M. L., FRIEDMAN, J. A. & HART, D. W.: Dissociation of esterolytic and clotting activities of thrombin by trypsin-binding macroglobulin. Proc. Soc. Exp. Biol. 121 (1966) p 444.

LANDABURU, R. H. & ALBADO, E.: Factor X precursor in purified bovine prothrombin preparations. Coagulation 2 (1969) p 269.

LANDABURU, R. H., ALBADO, E. & SANTILLÁN, R.: Prothrombin purification by chromatography. Thromb. Diath. Haemorrh. 19 (1968) p 316.

LARRIEU, M. J.: Action of fibrinogen degradation products and fibrin monomer soluble complexes on platelet aggregation. Scand. J. Haematol. Suppl. 13 (1971) p 273.

LARRIEU, M. J., CAEN, J. P., MEYER, D. O., VAINER, H., SULTAN, Y. & BERNARD, J.: Congenital bleeding disorders with long bleeding time and normal platelet count. II. von Willebrand's disease (report of thirty-seven patients). Amer. J. Med. 45 (1968) p 354.

LARRIEU, M. J., RIGOLLOT, C. & MARDER, V. J.: Comparative effects of fibrinogen degradation fragments D and E on coagulation. Brit. J. Haemat. 22 (1972) p 719.

LARSSON, S. O.: On coagulation and fibrinolysis in renal failure. Scand. J. Haematol. Suppl. 15 (1971) p 1.

LARSSON, S. O., HEDNER, U. & NILSSON, I. M.: a. On coagulation and fibrinolysis in conservatively treated chronic uraemia. Acta Med. Scand. 189 (1971) p 433.

LARSSON, S. O., HEDNER, U. & NILSSON, I. M.: b. On coagulation and fibrinolysis in acute renal insufficiency. Acta Med. Scand. 189 (1971) p 443.

LARSSON, S. O., HEDNER, U. & NILSSON, I. M.: c. On fibrinolytic split products in serum and urine in uraemia. Scand. J. Urol. Nephrol. 5 (1971) p 234.

LARSSON, S. O., LINDERGÅRD, B., HENRIKSSON, H., HEDNER, U. & NILSSON, I. M.: d. A case of acute glomerulonephritis and severe uraemia, treated with heparin and corticosteroids. Scand. J. Urol. Nephrol. 5 (1971) p 291.

LASCH, H. G.: a. Coagulation and disturbances in shock. Postgrad. Med. J. 45 (1969) p 539.

LASCH, H. G.: b. Therapeutic aspects of disseminated intravascular coagulation. Thromb. Diath. Haemorrh. Suppl. 36 (1969) p 281.

LASCH, H. G.: Klinik und Therapie disseminierter intravasculärer Gerinnungsvorgänge. XIII. Intern. Congr. Hematol., Munich (1970) p 121.

LASSEN, M.: Heat denaturation of plasminogen in the fibrin plate method. Acta Physiol. Scand. 27 (1952) p 371.

LATALLO, Z. S., WEGRZYNOWICZ, Z., BUDZYNSKI, A. Z. & KOPEČ, M.: Effect of protamine sulphate on the solubility of fibrinogen, its derivatives and other plasma proteins. Scand. J. Haematol. Suppl. 13 (1971) p 151.

LAURELL, C.-B.: Quantitative estimation of proteins by electrophoresis in agarose gel containing antibodies. Anal. Biochem. 15 (1966) p 45.

LAURITSEN, O. S.: Urokinase inhibitor in human plasma. Scand. J. Clin. Lab. Invest. 22 (1968) p 314.

LAZERSON, J.: Hemophilia home transfusion program. Effect on school attendance. J. Pediat. 81 (1972) p 330.

LECHLER, E., WEBSTER, W. P., ROBERTS, H. R. & PENICK, G. D.: The inheritance of Stuart disease: Investigation of a family with factor X deficiency. Amer. J. Med. Sci. 249 (1965) p 291.

LECHNER, K., LUDWIG, E., NIESSNER, H., THALER, E. & DEUTSCH, E.: Immunosuppressive treatment of patients with inhibitors of blood coagulation. III Congr. Internat. Society on Thrombosis and Haemostasis Washington (1972) p 118.

LECHNER, K., REGELE, H., WALDHÄUSL, W. & KAROBATH, H.: Verbrauchskoagulopathie bei metastasierenden Prostatakarzinom. Acta Haematol. 40 (1968) p 95.

LEE, L., PROSE, P. H. & COHEN, M. H.: The role of the reticuloendothelial system in diffuse, low grade intravascular coagulation. Thromb. Diath. Haemorrh. Suppl. 20 (1966) p 87.

LEGRAND, Y.: Collagen in experimental survey. In Platelet aggregation. Ed. J. P. Caen, Masson, Paris (1971).

LEHMANN, W. L.: Untersuchungen zu Thrombopathie (v. Willebrand-Jürgens) auf den Åland-Inseln (Finland). Acta Genet. Med. Suppl. 2. 8 (1959) p 38.

LEMOYNE, J. & LARRIEU, M. J.: Amygdalectomie pour hémorrhagies amygdaliennes chez un sujet atteint de maladie de Willebrand. Ann. Oto-Laryngol. 84 (1967) p 878.

LERNER, R. G., RAPAPORT, S. I., SIEMSEN, J. K. & SPITZER, J. M.: Disappearance of fibrinogen- 131I after endotoxin: effects of a first and second injection. Amer. J. Physiol. 214 (1968) p 532.

LESUK, A., TERMINIELLE, L. & TRAVER, J. H.: Crystalline human urokinase: some properties. Science 147 (1965) p 880.

LESUK, A., TERMINIELLE, L., TRAVER, J. H. & GROFF, J. L.: Biochemical and biophysical studies of human urokinase. Thromb. Diath. Haemorrh. 18 (1967) p 293.

LEVESON, J. E. & ESNOUF, M. P.: The inhibition of activated factor X with diisopropyl fluorophosphate. Brit. J. Haematol. 17 (1969) p 173.

LIEBERMANN, E.: Hemolytic-uremic syndrome. J. Pediat. 80 (1972) p 1.

LIPINSKI, B., WEGRZYNOWICZ, Z., BUDZYNSKI, A. Z., KOPEČ, M., LATALLO, Z. S. & KOWALSKI, E.: Soluble unclottable complexes formed in the presence of fibrinogen degradation products (FDP) during the fibrinogen-fibrin conversion and their potential significance in pathology. Throm. Diath. Haemorrh. 17 (1967) p 65.

LIPINSKI, B. & WOROWSKI, K.: Detection of soluble fibrin monomer complexes in blood by means of protamine sulphate test. Thromb. Diath. Haemorrh. 20 (1968) p 44.

LIPPMANN, W. & WISHNICK, M.: Effects of the administration of epsilon-amino caproic acid on catecholamine and serotonin levels in the rat and dog. J. Pharmacol. Exp. Therap. 150 (1965) p 196.

LITTLE, J. R.: Purpura fulminans treated successfully with anticoagulation. J A M A 169 (1969) p 36.

LJUNGQVIST, U., BERGENTZ, S.-E., LEANDOER, L. & NILSSON, I. M.: Coagulation and fibrinolysis after renal transplantation. Scand. J. Urol. Nephrol. 3 (1969) p 23.

LO, S. S., HITZIG, W. H. & FRICK, P. G.: Clinical experience with anticoagulant therapy in the management of disseminated intravascular coagulation in children. Acta Haematol. 45 (1971) p 1.

LOELIGER, E. A., v. d. ESCH, B., ter HAAR ROMENY-WACHTER, C. CH. & BOOIJ, H. I.: Factor VII: Its turnover rate and its possible role in thrombogenesis. Thromb. Diath Haemorrh. 4 (1960) p 196.

LOELIGER, E. A. & HEMKER, H. C.: Principles of the mode of action of coumarin congeners. 3. Intern. Pharmacol. Meet., Sao Paulo, 1966. In Drugs in Relation to Blood Coagulation, Haemostasis and Thrombosis. 6 (1968) p 13.

LOELIGER, E. A. & HENSEN, A.: a. Coagulation studies in a case of Hageman trait., Thromb. Diath. Haemorrh. 5 (1961) p 187.

LOELIGER, E. A. & HENSEN, A.: b. Substitution therapy in haemophilia B. Thromb. Diath. Haemorrh. 6 (1961) p 391.

LOELIGER, E. A., HENSEN, A., MATTERN, M. J., VELTKAMP, J. J., BRUNING, P. F. & HEMKER, H. C.: Treatment of haemophilia B with purified factor IX (PPSB). Folia Med. Neerl. 10 (1967) p 112.

LOELIGER, A. & HERS, J. F. P.: Chronic antithrombinaemia (antithrombin V) with haemorrhagic diathesis in a case of rheumatoid arthritis with hypergammaglobulinaemia. Thromb. Diath Haemorrh. 1 (1957) p 499.

LOEWY, A. G., DUNATHAN, K., KRIEL, R. & WOLFINGER, H. L. JR: Fibrinase. I. Purification of substrate and enzyme. J. Biol. Chem. 236 (1961) p 2625.

LÖPEZ, V., PFLÜGSHAUPT, R., WIRTHNER, H. & BÜTLER, R.: Hereditäre Faktor-V-Mangel (Pharahämophilie) in einer Schweizer Familie. Schweiz. Med. Wochenschr. 99 (1969) p 1354.

LORAND, L.: Fibrino-peptide. Biochem. J. 52 (1952) p 200.

LORAND, L.: Physiological crosslinking of fibrin. Thromb. Diath. Haemorrh. Suppl. 34 (1970) p 75.

LORAND, L.: Fibrinoligase: The fibrin-stabilizing factor system of blood plasma. Ann. N. Y. Acad. Sci. 202 (1972) p 6.

LORAND, L. & DICKENMAN, R. C.: Assay method for the "fibrin-stabilizing factor". Proc. Soc. Exp. Biol. N. Y. 89 (1955) p 45.

LORAND, L. & GOTOH, T.: Fibrinoligase. The fibrin stabilizing factor system. Methods in enzymology. Academic Press New York 19 (1970) p 770.

LORAND, L. & JACOBSEN, A.: Studies on the polymerization of fibrin. The role of the globulin: fibrin-stabilizing factor. J. Biol. Chem. 230 (1958) p 421.

LORAND, L., MALDONADO, N., FRADERA, J., ATENCIO, A. C., ROBERTSON, B. & URAYAMA, T.: Haemorrhagic syndrome of autoimmune origin with a specific inhibitor against fibrin stabilizing factor (factor XIII). Brit. J. Haemat. 23 (1972) p 17.

LORAND, L., URAYAMA, T., ATENCIO, A. C. & HSIA, D. Y. Y.: Inheritance of deficiency of fibrin-stabilizing factor (factor XIII). Amer. J. Hum. Genet. 22 (1970) p 89.

LORAND, K., URAYAMA, T., de KIEWIET, J. W. C. & NOSSEL, H. L.: Diagnostic and genetic studies on fibrin-stabilizing factor with a new assay based on amine incorporation. J. Clin. Invest. 48 (1969) p 1054.

LOSOWSKY, M. S. & WALLS, W. D.: Abnormal fibrin stabilization in renal failure. Thromb. Diath. Haemorrh. 22 (1969) p 216.

LUDWIG, H.: Experimentelle Untersuchungen zum diaplacentaren Übertritt von Streptokinase. Geburtsh. Frauenheilk. 26 (1966) p 736.

LUKE, R. G., SIEGEL, R. R., TALBERG, W. & HOLLAND, N.: Heparin treatment for postpartum renal failure with microangiopathic haemolytic anaemia. Lancet II (1970) p 750.

LUSHER, J. M., IYER, R. & EVANS, R. K.: Effective suppression of factor 8 antibody in patients with hemophilia A with cyclophosphamide. VIIth Congress of the World Federation of Haemophilia, Tehran-Iran May (1971) p 74.

LUSHER, J. M., SHUSTER, J., EVANS, R. K. & POULIK, M. D.: Antibody nature of an AHG (factor VIII) inhibitor. J. Pediat. 72 (1968) p 325.

LUSHER, J. M., ZUELZER, W. W. & EVANS, R. K.: Hemophilia A in chromosomal female subjects. J. Pediat. 74 (1969) p 265.

MCCLUSKEY, R. T., VASSALLI, P., GALLO, G. & BALDWIN, D. S.: An immunofluorescent study of pathogenic mechanisms in glomerular diseases. New Engl. J. Med. 274 (1966) p 695.

MCCRACKEN JR, G. H. & DICKERMAN, J. D.: Septicemia and disseminated intravascular coagulation. Amer. J. Dis. Child. 118 (1969) p 431.

MCDONAGH, J., MCDONAGH, R. P. JR, DELAGE, J. M. & WAGNER, R. H.: Factor XIII in human plasma and platelets. J. Clin. Invest. 48 (1969) p 940.

MCDONAGH, J., MCDONAGH, R. P. JR & DUCKERT, F.: Inheritance of factor XIII deficiency. International Society of Thrombosis and Haemostasis. II Congress Oslo, Norway July (1971) p 36.

MCDONAGH, J., MESSEL, H., MCDONAGH R. P. JR, MURANO, G. & BLOMBÄCK, B.: Molecular weight analysis of fibrinogen and fibrin chains by an improved sodium dodecyl sulfate gel electrophoresis method. Biochim. Biophys. Acta 257 (1972) p 135.

MCDONAGH, R. P. JR & FERGUSON, J. H.: Studies on the participation of Hageman factor in fibrinolysis. Thromb. Diath. Haemorrh. 24 (1970) p 1.

MACFARLANE, A. S., TODD, D. & CROMWELL, S.: Fibrinogen catabolism in humans. Clin. Sci. 26 (1964) p 415.

MACFARLANE, R. G.: The coagulant action of Russell's viper venom; The use of antivenom in defining its reaction with a serum factor. Brit. J. Haematol. 7 (1961) p 496.

MACFARLANE, R. G.: An enzyme cascade in the blood clotting mechanism, and its function as a biochemical amplifier. Nature 202 (1964) p 495.

MCGEHEE, W. G., RAPAPORT, S. I. & HJORT, P. F.: Intravascular coagulation in fulminant meningococcemia. Ann. Internal. Med. 67 (1967) p 250.

MCKAY, D. G.: Disseminated intravascular coagulation. An intermediary mechanism of disease. Hoeber Medical Division, Harper & Row, Publishers New York, Everton, London (1965).

MCKAY, D. G.: a. Progress in disseminated intravascular coagulation. Part I. Calif. Med. 111 (1969) p 186.

MCKAY, D. G.: b. Progress in disseminated intravascular coagulation. Part II. Calif. Med. 111 (1969) p 279.

MCKAY, D. G.: c. Tissue damage in disseminated intravascular coagulation—mechanisms of localization of thrombi in the microcirculation. Thromb. Diath. Haemorrh. Suppl. 36 (1969) p 67.

MCKENZIE, F. N., DHALL, D. P., ARFORS, K.-E., NORDLUND, S. & MATHESON, N. A.: Blood platelet behaviour during and after open-heart surgery. Brit. Med. J. 2 (1969) p 795.

MCKUSICK, V. A.: Heritable Disorders of Connective Tissue. 2nd ed. Mosby, St Louis (1960) p 171.

MCMILLAN, C. W., DIAMOND, K. L. & SURGENOR, D. M.: Treatment of classic hemophilia: the use of fibrinogen rich in factor VIII for hemorrhage and for surgery. New Engl. J. Med. 265 (1961) pp 224–230, 277–283.

MACMILLAN, D. C.: Secondary clumping effect in human citrated platelet-rich plasma produced by adenosine diphosphate and adrenaline. Nature 211 (1966) p 140.

MCNICOL, G. P., BARAKAT, A. A. & DOUGLAS, A. S.: Plasma fibrinolytic activity in renal disease. Scot. Med. J. 10 (1965) p 189.

MCNICOL, G. P., FLETCHER, A. P., ALKJAERSIG, N. & SHERRY, S.: The absorption, distribution, and excretion of ε-aminocaproic acid following oral or intravenous administration to man. J. Lab. Clin. Med. 59 (1962) p 15.

MCNICOL, G. P., PRENTICE, C. R. M., BRIGGS, J. D. & PIDGEON, C.: Fibrinogen degradation products in renal disease: Estimation and significance of FDP in urine. Scand. J. Haematol. Suppl. 13 (1971) p 329.

MAGNUSSON, S.: Thrombin and prothrombin. The Enzymes. Vol III, 3rd edition. Ed. P. D. Boyer. Academic Press (1971).

MALOFIEJEW, W.: The biological and pharmacological properties of some fibrinogen degradation products. Scand. J. Haemat. Suppl. 13 (1971) p 303.

MANDELLI, F., MARIANI, G., GANDOLFO, G. M. & ISACCHI, G.: Considérations sur deux cas d'hypoconvertinémie congénitale. Nouv. Rev. Franc. Hématol. 9 (1969) p 485.

MANNUCCI, P. M. & RUGGERI, Z. M.: Circulating anticoagulants in haemophilia. Lancet II (1970) p 1360.

MANSFIELD, A. O.: Alteration in fibrinolysis associated with surgery and venous thrombosis. Brit. J. Surg. 59 (1972) p 754.

MARCHESI, S. L., SHULMAN, N. R. & GRALNICK, H. R.: Studies on the purification and characterization of human factor VIII. J. Clin. Invest. 51 (1972) p 2151.

MARCINIAK, E. & TSUKAMURA, S.: Two progressive inhibitors of factor X_a in human blood. Brit. J. Haemat. 22 (1972) p 341.

MARCUS, A. J., BRADLOW, B. A., SAFIER, L. B. & ULLMAN, H. L.: Biochemical and physiological properties of isolated platelet membranes. Thromb. Diath. Haemorrh. Suppl. 26 (1967) p 43.

MARDER, V. J.: Fibrinogen and fibrin degradation products. Physiochemical and physiological consi-

derations. Thromb. Diath. Haemorrh. Suppl. 47 (1971) p 85.

MARDER, V. J. & SHULMAN, N. R.: Clinical aspects of congenital factor VII deficiency. Amer. J. Med. 37 (1964) p 182.

MARDER, V. J., SHULMAN, N. R. & CARROLL, W. R.: The importance of intermediate degradation products of fibrinogen in fibrinolytic hemorrhage. Trans. Assoc. Amer. Physicians. 80 (1967) p 156.

MARENGO-ROWE, A. J., MURFF, G., LEVESON, J. E. & COOK, J.: Hemophilia-like disease associated with pregnancy. Obstet. Gynec. 40 (1972) p 56.

MARGARETTEN, W., CSAVOSSY, I. & MCKAY, D. G.: An electron microscopic study of thrombin-induced disseminated intravascular coagulation. Blood 29 (1967) p 169.

MARGARETTEN, W., ELTING, J., ROTHENBERG, J. & MCKAY, D. G.: Experimental adrenal hemorrhage in the generalized Shwartzman reaction. Lab. Invest. 14 (1965) p 687.

MARGOLIS, J.: a. The role of Hageman factor on plasma surface reactions. In: Hemophilia and other Hemorrhagic States. Ed.: K. M. Brinkhous. The University of North Carolina Press, Chapel Hill (1959) p 208.

MARGOLIS, J.: b. Hageman factor and capillary permeability. Aust. J. Exp. Biol. Med. Sci. 37 (1959) p 239.

MARGOLIS, J.: The effect of colloidal silica on blood coagulation. Aust. J. Exp. Biol. Med. Sci. 39 (1961) p 249.

MARGOLIUS, A. JR, JACKSON, D. P. & RATNOFF, O. D.: Circulating anticoagulants: A study of 40 cases and a review of the literature. Medicine 40 (1961) p 145.

MARKWARDT, F., KLOCKING, H.-P. & LANDMANN, H.: Vergleichende Untersuchungen über Antifibrinolytika. Thromb. Diath. Haemorrh. 15 (1967) p 561.

MARTIN, M., SCHOOP, W. & ZEITLER, E.: Streptokinase in chronic arterial occlusive disease. J. Amer. Med. Ass. 211 (1970) p 1169.

MASON, B. J.: Circulating anticoagulant to factor VIII associated with rheumatoid arthritis. Brit. Med. J. 4 (1969) p 726.

MATHUR, K. S., GUPTA, D. K. & WAHAL, P. K.: Plasma fibrinolytic activity in cirrhosis of the liver. Blood 4 (1968) p 18.

MAYCOCK, W. D. A., EVANS, S., VALLET, L., COMBRIDGE, B., WOLF, P., MCGIBBON, N., FRENCH, E. E., WALLETT, L. H., DACIE, J. V., BIGGS, R., HANDLEY, D. & MACFARLANE, R. G.: Further experience with a concentrate containing human antihaemophilic factor. Brit. J. Haematol. 9 (1963) p 215.

MAZZA, J. J., BOWIE, E. J. W., HAGEDORN, A. B., DIDISHEIM, P., TASWELL, H. F., PETERSON, L. F. A. & OWEN, CH. A. JR: Antihemophilic factor VIII in hemophilia. Use of concentrates to permit major surgery. J. Amer. Med. Ass. 211 (1970) p 1818.

MEILI, E. O. & STRAUB, P. W.: Elevation of factor VIII in acute fatal liver necrosis. Thromb. Diath. Haemorrh. 24 (1970) p 161.

MEILI, E. O., STRAUB, P. W. & FRICK, P. G.: Zur Pathogenese und Behandlung der von Willebrandchen Krankheit. Schweiz. med. Wochenschr. 99 (1969) p 1805.

MELANDER, B. et al.: Biochemistry and toxicology of Amikapron® :, the antifibrinolytically active isomer of AMCHA. (A comparative study with ε-aminocaproic acid.) Acta Pharmacol. Toxicol. 22 (1965) p 340.

MELLIGER, E. J.: Detection of fibrinogen degradation products by use of antibody coated latex particles. The possibilities and limits of the method. Thromb. Diath. Haemorrh. 23 (1970) p 211.

MELLMAN, W. J., WOLMAN, I. J., WURZEL, H. A., MOORHEAD, P. S. & QUALLS, D. H.: A chromosomal female with haemophilia A. Blood 17 (1961) p 719.

MÉNACHÉ, D.: a. The turnover rate of the coagulation factors II, VII and IX under normal metabolic conditions. Thromb. Diath. Haemorrh. Suppl. 13 (1964) p 187.

MÉNACHÉ, D.: b. Constitutional and familial abnormal fibrinogen. Thromb. Diath. Haemorrh. Suppl. 13 (1964) p 173.

MÉNACHÉ, D.: Fraction I₀ prepared in Paris. Clinical use for surgery in hemophilic patients. Bibl. haematol. 29 (1968) p 1100.

MENON, I. S., MCCOLLUM, J. P. K. & GIBSON, A. L.: Blood fibrinolytic activity in deep-vein thrombosis. Lancet I (1971) p 242.

MERSKEY, C.: Diagnosis and treatment of intravascular coagulation. Brit. J. Haematol. 15 (1968) p 523.

MERSKEY, C. & JOHNSON, A. J.: Diagnosis and treatment of intravascular coagulation. Thromb. Diath. Haemorrh. Suppl. 21 (1966) p 555.

MERSKEY, C. & JOHNSON, A. J.: The clinical significance of fibrinogen-fibrin-related antigen in serum. Scand. J. Haematol. Suppl. 13 (1971) p 313.

MERSKEY, C., JOHNSON, A. J. & LALEZARI, P.: Tanned red cell hemagglutination inhibition immunoassay for fibrinogen-fibrin-related antigen ("fibrinolytic degradation products") in human serum. Scand. J. Haematol. Suppl. 13 (1971) p 83.

MERSKEY, C., KLEINER, G. J. & JOHNSON, A. J.: Quantitative estimation of split products of fibrinogen in human serum, relation to diagnosis and treatment. Blood 28 (1966) p 1.

MERSKEY, C., LALEZARI, P. & JOHNSON, A. J.: A rapid simple, sensitive method for measuring fibrinolytic split products in human serum. Proc. Soc. Exp. Biol. Med. 131 (1969) p 871.

MERSKEY, C. & MARCUS, A. J.: Lipids, blood coagulation and fibrinolysis. Ann. Rev. Med. 14 (1963) p 323.

MEYER, D., LARRIEU, M. J., CAEN, J. & BERNARD, J.: Critères et limites du diagnostic de la maladie de Willebrand. Nouv. Rev. Franc. Hematol. 7 (1967) p 115.

MEYER, D., LARRIEU, M. J. & DREYFUS, J. C.: Migration electrophoretique des facteurs de coagulation sur acetate de cellulose. Nouv. Rev. Franc. Hémat. 9 (1969) p 611.

MEYER, D., LAVERGNE, J.-M., LARRIEU, M.-J. & JOSSO, F.: Cross-reacting material in congenital factor VIII deficiencies (haemophilia A and von Willebrand's disease). Thromb. Res. 1 (1972) p 183.

MICHAEL, S. E. & TUNNAH, G. W.: The purification of factor VIII (antihaemophilic globulin). Brit. J. Haematol. 9 (1963) p 236.

MICHAL, F. & BORN, G. V. R.: Effect of the rapid shape change of platelets on the transmission and scattering of light through plasma. Nature New Biol. 231 (1971) p 220.

MILLER, G. A. H., SUTTON, G. C., KERR, I. H. GIBSON, R. V. & HONEY, M.: Comparison of streptokinase and heparin in treatment of isolated acute massive pulmonary embolism. Brit. Med. J. 2 (1971) p 681.

MILLER, L. L. & BALE, W. F.: Synthesis of all plasma protein fractions except gamma globulin by liver. J. Exp. Med. 99 (1954) p 125.

MILLER, S. P. & DAVISON, T.: Defibrination syndrome in cancer; treatment with heparin. New York J. Med. 67 (1967) p 452.

MOOLTEN, S. E., VROMAN, L. & VROMAN, G. M. S.: Adhesiveness of blood platelets in thromboembolism and hemorrhagic disorders. II. Diagnostic and prognostic significance of platelet adhesiveness. Amer. J. Clin. Pathol. 19 (1949) p 814.

MOOR-JANKOWSKI, J. K., HUSER, H. J., ROSIN, S., TRUOG, G., SCHNEEBERGER, M. & GEIGER, M.: Haemophilie B. Genetische, klinische und gerinnungsphysiologische Aspekte (Untersuchungen an einem weitverbreiteten Bluterstamm). Karger, Basel och New York (1958).

MOSESSON, M. W.: The preparation of human fibrinogen free of plasminogen. Biochim. Biophys. Acta 57 (1962) p 204.

MOSESSON, M. W., COLMAN, R. W. & SHERRY, S.: Chronic intravascular coagulation syndrome. Report of a case with special studies of an associated plasma cryoprecipitate ("cryofibrinogen"). New Engl. J. Med. 278 (1968) p 815.

MOSESSON, M. W., FINLAYSON, J. S., UMFLEET, R. A. & GALANAKIS, D.: a. Human fibrinogen heterogeneities. I. Structural and related studies of plasma fibrinogens which are high solubility catabolic intermediates. J. Biol. Chem. 247 (1972) p 5210.

MOSESSON, M. W., FINLAYSON, J. S. & UMFLEET, R. A.: b. Human fibrinogen heterogeneities. III. Identification of γchain variants. J. Biol. Chem. 247 (1972) p 5223.

van MOURIK, J. A. & MOCHTAR, I. A.: Purification of human antihemophilic factor (factor VIII) by gel chromatography. Biochim. Biophys. Acta 221 (1970) p 677.

MURPHY, S., OSKI, F. A., NAIMAN, J. L., LUSCH, C. J., GOLDBERG, S. & GARDNER, F. H.: Platelet size and kinetics in hereditary and acquired thrombocytopenia. New Engl. J. Med. 286 (1972) p 499.

MUSTARD, J. F. & PACKHAM, M. A.: Platelet phagocytosis. Series Haematol. 1 (1968) p 168.

MUSTARD, J. F. & PACKHAM, M. A.: Factors influencing platelet function: adhesion, release, and aggregation. Pharmacol. Rev. 22 (1970) p 97.

MÜLLER-BERGHAUS, G.: Pathophysiology of disseminated intravascular coagulation. Thromb. Diath. Haemorrh. Suppl. 36 (1969) p 45.

MÜLLERTZ, S.: Mechanism of activation and effect of plasmin in blood. Acta Physiol. Scand. 38, Suppl. 130 (1956).

MÜLLERTZ, S. & LASSEN, M.: An activator system in blood indispensable for formation of plasmin by streptokinase. Proc. Soc. Exp. Biol. Med. 82 (1953) p 264.

MYLLYLÄ, G., PELKONEN, R., IKKALA, E. & APAJALAHTI, J.: Hereditary thrombocytopenia. Report of three families. Scand J. Haematol. 4 (1967) p 441.

NACHMAN, R. L., MARCUS, A. J. & SAFIER, L. B.: Platelet thrombosthenin: Subcellular localization and function. J. Clin. Invest. 46 (1967) p 1380.

NAEYE, R. L.: Thrombotic disorders with increased levels of antiplasmin and antiplasminogen. New Engl. J. Med. 265 (1961) p 867.

NAJEAN, Y., ARDAILLOU, N. & DRESCH, C.: Platelet lifespan. Ann. Rev. Med. 20 (1969) p 47.

NEGUS, D., PINTO, D. J. & BROWN, N.: Platelet adhesiveness in postoperative deep-vein thrombosis. Lancet I (1969) p 220.

NEGUS, D., PINTO, D. J., LE QUESNE, L. P., BROWN, N. & CHAPMAN, M.: 125-I-labelled fibrinogen in the diagnosis of deep-vein thrombosis and its correlation with phlebography. Brit. J. Surg. 55 (1968) p 835.

NEMERSON, Y.: Characteristics and lipid requirements of coagulant proteins extracted from lung and brain: the specificity of the protein component of tissue factor. J. Clin. Invest. 48 (1969) p 322.

NEMERSON, Y. & PITLICK, F. A.: Purification and characterization of the protein component of tissue factor. Biochem. 9 (1970) p 5100.

NEWCOMB, T. & WATSON, M. E.: Elective surgery in hemophilia. II. Hematologic control. J. Amer. Med. Ass. 185 (1963) p 631.

NEWMAN, J., JOHNSON, A. J., KARPATKIN, M. H. & PUSZKIN, S.: Methods for the production of clinically effective intermediate- and high-purity factor-VIII concentrates. Brit. J. Haemat. 21 (1971) p 1.

de NICOLA, P., GIBELLI, A. & FRANDOLI, G.: Fibrinolysis in the aged: study in 196 arteriosclerotic subjects by means of the fibrin plate method. Clin. Sci. 7 (1964) p 139.

NICOLAIDES, A. N., DESAI, S., DOUGLAS, J. N., FOURIDES, G., DUPONT, P. A., LEWIS, J. D., DODSWORTH, H., LUCK, R. J. & JAMIESON, C. W.: Small doses of subcutaneous sodium heparin in preventing deep venous thrombosis after major surgery. Lancet II (1972) p 890.

NIEWIAROWSKI, S., BANKOWSKI, E. & ROGOWICKA, I.: Studies on the adsorption and activation of the Hageman factor (factor XII) by collagen and elastin. Thromb. Diath. Haemorrh. 14 (1965) p 387.

NIEWIAROWSKI, S. & KOWALSKI, E.: Formation of an antithrombinlike anticoagulant during proteolysis of fibrinogen. Bull. Acad. pol. Sci. 5 (1957) p 169.

NILÉHN, J.-E.: On symptomatic antihaemophilic globulin (AHF) deficiency. Acta Med. Scand. 171 (1962) p 491.

NILÉHN, J.-E.: a. Split products of fibrinogen after prolonged interaction with plasmin. Thromb. Diath. Haemorrh. 18 (1967) p 89.

NILÉHN, J.-E.: b. Separation and estimation of "split products" of fibrinogen and fibrin in human serum. Thromb. Diath. Haemorrh. 18 (1967) p 487.

NILÉHN, J.-E.: c. Influence of split products of fibrinogen on results of blood coagulation tests and platelet adhesiveness. Scand. J. Haematol 4 (1967) p 430.

NILÉHN, J.-E. & GANROT, P. O.: Plasmin, plasmin inhibitors and degradation products of fibrinogen in human serum during and after intravenous infusion of streptokinase. Scand. J. Clin. Lab. Invest. 20 (1967) p 113.

NILÉHN, J.-E. & GANROT, P. O.: Plasma prothrombin during treatment with dicumarol. I. Immunochemical determination of its concentration in plasma. Scand. J. Clin. Lab. Invest. 22 (1968) p 17.

NILÉHN, J.-E. & NILSSON, I. M.: Haemophilia B in a girl. Thromb. Diath. Haemorrh. 7 (1962) p 552.

NILÉHN, J.-E. & NILSSON, I. M.: Demonstration of fibrinolytic split products in human serum by an immunological method in spontaneous and induced fibrinolytic states. Scand. J. Haematol. 1 (1964) p 313.

NILÉHN, J.-E. & NILSSON, I. M.: Coagulation studies in different types of myeloma. Acta Med. Scand. Suppl. 445 (1966) p 194.

NILÉHN, J.-E. & ROBERTSON, B.: On the degradation products of fibrinogen or fibrin after infusion of streptokinase in patients with venous thrombosis. Scand. J. Haematol. 2 (1965) p 267.

NILSSON, I. M.: Ein Fall weiblicher Hämophilie und dessen Behandlung mit speziell hergestelltem, menschlichem Antihämophilieglobulin. In: Symposion über Nebenwirkungen von Arzneimitteln auf Blut und Knochenmark, Stuttgart, Germany. Schattauer, Stuttgart (1957) p 1.

NILSSON, I. M.: Blood Coagulation Studies in the Aged. In Age with a Future. Proc. VI Internat. Congr. Gerontology, Copenhagen. Munksgaard, Copenhagen (1964) p 629.

NILSSON, I. M.: Treatment of Haemophilia A and v. Willebrand's Disease. Proc. 10th Congr. int. Soc. Blood Transf. Sthlm 1964 (1965) p 1307.

NILSSON, I. M.: The development of thrombosis. Thule International Symposia Stroke, Nordiska Bokhandeln, Stockholm (1967) p 191.

NILSSON, I. M.: Fibrinolysis and fibrinolytic degradation products in renal disease. Coagulation 3 (1970) p 215.

NILSSON, I. M., AHLBERG, Å. & BJÖRLIN, G.: Clinical experience with a Swedish factor IX concentrate. Acta Med. Scand. 190 (1971) p 257.

NILSSON, I. M., ANDERSSON, L. & BJÖRKMAN, S. E.: Epsilon-aminocaproic acid (EACA) as a therapeutic agent. Based on 5 years' clinical experience. Acta Med. Scand. Suppl. 448 (1966).

NILSSON, I. M., BERGMAN, S., REITALU, J. & WALDENSTRÖM, J.: Haemophilia A in a "girl" with male sex-chromatin pattern. Lancet II (1959) p 264.

NILSSON, I. M. & BJÖRKMAN, S. E.: Experiences with ε-aminocaproic acid (ε-ACA) in the treatment of profuse menstruation. Acta Med. Scand. 177 (1965) p 445.

NILSSON, I. M. & BLOMBACK, M.: von Willebrand's disease in Sweden. Occurrence, pathogenesis and treatment. Thromb. Diath. Haemorrh. 9 (1963) p 103.

NILSSON, I. M., BLOMBÄCK, M. & AHLBERG, Å.: Our Experience in Sweden with Prophylaxis on Haemophilia. The Hemophilic and His World: Proc. 5th Congr. Wld Fed. Hemophilia. Montreal 1968: Bibl Haematol. 34 (1970) p 111.

NILSSON, I. M., BLOMBÄCK, M. & BLOMBÄCK, B.: v. Willebrand's disease in Sweden. Its pathogenesis and treatment. Acta Med. Scand. 164 (1959) p 263.

NILSSON, I. M., BLOMBÄCK, M. & von FRANCKEN, I.: On an inherited autosomal hemorrhagic diathesis with antihemophilic globulin (AHG) deficiency and prolonged bleeding time. Acta Med. Scand. 159 (1957) p 35.

NILSSON, I. M., BLOMBÄCK, M., JORPES, E., BLOMBÄCK, B. & JOHANSSON, S.-A.: v. Wilebrand's disease and its correction with human plasma fraction I-0. Acta Med. Scand. 159 (1957) p 179.

NILSSON, I. M., BLOMBÄCK, M. & RAMGREN, O.: Haemophilia in Sweden. I. Coagulation studies. Acta Med. Scand. 170 (1961) p 665.

NILSSON, I. M., BLOMBÄCK, M. & RAMGREN, O.: Haemophilia in Sweden. VI. Treatment of haemophilia A with the human antihaemophilic factor preparation (fraction I-0). Acta Med. Scand. Suppl. 379 (1962) p 61.

NILSSON, I. M., BLOMBÄCK, M. & RAMGREN, O.: Investigations on hemophilia A and B carriers. Bibl. Haematol. 26 (1966) p 26.

NILSSON, I. M., BLOMBÄCK, M., RAMGREN, O. & von FRANCKEN, I.: Haemophilia in Sweden. II. Carriers of haemophilia A and B. Acta Med. Scand. 171 (1962) p 223.

NILSSON, I. M., BLOMBÄCK, M., THILÉN, A. & von FRANCKEN, I.: Carriers of hemophilia A. A laboratory study. Acta Med. Scand. 165 (1959) p 357.

NILSSON, I. M. & HEDNER, U.: Partial purification of an activator inhibitor in serum. J. Clin. Path. 25 (1972) p 621.

NILSSON, I. M., HEDNER, U. & HOLMBERG,

L.: a. Suppression of factor VIII antibody by combined factor VIII and cyclophosphamide. Acta Med. Scand. (1973)

NILSSON, I. M., HEDNER, U. & BJÖRLIN, G.: b. Suppression of factor IX antibody in haemophilia B by factor IX and cyclophosphamide. Ann. Intern. Med. 78 (1973) p 91.

NILSSON, I. M., HEDNER, U., EKBERG, M. & DENNEBERG, T.: A circulating anticoagulant against factor V and penicillin allergy. Acta Med. Scand. (1973) In Press.

NILSSON, I. M., KROOK, H., STERNBY, N.-H., SÖDERBERG, E. & SÖDERSTRÖM, N.: Severe thrombotic disease in a young man with bone marrow and skeletal changes and with a high content of an inhibitor in the fibrinolytic system. Acta Med. Scand. 169 (1961) p 323.

NILSSON, I. M., MAGNUSSON. S. & BORCH-GREVINK, CHR.: The Duke and Ivy methods for determination of the bleeding time. Thromb. Diath. Haemorrh. 10 (1963) p 223.

NILSSON, I. M., NILÉHN, J.-E., CRONBERG, S. & NORDÉN, G.: Hypofibrinogenaemia and massive thrombosis. Acta Med. Scand. 180 (1966) p 65.

NILSSON, I. M. & OLOW, B.: a. Fibrinolysis induced by streptokinase in man. Acta Chir. Scand. 123 (1962) p 247.

NILSSON, I. M. & OLOW, B.: b. Determination of fibrinogen and fibrinogenolytic activity. Thromb. Diath. Haemorrh. 8 (1962) p 297.

NILSSON, I. M. & PANDOLFI, M.: Fibrinolytic response of the vascular wall. Thromb. Diath. Haemorrh. Suppl. 40 (1970) p 231.

NILSSON, I. M., PANDOLFI, M. & ROBERT-SON, B.: Properties of fibrinolytic activators appearing after venous stasis and intravenous injection of nicotinic acid. Coagulation 3 (1970) p 13.

NILSSON, I. M. & ROBERTSON, B.: Effect of venous occlusion on coagulation and fibrinolytic components in normal subjects. Thromb. Diath. Haemorrh. 20 (1968) p 397.

NILSSON, L. & RYBO, G.: Treatment of menorrhagia with an antifibrinolytic agent, tranexamic acid (AMCA). Acta Obstet. Gynecol. Scand. 46 (1967) p 572.

NILSSON, I. M., SJOERDSMA, A. & WAL-DENSTROM, J.: Antifibrinolytic activity and metabolism of E-aminocaproic acid in man. Lancet I (1960) p 1322.

NILSSON, I. M., SKANSE, B. & GYDELL, K.: Circulating anticoagulant after pregnancy and its response to ACTH. Acta Haematol. 19 (1958) p 40.

NILSSON, I. M. & WENCKERT, A.: Demonstra-

tion of a heparin-like anticoagulant in normal blood. I. Human blood. Acta Med. Scand. 150, Suppl. 297 (1954).

NORDENFELT, E. & NILSSON, I. M.: Antibodies against Australia-antigen in haemophiliacs. Europ. J. Clin. Biol. Res. 16 (1971) p 151.

NORMAN, J. C., COVELLI, V. H. & SISE, H. S.: Transplantation of the spleen: Experimental cure of hemophilia. Surgery 64 (1968) p 1.

NORMAN, J. C., LAMBILLIOTTE, J. P., KOJIMA, Y. & SISE, H. S.: Antihemophilic factor release by perfused liver and spleen. Relationship to hemophilia. Science 158 (1967) p 1060.

NOSSEL, H. L.: The contact phase of blood coagulation. Blackwell, Oxford (1964).

NUSSBAUM, M. & MORSE, B. S.: Plasma fibrin stabilizing factor activity in various diseases. Blood 23 (1964) p 669.

NYE, S. W., GRAHAM, J. B. & BRINKHOUS, K. M.: The partial thromboplastin time as a screening test for the detection of latent bleeders. Amer. J. Med. Sci. 243 (1962) p 55/279.

OBER, W. B., REID, D. E., ROMNEY, S. L. & MERRILL, J. P.: Renal lesions and acute renal failure in pregnancy. Amer. J. Med. 21 (1956) p 781.

O'BRIEN, E. T.: The fibrinolytic system in arteriosclerosis. J. Irish Med. Ass. 62 (1969) p 203.

O'BRIEN, J. R.: Platelets: a Portsmouth syndrome? Lancet II (1967) p 258.

O'BRIEN, J. R.: Effects of salicylates on human platelets. Lancet I (1968) p 1431.

O'CONNELL, R. A., GROSSI, C. E. & ROUS-SELOT, L. M.: Role of inhibitors of fibrinolysis in hepatic cirrhosis. Lancet II (1964) p 990.

OGSTON, D., MCANDREW, G. M. & OGSTON, C. M.: Fibrinolysis in leukaemia. J. Clin. Path. 21 (1968) p 136.

OGSTON, D., OGSTON, C. M. & FULLERTON, H. W.: The plasminogen content of thrombi. Thromb. Diath. Haemorrh. 15 (1966) p 220.

OHLSSON, K.: Preparation of human fibrinogen free from plasminogen by an immunochemical technique. Clin. Chim. Acta 25 (1969) p 221.

OKAMOTO, S. & OKAMOTO, U.: Aminomethyl-cyclohexane-carboxylic acid: AMCHA. A new potent inhibitor of the fibrinolysis. Keio J. Med. 11 (1962) p 105.

OKAMOTO, S., OSHIBA, S., MIHARA, H. & OKAMOTO, U.: Synthetic inhibitors of fibrinolysis: in vitro and in vivo mode of action. Ann. N. Y. Acad. Sci. 146 (1968) p 414.

OLLENDORFF, P.: Initiation of blood clotting and glass activation followed with a three-stage technique. Scand. J. Clin. Lab. Invest. 14 (1962) p 641.

OLOW, B.: Effect of streptokinase on postoperative changes in some coagulation factors and the fibrinolytic system. Acta Chir. Scand. 126 (1963) p 197.

OLOW, B., JOHANSSON, C., ANDERSSON, J. & EKLÖF, B.: Deep venous thrombosis treated with a standard dosage of streptokinase. Acta Chir. Scand. 136 (1970) p 181.

OLSSON, P.: Variations in antithrombin activity in plasma after major surgery. Acta Chir. Scand. 126 (1963) p 24.

O'MEARA, R. A.: Coagulative properties of cancers. Irish J. Med. Sci. 394 (1958) p 474.

O'REILLY, R. A.: The second reported kindred with hereditary resistance to oral anticoagulant drugs. New Engl. J. Med. 282 (1970) p 1448.

OWEN, C. A. JR, AMUNDSEN, M. A., THOMPSON, J. H. JR, SPITTELL, J. A. JR, BOWIE, E. J. W., STILWELL, G. G., HEWLETT, J. S., MILLS, S. D., SAUER, W. G. & GAGE, R. P.: Congenital deficiency of factor VII (hypoproconvertinemia). Amer. J. Med. 37 (1964) p 71.

OWEN, C. A. JR, BOWIE, E. J. W., DIDISHEIM, P. & THOMPSON, J. H. JR.: The Pathophysiology of von Willebrand's Disease. Haemophilia and New Haemorrhagic States. International Symposium New York 1970. Ed. K. M. Brinkhous. The University of North Carolina Press, Chapel Hill. p 187.

OWEN, C. A. JR, OELS. H. C., BOWIE, E. J. W., DIDISHEIM, P. & THOMPSON, J. H. JR: Chronic intravascular coagulation (ICF) syndrome. Thromb. Diath. Haemorrh. Suppl. 36 (1969) p 197.

OWEN, W. G. & WAGNER, R. H.: Antihemophilic factor. A new method for purification. Thromb. Res. 1 (1972) p 71.

OWREN, P. A.: The coagulation of blood; investigations on a new clotting factor. Acta Med. Scand. Suppl. 194 (1947).

OWREN, P. A.: The fifth coagulation factor ("factor V"). Preparation and properties. Biochem. J. 43 (1948) p 136.

OWREN, P. A.: The diagnostic and prognostic significance of plasma prothrombin and factor V levels in parenchymatous hepatitis and obstructive jaundice. Scand. J. Clin. Lab. Invest. 1 (1949) p 131.

OWREN, P. A.: The function of proconvertin in blood clotting and the quantitative determination of prothrombin and proconvertin. Int. Congr. Clin. Pathol. London 1951. Lancet II (1951) p 169.

OWREN, P. A.: La proconvertine. Rev. Hématol. 7 (1952) p 147.

OWREN, P. A.: The present state of the converting and accelerator factors in prothrombin conversion. Thrombose and Embolie. I. Internationale Tagung Basel 1954. Schwabe, Basel (1954) p 65.

OWREN, P. A.: Coronary thrombosis. Its mechanism and possible prevention by linolenic acid. Ann. Intern. Med. 63 (1965) p 167.

OWREN, P. A. & AAS, K.: The control of dicumarol therapy and the quantitative determination of prothrombin and proconvertin. Scand. J. Clin. Lab. Invest. 3 (1951) p 201.

PACHTER, M. R., JOHNSON, S. A., NEBLETT, T. R. & TRUANT, J. P.: Bleeding, platelets and macroglobulinemia. Amer. J. Clin. Path. 31 (1959) p 467.

PANDOLFI, M.: Studies on fibrinolysis in some tissues and in aqueous humor. Thesis. Berlingska Boktryckeriet (1969) Lund.

PANDOLFI, M.: Persistence of fibrinolytic activity in fragments of human veins cultured in vitro. Thromb. Diath. Haemorrh. 24 (1970) p 43.

PANDOLFI, M., AHLBERG, Å., TRALDI, A. & NILSSON, I. M.: Fibrinolytic activity of human synovial membranes in health and in haemophilia. Scand. J. Haemat. 9 (1972) p 572.

PANDOLFI, M., BERGENTZ, S.-E., CLAES, G. & LJUNGQVIST, U.: Localization of fibrinolytic activity in healthy and diseased renal tissue. 6th Europ. Conf. Microcirculation, Aalborg 1970 (1971) p 88.

PANDOLFI, M., BJERNSTAD, A. & NILSSON, I. M.: Technical remarks on the microscopical demonstration of tissue plasminogen activator. Thromb. Diath. Haemorrh. 27 (1972) p 88.

PANDOLFI, M., ISACSON, S. & NILSSON, I. M.: Low fibrinolytic activity in the walls of veins in patients with thrombosis. Acta Med. Scand. 186 (1969) p 1.

PANDOLFI, M., NILSSON, I. M. & HEDNER, U.: Bilateral occlusion of the retinal veins in a patient with inhibition of fibrinolysis. Ann. Ophthal. 2 (1970) p 481.

PANDOLFI, M., NILSSON, I. M., ROBERTSON, B. & ISACSON, S.: Fibrinolytic activity of human veins. Lancet II (1967) p 127.

PANDOLFI, M., ROBERTSON, B., ISACSON, S. & NILSSON, I. M.: Fibrinolytic activity of human veins in arms and legs. Thromb. Diath. Haemorrh. 20 (1968) p 247.

PAPAHADJOPOULOS, D. & HANAHAN, D. J.: Observations on the interaction of phospholipids and certain clotting factors in prothrombin activator formation. Biochim. Biophys. Acta 90 (1964) p 436.

PARASKEVAS, M., NILSSON, I. M. & MAR-

TINSSON, G.: A method for determining serum inhibitors of plasminogen activation. Scand. J. Clin. Lab. Invest. 14 (1962) p 138.

PATEK, A. J. JR & TAYLOR, F. H. L.: The blood in hemophilia. Science 84 (1936) p 271.

PAULSSEN, M.M.P., WOUTERLOOD, A.C.M. G.B. & SCHEFFERS, H.L.M.A.: Purification of the antihemophilic factor by gel filtration on agarose. Thromb. Diath. Haemorrh. 22 (1969) p 577.

PECHET, L.: Fibrinolysis. New Engl. J. Med. 273 (1965) p 966.

PENICK, G. D. & BRINKHOUS, K. M.: Relative stability of plasma antihemophilic factor (AHF) under different conditions of storage. Amer. J. Med. Sci. 232 (1956) p 434.

PENICK, G. D., DEJANOV, I. I., REDDICK, k. L. & ROBERTS, H. R.: Predisposition to intravascular coagulation. Thromb. Diath. Haemorrh. 21 (1966) p 543.

PENICK, G. D., WEBSTER, W. P., PEACOCK, E. E., HUTCHIN, P. & ZUKOSKI, C. F.: Organ Transplantation in Animal Hemophilia. Hemophilia and New Hemorrhagic States. Internat. Symp. Ed. K. M. Brinkhous. Univ. North Carolina Press, Chapel Hill (1970) p 97.

PERKINS, H. A.: Correction of the hemostatic defects in von Willebrand's disease. Blood 30 (1967) p 375.

PERKINS, H. A., MACKENZIE, M. R. & FUDENBERG, H. H.: Hemostatic defects in dysproteinemias. Blood 35 (1970) p 695.

PERRY, S.: Coagulation factors in patients with plasma protein disorders. J. Lab. Clin. Med. 61 (1963) p 411.

PERT, J. H., JOHNSON, A. J. & WICKERHAUSER, M.: Preparation of Factors II, VII, IX and X Concentrates and Other Blood Components from Blood Collected in ACD (A) Anticoagulant. Hemophilia and New Hemorrhagic States. International Symposium, New York. Ed. K. M. Brinkhous. The University of North Carolina Press, Chapel Hill (1970) p 39.

PETERSON, H.-I.: Experimental studies on fibrinolysis in growth and spread of tumour. Acta Chir. Scand. Suppl. 394 (1968).

PFEIFER, G. W.: Experimentelle Untersuchungen zur frage eines diaplacentaren Effektes von Streptokinase. Klin. Wschr. 43 (1965) p 775.

PFEIFER, G. W.: The use of thrombolytic therapy in obstetrics and gynaecology. Aust. Ann. Med. 19, Suppl. 1 (1970) p 28.

PFEIFER, G. W., DOERR, F. & BROD, K. H.: Zur Pharmakokinetik von 131J-Streptokinase am Menschen. Klin. Wochenschr. 47 (1969) p 482.

PHILLIPS, L. L., SKRODELIS, V. & WOLFF, J. A.: Normal fibrinolytic system in two cases of familial hypofibrinogenemia. Acta Haematol. 30 (1963) p 244.

PIEL, C. F. & PHIBBS, R. H.: The hemolytic-uremic syndrome. Pediat. Clin. N. Amer. 13 (1966) p 295.

PISANO, J. J., FINLAYSON, J. S., BRONZERT, T. J. & PEYTON, M. P.: ε-(g-glutamyl) lysine crosslink formation in fibrin prepared under various conditions. International Soc. of Thrombosis and Haemostasis, Washington (1972).

PITNEY, W. R.: The assay of antihaemophilic globulin (AHG) in plasma. Brit. J. Haemat. 2 (1956) p 250.

PITNEY, W. R.: Disseminated intravascular coagulation. Sem. Hemat. 8 (1971) p 65.

PITNEY, W. R., BELL, W. R. & BOLTON, G.: a. Blood fibrinolytic activity during Arvin therapy. Brit. J. Haematol. 16 (1969) p 165.

PITNEY, W. R., BRAY, C., HOLT, P.J.L. & BOLTON, G.: b. Acquired resistance to treatment with Arvin. Lancet I (1969) p 79.

PITTMAN, G. R., SENHAUSER, D. A. & LOWNEY, J. F.: Acute promyelocytic leukemia: A report of 3 autopsied cases. Amer. J. Clin. Path. 46 (1966) p 214.

PIZZO, S. V., SCHWARTZ, M. L., HILL, R. L. & MCKEE, P. A.: The effect of plasmin on the subunit structure of human fibrinogen. J. Biol. Chem. 247 (1972) p 636.

POLIWODA, H.: In H. Hess (ed.): Thrombolytische Therapie. Symposion der Deutschen Gesellschaft für Angiologie. München, Oktober 1966. Schattauer, Stuttgart (1967) p 79.

PONN, R. B., KELLOGG, E. A., KORFF, J. M. et al.: The role of the splenic macrophage in antihemophilic (factor VIII) synthesis. Arch. Surg. 103 (1971) p 398,

POOL, J. G.: The effect of several variables on cryoprecipitated factor VIII (AHG) concentrates. Transfusion 7 (1967) p 165.

POOL, J. G.: Cryoprecipitated factor VIII concentrate. Thromb. Diath. Haemorrh. Suppl. 35 (1969) p 35.

POOL, J. G.: HERSHGOLD, E. J. & PAPPENHAGEN, A. R.: High potency antihemophilic factor concentrate prepared from cryoglobulin precipitate. Nature 203 (1964) p 312.

POOL, J. G. & ROBINSON, J.: Observations on plasma banking and transfusion procedures for haemophilic patients using a quantitative assay for antihemophilic globulin (AHG). Brit. J. Haematol. 5 (1959) p 24.

POOL, J. G. & SHANNON, A. E.: Production of high-potency concentrates of antihaemophilic globulin in a closed-bag system. New Engl. J. Med. 273 (1965) p 1443.

POOL, J. G. & SPAET, T. H.: Ethionine-induced

depression of plasma antihemophilic globulin in the rat. Proc. Soc. Exp. Biol. Med. 87 (1954) p 54.

da PRADA, M., PLETSCHER, A., TRANZER, J. P. & KNUCHEL, H.: Subcellular localization of 5-hydroxytryptamine and histamine in blood platelets. Nature 216 (1967) p 1315.

PRENTICE, C. R. M., BRECKENRIDGE, R. T. & RATNOFF, O. D.: Studies on the conversion of prothrombin to thrombin: With notes on the cation requirement for this reaction. J. Lab. Clin. Med. 69 (1967) p 229.

PRENTICE, C.R.M., LINDSAY, R. M., BARR, R. D., FORBES, C. D., KENNEDY, A. C., MCNICOL, G. P. & DOUGLAS, A. S.: Renal complications in haemophilia and Christmas disease. Quart. J. Med. 40 (1971) p 47.

PRENTICE, C. R. M. & RATNOFF, O. D.: The action of Russell's viper venom on factor V and the prothrombin-converting principle. Brit. J. Haematol. 16 (1969) p 291.

PRENTICE, C. R. M., TURPIE, A. G. G., HASSANEIN, A. A., MCNICOL, G. P. & DOUGLAS. A. S.: Changes in platelet behaviour during arvin therapy. Lancet I (1969) p 644.

PRESTON, F. E., MALIA, R. G., BLACKBURN, E. K. & PLATTS, M.: FDP in glomerulonephritis. Brit. Med. J. 4 (1971) p 171.

PRICHARD, R. W. & VANN, R. L.: Congenital afibrinogenemia. Report on a child without fibrinogen and review of the literature. Amer. J. Dis. Child. 88 (1954) p 703.

PROCTOR, R. R. & RAPAPORT, S. I.: The partial thromboplastin time with kaolin. A simple screening test for first stage plasma clotting factor deficiencies. Amer. J. Clin. Pathol. 36 (1961) p 212.

PRYDZ, H.: b. Studies on proconvertin (factor VII). II. Purification. Scand. J. Clin. Lab. Invest. 16 (1964) p 101.

PRYDZ, H.: a. Studies on proconvertin (factor VII). IV. The adsorption on barium sulphate. Scand. J. Clin. Lab. Invest. 16 (1964) p 409.

PRYDZ, H.: a. Studies on proconvertin (factor VII). VI. The production in rabbits of an antiserum against factor VII. Scand. J. Clin. Lab. Invest. 17 (1965) p 66.

PRYDZ, H.: b. Studies on proconvertin (factor VII). VII. Further studies on the biosynthesis of factor VII in rat cell suspensions. Scand. J. Clin. Lab. Invest. 17 (1965) p 143.

PRYDZ, H.: c. Some characteristics of purified factor VII preparations. Scand. J. Clin. Lab. Invest. Suppl. 84 (1965) p 78.

PRYDZ, H. & GLADHAUG, A.: Factor X. Immunological studies. Thromb. Diath. Haemorrh. 25 (1971) p 157.

QUICK, A. J.: The prothrombin in hemophilia

and in obstructive jaundice. J. Biol. Chem. 109 (1935) p 73.

QUICK, A. J.: The hemorrhagic diseases and the physiology of hemostasis. Thomas, Springfield (1942).

QUICK, A. J.: The Minot-von Willebrand syndrome. Amer. J. Med. Sci. 253 (1967) p 520.

RABINER, S. F., GOLDFINE, I. D., HART, A., SUMMARIA, L. & ROBBINS, K. C.: Radioimmunoassay of human plasminogen and plasmin. J. Lab. Clin. Med. 74 (1969) p 265.

RABINER, S. F., TELFER, M. & FAJARDO, R.: Home transfusions of hemophiliacs. J A M A 221 (1972) p 885.

RAFELSON, M. E. JR & BOOYSE, F.: Molecular aspects of platelet aggregation. Platelet aggregation. Ed. J. P. Caen. Masson, Paris (1971).

RAKE, M. O., SHILKIN, K. B., WINCH, J., FLUTE, P. T., LEWIS, M. L. & WILLIAMS, R.: Early and intensive therapy of intravascular coagulation in acute liver failure. Lancet II (1971) p 1215.

RAMGREN, O.: a. Haemophilia in Sweden. V. Medico-social aspects. Acta Med. Scand. 171, Suppl. 379 (1962) p 37.

RAMGREN, O.: b. A clinical and medico-social study of haemophilia in Sweden. Acta Med. Scand. Suppl. 379 (1962) p 114.

RAMGREN, O., NILSSON, I. M. & BLOMBÄCK, M.: Haemophilia in Sweden. IV. Hereditary investigations. Acta Med. Scand. 171 (1962) p 759.

RAPAPORT, S. I.: Plasma thromboplastin antecedent levels in patients receiving coumarin anticoagulants and in patients with Laennec's cirrhosis. Proc. Soc. Exp. Biol. Med. 108 (1961) p 115.

RAPAPORT, S. I., AMES, S. B. & MIKKELSEN, S.: The levels of antihemophilic globulin and proaccelerin in fresh and bank blood. Amer. J. Clin. Pathol. 31 (1959) p 297.

RAPAPORT, S. I., AMES, S. B., MIKKELSEN, S. & GOODMAN, J. R.: Plasma clotting factors in chronic hepatocellular disease. New Engl. J. Med. 263 (1960) p 278.

RAPAPORT, S. I. & HJORT, P. F.: The blood clotting properties of rabbit peritoneal leukocytes in vitro. Thromb. Diath. Haemorrh. 17 (1967) p 222.

RAPAPORT, S. I., PROCTOR, R. R., PATCH, M. J. & YETTRA, M.: The mode of inheritance of PTA deficiency: Evidence for the existence of major PTA deficiency and minor PTA deficiency. Blood 18 (1961) p 149.

RATNOFF, O. D.: A familial trait characterized by deficiency of a clot-promoting fraction of plasma. J. Lab. Clin. Med. 44 (1954) p 915.

RATNOFF, O. D.: a. Bleeding syndromes. Thomas, Springfield (1960) p 278.

RATNOFF, O. D.: b. "Hageman trait". Thromb. Diath. Haemorrh. Suppl. 1 (1960) p 116.

RATNOFF, O. D.: PTA deficiency and Hageman trait. Series Haematol. 7 (1965) p 29.

RATNOFF, O. D.: Disseminated intravascular coagulation: new bottles for an old wine. Calif. Med. 111 (1969) p 224.

RATNOFF, O. D., BUSSE, R. J. JR & SHEON, R. P.: Medical intelligence. The demise of John Hageman. New Engl. J. Med. 279 (1968) p 760.

RATNOFF, O. D. & COLOPY, J. E.: A familial hemorrhagic trait associated with deficiency of a clot-promoting fraction of plasma. J. Clin. Invest. 34 (1955) p 602.

RATNOFF, O. D. & DAVIE, E. W.: The purification of activated Hageman factor (activated factor XII). Biochemistry 1 (1962) p 967.

RATNOFF, O. D., KASS, L. & LANG, P. D.: Studies on the purification of antihemophilic factor (factor VIII). II. Separation of partially purified antihemophilic factor by gel filtration of plasma. J. Clin. Invest. 48 (1969) p 957.

RAYNER, H., PARASKEVAS, F., ISRAELS, L. G. & ISRAELS, E. D.: Fibrinogen breakdown products: Identification and assay in serum and urine. J. Lab. Clin. Med. 74 (1969) p 586.

REDDY, K. N. N. & MARKUS, G.: Mechanism of activation of human plasminogen by streptokinase. Presence of active center in streptokinase-plasminogen complex. J. Biol. Chem. 247 (1972) p 1683.

REID, H. A.: Maintenance dose of Arvin. Lancet I (1969) p 1048.

REID, H. A., THEAN, P. C., CHAN, K. E. & BAHAROM, A. R.: Clinical effects of bites by malayan viper (ancistrodon rhodostoma). Lancet I (1963) p 617.

de RENZO, E. C., BOGGIANO, E. & HUMMEL, B. C. W.: Interaction of streptokinase with human plasminogen and human plasmin. Fed. Proc. 24 (1965) p 260.

RIMON, A., SHAMASH, Y. & SHAPIRO, B.: The plasmin inhibitor of human plasma. J. Biol. Chem. 241 (1966) p 5102.

RIZZA, C. R. & BIGGS, R.: Treatment of congenital deficiencies of factor VIII and factor IX. Thromb. Diath. Haemorrh. Suppl. 35 (1969) p 73.

ROBBINS, K. C. & SUMMARIA, I.: Biochemistry of fibrinolysis. Thromb. Diath. Haemorrh. Suppl. 47 (1971) p 9.

ROBBINS, K. C., SUMMARIA, L., ELWYN, D. & BARLOW, G. H.: Further studies on the purification and characterization of human plasminogen and plasmin. J. Biol. Chem. 240 (1965) p 541.

ROBBINS, K. C., SUMMARIA, L., HSIEH, B. & SHAH, R. H.: The peptide chains of human plasmin. Mechanism of activation of human plasminogen to plasmin. J. Biol. Chem. 242 (1967) p 2333.

ROBBOY, S. J., COLMAN, R. W. & MINNA, J. D.: Pathology of disseminated intravascular coagulation (DIC). Analysis of 26 cases. Human Path. 3 (1972) p 327.

ROBBOY, S. J., LEWIS, E. J., SCHUR, P. H. & COLMAN, R. W.: Circulating anticoagulants to factor VIII. Immunochemical studies and clinical response to factor VIII concentrates. Amer. J. Med. 49 (1970) p 742.

ROBERTS, H. R., GRIZZLE, J. E., MCLESTER, W. D. & PENICK, G. D.: Genetic variants of hemophilia B: Detection by means of a specific PTC inhibitor. J. Clin. Invest. 47 (1968) p 360.

ROBERTS, H. R., SCALES, M. B., MADISON, J. T., WEBSTER, W. P. & PENICK, G. D.: A clinical and experimental study of acquired inhibitors of factor VIII. Blood 26 (1965) p 805.

ROBERTSON, B. R.: a. Effect of nicotinic acid on fibrinolytic activity in health, in thrombotic disease and in liver cirrhosis. Acta Chir. Scand. 137 (1971) p 643.

ROBERTSON, B. R.: b. On thrombosis, thrombolysis, and fibrinolysis. I. Thrombolytic therapy of deep venous thrombosis. II. Assay of individual fibrinolytic response. Acta Chir. Scand. (1971) Suppl. 421.

ROBERTSON, B. R., NILSSON, I. M. & NYLANDER, G.: Value of streptokinase and heparin in treatment of acute deep venous thrombosis. Acta Chir. Scand. 134 (1968) p 203.

ROBERTSON, B. R., NILSSON, I. M. & NYLANDER, G.: Thrombolytic effect of streptokinase as evaluated by phlebography of deep venous thrombi of the leg. Acta Chir. Scand. 136 (1970) p 173.

ROBERTSON, B. R., NILSSON, I. M., NYLANDER, G. & OLOW, B.: Effect of streptokinase and heparin on patients with deep venous thrombosis. A coded examination. Acta Chir. Scand. 133 (1967) p 205.

ROBERTSON, B. R., PANDOLFI, M. & NILSSON, I. M.: a. Response of local fibrinolytic activity to venous occlusion of arms and legs in healthy volunteers. Acta Chir. Scand. 138 (1972) p 437.

ROBERTSON, B. R., PANDOLFI, M. & NILSSON, I. M.: b. "Fibrinolytic capacity" in healthy volunteers as estimated from effect of venous occlusion of arms. Acta Chir. Scand. 138 (1972) p 429.

ROBERTSON, B. R., PANDOLFI, M. & NILSSON, I. M.: c. "Fibrinolytic capacity" in healthy volunteers at different ages as studied by standardized venous occlusion of arms and legs Acta Med. Scand. 191 (1972) p 199.

RODRIGUEZ-ERDMANN, F.: Production of the Sanarelli-Shwartzman phenomenon by platelet-factor 3. Thromb. Diath. Haemorrh. Suppl. 36 (1969) p 63.

RODRIGUEZ-ERDMANN, F. & GUTTMANN, R. D.: Coagulation in renal allograft rejection. New Engl. J. Med. 281 (1969) p 1428.

ROSENBERG, J. C., BROERSMA, R. J., BULLEMER, G., MARUMELL, E. F., LENAGHAN, R. & ROSENBERG, B. F.: Relationship of platelets, blood coagulation and fibrinolysis to hyperacute rejection of renal xenografts. Transplantation 8 (1969) p 152.

ROSENMANN, E., KANTER, A., BACANI, R. A., PIRANI. C. L. & POLLAK, V. E.: Fatal late post-partum intravascular coagulation with acute renal failure. Amer. J. Med. Sci. 257 (1969) p 259.

ROSENTHAL, R. L.: Properties of plasma thromboplastin antecedent (PTA) in relation to blood coagulation. J. Lab. Clin. Med. 45 (1955) p 123.

ROSENTHAL, R. L.: Plasma thromboplastin antecedent (PTA) activity. Thromb. Diath. Haemorrh. Suppl. 3 (1961) p 379.

ROSENTHAL, R. L., DRESKIN, O. H. & ROSENTHAL, N.: New hemophilia-like disease caused by deficiency of a third plasma thromboplastin factor. Proc. Soc. Exp. Biol. Med. 82 (1953) p 171.

ROSENTHAL, R. L. & SLOAN, E.: PTA (factor XI) levels and coagulation studies after plasma infusions in PTA-deficient patients. J. Lab. Clin. Med. 66 (1965) p 709.

ROSNER, F. & RITZ, N. D.: The defibrination syndrome. Arch. Intern. Med. 117 (1966) p 17.

ROSSI, E. C. & GREEN, D.: A study of platelet retention by glass bead columns ('platelet adhesiveness' in normal subjects). Brit. J. Haemat. 23 (1972) p 47.

RUDENSTAM, C.-M.: Experimental studies on trauma and metastasis formation. Acta Chir. Scand. Suppl. 391 (1968).

RYBO, G.: Plasminogen activators in the endometrium. Clinical aspects. Acta Obstet. Gynecol. Scand. 45 (1966) p 429.

SAHUD, M. A. & AGGELER, P. M.: Platelet dysfunction—differentiation of a newly recognized primary type from that produced by aspirin. New Engl. J. Med. 280 (1969) p 453.

SAITO, H., SHIOYA, M., KOIE, K., KAMIYA, T. & KATSUMI, O.: Congenital combined deficiency of factor V and factor VIII. A case report and the effect of transfusion of normal plasma and hemophilic blood. Thromb. Diath. Haemorrh. 22 (1969) p 316.

SALZMAN, E. W.: Measurement of platelet adhesiveness. A simple in vitro technique demonstrating an abnormality in von Willebrand's disease. J. Lab. Clin. Med. 62 (1963) p 724.

SALZMAN, E. W.: Does intravascular coagulation occur in hemorrhagic shock in man? J. Trauma 8 (1968) p 867.

SAWYER, W. D., ALKJAERSIG, N., FLETCHER, A. P. & SHERRY, S.: Thrombolytic therapy. Basic and therapeutic consideration. Arch. Internal. Med. 107 (1961) p 274.

SCHIFFMAN, S., THEODOR, I. & RAPAPORT, S. I.: Separation from Russell's viper venom of one fraction reacting with factor X and another reacting with factor V. Biochemistry 8 (1969) p 1397.

SCHMUTZLER, R.: Thrombolytic treatment of acute peripheral arterial and venous occlusions. Angiologica 5 (1968) p 119.

SCHMUTZLER, R.: Klinik der thrombolytischen Behandlung. Internist 10 (1969) p 21.

SCHNEIDER, C. L.: "Fibrin embolism" (disseminated intravascular coagulation) with defibrination as one of the end results during placenta abruptio. Surg. Gynecol. Obstet. 92 (1951) p 27.

SCHNEIDER, C. L.: When patients hemorrhage at delivery. Postgrad. Med. 43 (1968) p 133.

SCHOENMAKERS, J. G. G., KURSTJENS, R. M., HAANEN, C. & ZILLIKEN, F.: Purification of activated bovine Hageman factor. Thromb. Diath. Haemorrh. 9 (1963) p 546.

SCHOENMAKERS, J. G. G., MATZE, R., HAANEN C. & ZILLIKEN, F.: Hageman factor, a novel sialoglycoprotein with esterase activity. Biochim. Biophys. Acta 101 (1965) p 166.

SCHULMAN, I., SMITH, C. H., ERLANDSON, M. & FORT, E.: Vascular hemophilia: A familial hemorrhagic disease in males and females characterized by combined antihemophilic globulin deficiency and vascular abnormality. Amer. J. Dis. Child. 90 (1955) p 526.

SCHWARZ, M. L., PIZZO, S. V., HILL, R. L. & MCKEE, P. A.: The subunit structures of human plasma and platelet factor XIII (fibrin stabilizing factor). J. Biol. Chem. 246 (1971) p 5851.

SCHWARZ, M. L., PIZZO, S. V., HILL, R. L. & MCKEE, P. A.: Molecular weight and subunit structure of plasma and platelet factor XIII. International Soc. of Thrombosis and Haemostasis, Washington (1972).

SCHWICK, H. G. & HEIMBURGER, N.: Biochemie der Fibrinolyse. Thromb. Diath. Haemorrh. Suppl. 32 (1969) p 9.

SEEGERS, W. H.: Purification of prothrombin and thrombin: Chemical properties of purified preparations. J. Biol. Chem. 136 (1940) p 103.

SEEGERS, W. H.: Coagulation of the blood. Harvey Lect. 47 (1951–52) p 180.

SEEGERS, W. H.: Prothrombin. Published for The Commonwealth Fund by Harvard University Press. Cambridge, Mass. (1962).

SEEGERS, W. H.: Enzyme theory of blood clotting. Fed. Proc. 23 (1964) p 749.

SEEGERS, W. H.: Use and regulation of the blood clotting mechanisms. Blood clotting enzymology. Ed. Walter T. Seegers. Academic Press, New York and London, Chapter 1 (1967) p 1.

SEEGERS, W. H., MCCOY, L. & MARCINIAK, E.: Blood-clotting enzymology. Three basic reactions. Clin. Chem. 14 (1968) p 97.

SEEGERS, W. H., MURANO, G. & MCCOY, L.: Structural changes in prothrombin during activation: A theory. Thromb. Diath. Haemorrh. 23 (1970) p 26.

SEEGERS, W. H., SCHRÖER, H. & MARCINIAK, E.: Activation of prothrombin. Blood clotting enzymology. Ed. Walter H. Seegers. Academic Press, New York and London (1967) p 104.

SEIP, M. & KJAERHEIM, Å.: A familial platelet disease—hereditary thrombasthenic—thrombopathic thrombocytopenia. Scand. J. Clin. Lab. Invest. Suppl. 84, 17 (1965) p 159.

SELIGSOHN, U. & RAMOT, B.: Combined factor-V and factor-VIII deficiency: Report of four cases. Brit. J. Haematol. 16 (1969) p 475.

SEN, N. N., SEN, R., DENSON, K. W. E. & BIGGS, R.: A modified method for the assay of factor IX. Thromb. Diath. Haemorrh. 18 (1967) p 241.

SHAMASH, Y. & RIMON, A.: The plasmin inhibitors of plasma. I. A method for their estimation. Thromb. Diath. Heamorrh. 12 (1964) p 119.

SHANBERGE, J. N., SARELIS, A. & REGAN, E. E.: The effect of heparin on plasma thromboplastin formation. J. Lab. Clin. Med. 54 (1959) p 501.

SHANBROM, E.: Clinical experience with factor IX concentrates (prothrombin complex). Hemophilia and New Hemorrhagic States. International Symposium, New York. Ed. K. M. Brinkhous. The University of North Carolina Press, Chapel Hill (1970) p 27.

SHANBROM, E. & THELIN, M.: Experimental prophylaxis of severe haemophilia with a factor VIII concentrate. J A M A 208 (1969) p 1853.

SHAPIRO, S. S.: The immunological character of acquired inhibitors of antihaemophilic globulin (factor VIII) and the kinetics of their interaction with factor VIII. J. Clin. Invest. 46 (1967) p 147.

SHAPIRO, S. S. & CARROLL, K. S.: Acquired factor VIII antibodies: Further immunologic and electrophoretic studies. Science 160 (1968) p 786.

SHAPIRO, S. S. & MARTINEZ, J.: Human prothrombin metabolism in normal man and in hypocoagulable subjects. J. Clin. Invest. 48 (1969) p 1292.

SHERMAN, L. A., GOLDSTEIN, M. A. & SISE, H. S.: Circulating anticoagulant (antifactor VIII) treated with immunosuppressive drugs. Thromb. Diath. Haemorrh. 21 (1969) p 249.

SHERRY, S.: a. Fibrinolysis. Ann. Rev. Med. 19 (1968) p 247.

SHERRY, S.: b. Urokinase. Internal. Med. 69 (1968) p 415.

SHERRY, S.: Urokinase pulmonary embolism trial. Phase 1. Results. J. Amer. Med. Ass. 214 (1970) p 2163.

SHERRY, S., ALKJAERSIG, N. & FLETCHER, A. P.: Activity of plasmin and streptokinase-activator on substituted arginine and lysine esters. Thromb. Diath. Haemorrh. 16 (1966) p 18.

SHERRY, S., FLETCHER, A. P. & ALKJAERSIG, N.: Fibrinolysis and fibrinolytic activity in man. Physiol. Rev. 39 (1959) p 343.

SHERRY, S., FLETCHER, A. P. & ALKJAERSIG, N.: Fibrinolytic bleeding and its management. Ann. N. Y. Acad. Sci. 115 (1964) p 481.

SHULMAN, S., LANDABURU, R. H. & SEEGERS, W. H.: Biophysical studies on platelet cofactor I preparations. Thromb. Diath. Haemorrh. 4 (1960) p 336.

SIBINGA, C. Th. S., GÖKEMEYER, J. D. M., ten KATE, L. P. & BOS-VAN ZWOL, F.: Combined deficiency of factor V and factor VIII: Report of a family and genetic analysis. Brit. J. Haemat. 23 (1972) p 467.

SIGG, P. E. & DUCKERT, F.: Ein neuer Test zur Bestimmung des fibrinstabilisierenden Faktors. Schw. med. Wochenschr. 93 (1963) p 1455.

SIGSTAD, H. & LAMVIK, J.: Haemorrhagic diathesis, fibrinolysis and fibrinogenopenia in prostatic cancer: Report of a case. Acta Med. Scand. 173 (1963) p 215.

SILWER, J.: von Willebrand's disease in Sweden. Acta Pediat. Scand. Suppl. 238 (1973).

SILWER, J. & NILSSON, I. M.: On a Swedish family with v. Willebrand's disease with 51 affected members. Acta Med. Scand. 175 (1964) p 627.

SIMMONS, A., SCHWABBAUER, M. L. & EARHART, C. A.: Automated platelet counting with the autoanalyser. J. Lab. Clin. Med. 77 (1971) p 656.

SIMSON, L. R., OBERMAN, H. A. & PENNER, J. A.: Clinical evaluation of cryoprecipitated factor VIII. J. Amer. Med. Ass. 199 (1967) p 554.

SINGER, K. & RAMOT, B.: Pseudohemophilia type B. Hereditary hemorrhagic diathesis characterized by prolonged bleeding time and decrease in antihemophilic factor. Arch Internal. Med. 97 (1956) p 715.

SIRRIDGE, M. S.: Waldenström's macroglobulinemia with cryoglobulinemia. Ann. Internal. Med. 53 (1960) p 380.

SKJÖRTEN, F.: Generalized Shwartzman reaction. Acta Path. Microbiol. Scand. 68 (1966) p 517.

SMINK, M. MCL., DANIEL, T. M., RATNOFF, O. D. & STAVITSKY, A. B.: Immunologic demonstration of a deficiency of Hageman factor-like material in Hageman trait. J. Lab. Clin. Med. 69 (1967) p 819.

SMITH, C. M., MILLER, G. E. & BRECKEN-RIDGE, R. T.: Factor VIII concentrates in outpatient therapy. J A M A 220 (1972) p 1352.

SOMER, J. B. & CASTALDI, P. A.: Coagulation factor IX in normal and haemophilia B plasma. Brit. J. Haematol. 18 (1970) p 147.

SORIA, J., SORIA, C., SAMAMA, M., COUPIER, J., GIRARD, M. L., BOUSSER, J. & BILSKI-PASQUIER, G.: Dysfibrinogénémies acquises dans les atteintes hépatiques sévères. Coagulation 3 (1970) p 37.

SOULIER, J. P., BLATRIX, C. & STEINBUCH, M.: Fractions "coagulantes" contenant les facteurs de coagulation absorbables par le phosphate tricalcique. Presse Méd. 72 (1964) p 1223.

SOULIER, J. P., LARRIEU, M. J., DUBRISAY, J. & MAHOUDEAU, D.: Étude biologique de deux cas d'afibrinogénémie congénitale. Rev. Hématol. 10 (1955) p 689.

SOULIER, J. P., MÉNACHÉ, D., STEINBUCH, M., BLATRIX, CH. & JOSSO, F.: Preparation and clinical use of P. P. S. B. (factors II, VII, X and IX concentrate). Thromb. Diath. Haemorrh. Suppl. 35 (1969) p 61.

SOULIER, J. P. & PROU-WARTELLE, O.: Nouvelles données sur les facteurs Hageman et P. T. A. et sur le "contact". Rev. Franc. Etud. Clin. Biol. 4 (1959) p 932.

SOULIER, J. P., PROU-WARTELLE, O. & MÉNACHÉ, D.: Hageman trait and PTA deficiency. The role of contact of blood with glass. Brit. J. Haematol. 5 (1959) p 121.

SPAET, T. H. & ERICHSON, R. B.: The Vascular Wall in the Pathogenesis of Thrombosis. Proc. 2nd Internat. Conf. Thrombosis, Basel (1965) p 67.

SPEER, R. J., RIDGWAY, H. & HILL, J. M.: Activated human Hageman factor (XII). Thromb. Diath. Haemorrh. 14 (1965) p 1.

STARR, K. J. & PETRIE, J. C.: Drug interactions in patients on long-term oral anticoagulant and antihypertensive, adrenergic neuron-blocking drugs. Brit. Med. J. 4 (1972) p 133.

STAVEM, P., JEREMIC, M., HJORT, P. F., WISLÖFF, F., VOGT, E., ÖYEN, R., ABRA-HAMSEN, A. F. & SÖVDE, A.: Hereditary thrombocytopenia with excessively prolonged bleeding time. Scand. J. Haematol. 6 (1969) p 250.

STEFANINI, M., EWBANK, R. L. & ANDRACKI, E. G.: Deficiency of fibrin stabilizing factor: Report of a case, probably congenital, with observations on the effects of treatment with ε-aminocaproic acid and with prednisone. Amer. J. Clin. Path. 57 (1972) p 364.

STEICHELE, D. F.: Consumption coagulopathy in obstetrics and gynecology. Thromb. Diath. Haemorrh. Suppl. 36 (1969) p 177.

STEIN, I. M., COHEN, B. D. & KORNHAUSER, R. S.: Guanidinosuccinic acid in renal failure, experimental azotemia and inborn errors of the urea cycle. New Engl. J. Med. 280 (1969) p 926.

STEINBUCH, M., BLATRIX, CH. & JOSSO, F.: Activité antiplasmine, antitrypsine et anti-thrombine de l'alpha$_2$-macroglobuline. Transfusion (Paris) 10 (1967) p 103.

STEINBUCH, M., QUENTIN, M. & PEJAUDIER, L.: Specific technique for the isolation of human α_2-macroglobulin. Nature 205 (1965) p 1227.

STENFLO, J.: a. Vitamin K and the biosynthesis of prothrombin. I. Identification and purification of a dicoumarol-induced abnormal prothrombin from bovine plasma. J. Biol. Chem. 247 (1972) p 8160.

STENFLO, J.: b. Vitamin K and the biosynthesis of prothrombin. II. Structural comparison of normal and dicoumarol-induced bovine prothrombin. J. Biol. Chem. 247 (1972) p 8167.

STIEHM, E. R., KUPLIC, L. S. & UEHLING, D. T.: Urinary fibrin split products in human renal disease. J. Lab. Clin. Med. 77 (1971) p 843.

STITES, D. P., HERSHGOLD, E. J., PERLMAN, J. D. & FUDENBERG, H. H.: Factor VIII detection by hemagglutination inhibition: haemophilia A and von Willebrand's disease. Science 171 (1971) p 196.

STORM, O., OLLENDORFF, P., DREWSEN, E. & TANG, P.: Deep Venous Thrombosis Treated with Plasmin. Results of a Double Blind Trial, International Society on Thrombosis and Haemostasis. II. Congress Oslo, Norway (1971) p 136.

STRAUB, P. W.: A study of fibrinogen production by human liver slices *in vitro* by an immunoprecipitin method. J. Clin. Invest. 42 (1963) p 130.

STRAUB, P. W. & FRICK, P. G.: The coagulation disorder in promyelocytic leukemia. Helv. med. Acta 34 (1967) p 44.

STRAUSS, H. S.: Acquired circulating anticoagulants in hemophilia A. New Engl. J. Med. 281 (1969) p 866.

STRAUSS, H. S. & BLOOM, G. E.: von Willebrand's disease. Use of platelet adhesiveness test in diagnosis and family investigation. New Engl. J. Med. 273 (1965) p 171.

STRAUSS, H. S. & MERLER, E.: Characterization and properties of an inhibitor of factor VIII in the plasma of patients with hemophilia A following repeated transfusions. Blood 30 (1967) p 137.

SUOMELA, H.: Preparation of a highly purified human factor IX. IVth International Congress on Thrombosis and Haemostasis Vienna (1973) p 140.

SURGENOR, D. M., WILSON, N. A. & HENRY, A. S.: Factor V from human plasma. Thromb. Diath. Haemorrh. 5 (1961) p 1.

SWAN, C. H. J., ALEXANDER-WILLIAMS, J. & COOKE, W. T.: Fibrinolysis in colonic disease. Gut 11 (1970) p 588.

SVANBERG, L., HEDNER, U. & ÅSTEDT, B.: Value of determination of F. D. P. during pregnancy with an immunochemical and a latex agglutination inhibition method. Acta Obstet. Gynec. Scand. 53 (1974) p 81.

TAKADA, A., TAKADA, Y. & AMBRUS, J. L.: Proactivators in the fibrinolysin system. Thromb. Diath. Haemorrh. Suppl. 47 (1971) p 37.

TAKADA, A., TAKADA, Y. & AMBRUS, J. L.: Further studies of plasminogen proactivator. Biochim. Biophys. Acta 263 (1972) p 610.

TAKASHIMA, S., KOGA, M. & TANAKA, K.: Fibrinolytic activity of human brain and cerebrospinal fluid. Brit. J. Exp. Pathol. 50 (1969) p 533.

TAVENNER, R. W. H.: Use of tranexamic acid in control of haemorrhage after extraction of teeth in haemophilia and Christmas disease. Brit. Med. J. 2 (1972) p 314.

TAYLOR, L. M. JR, SLADE, C. L., PIZZO, S. V., HILL, R. L. & MCKEE, P. A.: The equivalence of fragment E from human fibrinogen and fibrin. Internat. Soc. on Thrombosis and Haemostasis, Washington 1972.

TELFER, T. P., DENSON, K. W. & WRIGHT, D. R.: A "new" coagulation defect. Brit. J. Haematol. 2 (1956) p 308.

THOMAS, D. P., NIEWIAROWSKI, S., MYERS, A. R., BLOCH, K. J. & COLMAN, R. W.: A comparative study of four methods for detecting fibrinogen degradation products in patients with various diseases. New Engl. J. Med. 283 (1970) p 663.

THOMAS, D. P. & WESSLER, S.: Stasis thrombi induced by bacterial endotoxin. Circ. Res. 14 (1964) p 486.

TOCANTINS, L. M., CARROLL, R. T. & MC BRIDE, I. J.: A lipid anticoagulant from brain tissue. Proc. Soc. Exp. Biol. Med. 68 (1948) p 110.

TODD, A. S.: The histological localization of fibrinolysin activator. J. Path. Bact. 78 (1959) p 281.

TODD, A. S. & NUNN, A.: Fibrinolytic activity in tissues and thrombi. Acta of the First International Symposium on Tissue Factors in the Homeostasis of the Coagulation-Fibrinolysis System. Florence (1967) p 57.

TODD, M. & WRIGHT, I. S.: Factor XI (P.T.A.) deficiency with no hemorrhagic symptoms. Thromb. Diath. Haemorrh. 11 (1964) p 187.

TOMAR, R. H. & TAYLOR, F. B.: The streptokinase-human plasminogen activator complex. Composition and identity of a subcomponent with activator activity. Biochem. J. 125 (1971) p 793.

TOVI, D.: Studies on fibrinolysis in the central nervous system with special reference to intracranial haemorrhages and to the effect of antifibrinolytic drugs. Umeå University Medical Dissertations, No. 8 (1972).

TOVI, D., NILSSON, I. M. & THULIN, C.-A.: b. a. Fibrinolytic activity of the cerebrospinal fluid after subarachnoid haemorrhage. Acta Neurol. Scand. 49 (1972) p 1.

TOVI, D., NILSSON, I. M. & THULIN, C.-A.: Fibrinolysis and subarachnoid haemorrhage. Inhibitory effect of tranexamic acid. A clinical study. Acta Neurol. Scand. 48 (1972) p 393.

TULLIS, J. L.: Clinical Experience with Factor IX Concentrates. Hemophilia and New Hemorrhagic States. International Symposium, New York. Ed. K. M. Brinkhous. The University of North Carolina Press, Chapel Hill (1970) p 35.

TULLIS, J. L., MELIN, M. & JURGIAN, P.: Clinical use of human prothrombin complexes. New Engl. J. Med. 273 (1965) p 667.

TYTGAT, G., COLLEN, D. & DE VREKER, R. A.: La diathése hémorragique en cas de cirrhose du foie. Coagulation 1 (1968) p 43.

URAYAMA, T.: Haemorrhagic syndrome of autoimmune origin with a specific inhibitor against fibrin stabilizing factor (factor XIII). Brit. J. Haemat. 23 (1972) p 17.

VASSALLI, P., MORRIS, R. H. & MCCLUSKEY, R. T.: The pathogenic role of fibrin deposition in the glomerular lesions of toxemia of pregnancy. J. Exp. Med. 118 (1963) p 467.

VEDER, H. A.: Further purification of the anti-haemophilic factor (AHF). Thromb. Diath. Haemorrh. 16 (1966) p 738.

VELTKAMP, J. J., DRION, E. F. & LOELIGER, E. A.: a. Detection of the carrier state in hereditary coagulation disorders. I. Thromb. Diath. Haemorrh. 19 (1968) p 279.

VELTKAMP, J. J., DRION, E. F. & LOELIGER, E. A.: b. Detection of the carrier state in hereditary coagulation disorders. II. Thromb. Diath. Haemorrh. 19 (1968) p 403.

VELTKAMP, J. J., LOELIGER, E. A. & HEMKER, H. C.: The biological half-time of Hageman factor. Thromb. Diath. Haemorrh. 18 (1965) p 1.

VELTKAMP, J. J., MEILOF, J., REMMELTS, H. G., van der VLERK, D. & LOELIGER, E. A.: Another genetic variant of haemophilia B: Haemophilia B Leyden. Scand. J. Haematol. 7 (1970) p 82.

VELTKAMP, J. J., SCHALM, S. W., van de TORREN, K. & TERPSTRA, J. L.: Transplantation in Canine Haemophilia. VIIth Congress of the World Federation of Haemophilia, Tehran-Iran May 17–20 (1971) p 32.

VERHAEGHE, R., van DAMME, B., MOLLA, A. & VERMYLEN, J.: Dysfibrinogenaemia associated with primary hepatoma. Scand. J. Haemat. 9 (1972) p 451.

VERMYLEN, K., DOTREMONT, G., DONATI, M. B., MOLLA, A. & MICHIELSEN, P.: Urinary excretion of fibrinogen-fibrin related antigen in glomerulonephritis: effect of Indomethacin. Internat. Soc. on Thrombosis and Haemostasis Washington (1972).

VERSTRAETE, M., OLISLAEGERS, P., van ITTERBEEK, H., WAUMAN, P. & LUST, A.: Human plasma and plasma fractions as sources of factor VIII (antihemophilic factor). Vox Sang 16 (1969) p 382.

VERSTRAETE, M. & VERMYLEN, J.: Acute and chronic "defibrination" in obstetrical practice. Thromb. Diath. Haemorrh. 20 (1968) p 443.

VERSTRAETE, M., VERMYLEN, J., AMERY, A. & VERMYLEN, C.: Thrombolytic therapy with streptokinase using a standard dosage scheme. Brit. Med. J. 1 (1966) p 454.

VERSTRAETE, M., VERMYLEN, C., VERMYLEN, J. & VANDENBROUCKE, J.: Excessive consumption of blood coagulation components as cause of hemorrhagic diathesis. Amer. J. Med. 38 (1965) p 899.

VIGLIANO, E. M. & HOROWITZ, H. I.: Bleeding syndrome in a patient with IgA myeloma: interaction of protein and connective tissue. Blood 29 (1967) p 823.

VILLASANTA, U.: Therapy in antepartum thrombophlebitis. Obstet. Gynecol. 26 (1965) p 534.

VINNICOMBE, J. & SHUTTLEWORTH, K. E. D.: Aminocaproic acid in the control of haemorrhage after prostatectomy. Safety of aminocaproic acid—a controlled trial. Lancet I (1966) p 232.

VOLKERT, M.: Studies on the antithrombin content of the blood and its relation to heparin. Acta Physiol. Scand. Suppl. 15 (1942).

VREEKEN, J., BOOMGARD, J. & DEGGELLER, K.: Urokinase excretion in patients with renal diseases. Acta Med. Scand. 180 (1966) p 153.

de VRIES, S. I. & BRAAT-van STRAATEN, M. A. J.: Haemorrhagic diathesis as the result of severe deficiency of plasma thromboplastin antecedent (PTA, factor XI). Thromb. Diath. Haemorrh. 11 (1964) p 167.

WAALER, B. A.: Contact activation in the intrinsic blood clotting system. Studies on a plasma product formed on contact with glass and similar surfaces. Scand. J. Clin. Lab. Invest. 11, Suppl. 37 (1959) p 1.

WAGNER, R. H., MCLESTER, W. D., SMITH, M. & BRINKHOUS, K. M.: Purification of antihemophilic factor (factor VIII) by aminoacid precipitation. Thromb. Diath. Haemorrh. 11 (1964) p 64.

WAGNER, R. H., ROBERTS, H. R., WEBSTER, W. P., SHANBROM, E. & BRINKHOUS, K. M.: Glycine-precipitated antihemophilic factor concentrates and their clinical use. Thromb. Diath. Haemorrh. Suppl. 35 (1969) p 41.

WALLÉN, P.: Plasmic degradation of fibrinogen. Scand. J. Haemat. Suppl. 13 (1971) p 3.

WALLÉN, P. & BERGSTRÖM, K.: Purification of human plasminogen on DEAE-cellulose. Acta Chem. Scand. 14 (1960) p 217.

WALLÉN, P. & WIMAN, B.: Characterization of human plasminogen. I. On the relationship between different molecular forms of plasminogen demonstrated in plasma and found in purified preparations. Biochim. Biophys. Acta 221 (1970) p 20.

WALLÉN, P. & WIMAN, B.: Characterization of human plasminogen. II. Separation and partial characterization of different molecular forms of human plasminogen. Biochim. Biophys. Acta 257 (1972) p 122.

WALLS, W. A. & LOSOWSKY, M. S.: Plasma fibrin stabilizing factor (F.S.F.) activity in normal subjects and patients with chronic liver disease. Thromb. Diath. Haemorrh. 21 (1969) p 134.

WALSH, P. N.: Platelet adhesiveness in Hageman trait. Lancet II (1970) p 575.

WALSH, P. N.: The effects of collagen and kaolin on the intrinsic coagulant activity of platelets. Brit. J. Haemat. 22 (1972) p 393.

WALSH, R, T. & BARNHART, M. I.: Clearance of coagulation and fibrinolysis products by the reticuloendothelial system. Thromb. Diath. Haemorrh. Suppl. 36 (1969) p 83.

WARDLE, E. N. & TAYLOR, G.: Fibrin breakdown products and fibrinolysis in renal disease. J. Clin. Path. 21 (1968) p 140.

WARE, A. G. & SEEGERS, W. H.: Plasma accelerator globulin: partial purification, quantitative determination, and properties. J. Biol. Chem. 172 (1948) p 699.

WARLOW, C. P., MCNEILL, A., OGSTON, D. & DOUGLAS, A. S.: Platelet adhesiveness, coagulation and fibrinolytic activity in obesity. J. Clin. Path. 25 (1972) p 484.

WARNER, E. D., BRINKHOUS, K. M. & SMITH, H. P.: A quantitative study on blood clotting. Prothrombin fluctuations under experimental conditions. Amer. J. Physiol. 114 (1936) p 667.

WASASTIERNA, C.: Cyclic thrombocytopenia of acute type. Scand. J. Haematol. 4 (1967) p 380.

WEAVER, R. A. & LANGDELL, R. D.: Antihemophilic factor (AHF) stability in fresh frozen blood bank plasma. Transfusion 6 (1966) p 224.

WEAVER, R. A., PRICE, R. E. & LANGDELL, R. D.: Antihemophilic factor in cross-circulated normal and hemophilic dogs. Amer. J. Physiol. 206 (1964) p 335.

WEBB, A. T., MEYER, F. L. & LONSER, E. R.: Hemorrhagic thrombocythemia. Response to Busulfan. Arch. Intern. Med. 111 (1963) p 280.

WEBSTER, W. P., MCMILLAN, C. W., LUCAS, O. N. & ROBERTS, H. R.: Dental management of bleeder patient. VIIth Congr. World Federation of Haemophilia Teheran-Iran, May (1971).

WEBSTER, W. P., PENICK, G. D. & MANDELL, S. R.: Orthotopic and Heterotopic Organ Transplantation in Canine Hemophilia. VIIth Congress of the World Federation of Haemophilia, Tehran-Iran, May 17–20 (1971) p 34.

WEBSTER, W. P., ROBERTS, H. R. & PENICK, G. D.: Hemostasis in factor V deficiency. Amer. J. Med. Sci. 248 (1964) p 194.

WEBSTER, W. P., ROBERTS, H. R., THELIN, G. M., WAGNER, R. H. & BRINKHOUS, K. M.: Clinical use of a new glycine-precipitated antihaemophilic fraction. Amer. J. Med. Sci. 250 (1965) p 643.

WEINER, M., REDISCH, W. & STEELE, J. M.: Occurrence of fibrinolytic activity following administration of nicotinic acid. Proc. Soc. Exp. Biol. Med. 98 (1958) p 755.

WEISS, H. J., CHERVENICK, P. A., ZALUSKY, R. & FACTOR, A.: A familial defect in platelet function associated with impaired release of adenosine diphosphate. New Engl. J. Med. 281 (1969) p 1264.

WEISS, H. J. & KOCHWA, S.: Antihaemophilic globulin (AHG) in multiple myeloma and macroglobulinaemia. Brit. J. Haematol. 14 (1968) p 205.

WEISS, H. J. & KOCHWA, S.: Molecular forms of antihaemophilic globulin in plasma, cryoprecipitate and after thrombin activation. Brit. J. Haemat. 18 (1970) p 89.

WESSLER, S. & DEYKIN, D.: Theory and practice in acute venous thrombosis. A reappraisal. Circulation 8 (1958) p 1190.

WESSLER, S. & STEHBENS, W. E.: Thrombosis. Thrombosis and bleeding disorders. Theory and methods. Thieme, Stuttgart; Academic Press, New York (1971) p 488.

WHISSELL, D. Y., HOAG, M. S., AGGELER, P. M., KROPATKIN, M. & GARNER, E.: Hemophilia in a woman. Amer. J. Med. 38 (1965) p 119.

WHITE, J. G. & KRIVIT, W.: The ultrastructural localization and release of platelet lipids. Blood 27 (1966) p 167.

WHITE, J. G., YUNIS, E., COLLIANDER, M. & KRIVIT, W.: Prolonged bleeding time in a patient with plasma thromboplastin antecedent deficiency: Observations on correction of the bleeding time by platelet transfusion. J. Pediat. 63 (1963) p 1081.

WHITE, W. F., BARLOW, G. H. & MOZEN, M. M.: The isolation and characterization of plasminogen activators (urokinase) from human urine. Biochem. 5 (1966) p 2160.

WILLIAMS, W. J. & ESNOUF, M. P.: The fractionation of Russell's-viper (Vipera russellii) venom with special reference to the coagulant protein. Biochem. J. 84 (1962) p 52.

WILNER, G. D., NOSSEL, H. L. & LEROY, E. C.: Activation of Hageman factor by collagen. J. Clin. Invest. 47 (1968) p 2616.

WITTE, S., SCHRICKER, K. T. & SCHMID, E.: Mikroskipische Befunde über die Blutstillung bei Serotoninausschaltung. Thromb. Diath. Haemorrh. 5 (1961) p 505.

WOLF, P.: A modification for routine laboratory use of Stefanini's method of estimating factor V activity in human oxalated plasma. J. Clin. Pathol. 6 (1953) p 34.

WOODFIELD, D. G., COLE, S. K., ALLAN, A. G. E. & CASH, J. D.: Serum fibrin degradation products throughout normal pregnancy. Brit. Med. J. 4 (1968) p 665.

WRIGHT, H. P.: The adhesiveness of blood platelets in normal subjects and with varying concentrations of anticoagulants. J. Path. Bact. 53 (1941) p 255.

WRIGHT, I. S.: Zusammenfassung der Eigenschaften der beiden neuen, mit internationalen Symbolen versehenen Gerinnungsfaktoren. Blut 8 (1962) p 102.

YIN, E. T., WESSLER, S. & STOLL, P. J.: Identity of plasma-activated factor X inhibitor with antithrombin III and heparin cofactor. J. Biol. Chem. 246 (1971) p 3712.

ZETTERQVIST, E. & v. FRANCKEN, I.: Coagulation disturbances with manifest bleeding in extrahepatic portal hypertension and in liver cirrhosis. Preliminary results of heparin treatment. Acta Med. Scand. 173 (1963) p 753.

ZIMMERMAN, T. S., RATNOFF, O. D. & LITTELL, A. S.: b. Detection of carriers of classic hemophilia using an immunologic assay for antihemophilic factor (factor VIII). J. Clin. Invest. 50 (1971) p 255.

ZIMMERMAN, T. S., RATNOFF, O. D. & POWELL, A. E.: a. Immunologic differentiation of classic hemophilia (factor VIII deficiency) and von Willebrand's disease. With observations on combined deficiencies of antihemophilic factor and proaccelerin (factor V) and on an acquired circulating anticoagulant against antihemophilic factor. J. Clin. Invest. 50 (1971) p 244.

ZUCKER, M. B.: In vitro abnormality of the blood in von Willebrand's disease correctable by normal plasma. Nature 197 (1963) p 601.

ZUCKER, M. B. & PETERSON, J.: Inhibition of adenosine diphosphate-induced secondary aggregation and other platelet functions by acetyl-salicylic acid ingestion. Proc. Soc. Exp. Biol. Med. 127 (1968) p 547.

ÅBERG, H. & NILSSON, I. M.: Recurrent thrombosis in a young woman with a circulating anticoagulant directed against factors XI and XII. Acta Med. Scand. 192 (1972) p 419.

ÅSTEDT, B.: On fibrinolysis. A. In pregnancy, labour, puerperium and during treatment with sex hormones. B. In human ontogenesis and in human organ culture. Acta Obstet. Gynec. Scand. Suppl. 18 (1972).

ÅSTEDT, B., ISACSON, S., NILSSON, I. M. & PANDOLFI, M.: Fibrinolytic activity of veins during pregnancy. Acta Obstet. Gynec. Scand. 49 (1970) p 171.

ÅSTEDT, B. & PANDOLFI, M.: On release and synthesis of fibrinolytic activators in human organ culture. Rev. Europ. Etudes Clin. Biol. 17 (1972) p 743.

ÅSTEDT, B., PANDOLFI, M. & NILSSON, I. M.: a. Quantitation of fibrinolytic agents released in tissue culture. Experientia 27 (1971) p 358.

ÅSTEDT, B., SVANBERG, L. & NILSSON, I. M.: b. Fibrin degradation products and ovarian tumours. Brit. Med. J. 4 (1971) p 458.

ÅSTEDT, B., SVANBERG, L. NILSSON, I. M.: FDP. Lancet II (1972) p 1312.

ODEGAARD, A. E., SKÅLHEGG, B. A. & HELLEM, A. J.: ADP-induced platelet adhesiveness as a diagnostic test in von Willebrand's disease. Thromb. Diath. Haemorrh. 11 (1964) p 23.

ÖSTERLIND, G. & NILSSON, I. M.: Extraction of cataract in a patient with severe haemophilia A. Acta Ophthal. 46 (1968) p 176.

ÖSTERUD, B.: Purification and some characteristics of human factor IX. IVth International Congress on Thrombosis and Haemostasis Vienna (1973) p 141.

ÖSTERUD, B., BERRE, Å., OTNAESS, A. B., BJÖRKELID, E. & PRYDZ, H.: Activation of the coagulation factor VII by tissue thromboplastin and calcium. Biochemistry 11 (1972) p 2853.

Index